Connective Tissue Disea

Connective Tissue Diseases

GRAHAM R. V. HUGHES

MD, FRCP
Consultant Rheumatologist,
Department of Rheumatology,
St Thomas' Hospital, London;
and Head,
Lupus Arthritis Research Unit,
The Rayne Institute,
St Thomas' Hospital, London

Fourth Edition

OXFORD

BLACKWELL SCIENTIFIC PUBLICATIONS

LONDON EDINBURGH BOSTON
MELBOURNE PARIS BERLIN VIENNA

© 1971, 1979, 1987, 1994 by
Blackwell Scientific Publications
Editorial Offices:
Osney Mead, Oxford OX2 OEL
25 John Street, London WC1N 2BL
23 Ainslie Place, Edinburgh EH3 6AJ
238 Main Street, Cambridge
  Massachusetts 02142, USA
54 University Street, Carlton
  Victoria 3053, Australia

Other Editorial Offices:
Librairie Arnette SA
1, rue de Lille
75007 Paris
France

Blackwell Wissenschafts-Verlag GmbH
Düsseldorfer Str. 38
D-10707 Berlin
Germany

Blackwell MZV
Feldgasse 13
A-1238 Wien
Austria

First published 1971
Second edition 1979
Third edition 1987
Fourth edition 1994

Set by Setrite Typesetters, Hong Kong
Printed and bound in Great Britain
at the University Press, Cambridge

DISTRIBUTORS

  Marston Book Services Ltd
  PO Box 87
  Oxford OX2 ODT
  (*Orders*: Tel: 0865 791155
         Fax: 0865 791927
         Telex: 837515)

USA
  Blackwell Scientific Publications, Inc.
  238 Main Street
  Cambridge, MA 02142
  (*Orders*: Tel: 800 759−6102
         617 876−7000)

Canada
  Times Mirror Professional Publishing, Ltd
  130 Flaska Drive
  Markham, Ontario L6G 1B8
  (*Orders*: Tel: 800 268−4178
         416 470−6739)

Australia
  Blackwell Scientific Publications Pty Ltd
  54 University Street
  Carlton, Victoria 3053
  (*Orders*: Tel: 03 347−5552)

A catalogue record for this title
is available from the British Library
and the Library of Congress

ISBN 0−632−03752−0

Contents

Preface

TO THE FOURTH EDITION

In a 1992 review of recommended rheumatology reading (*British Medical Journal* **305**, 375) *Connective Tissue Diseases* was awarded a rosette (for which many thanks, Robert Bernstein) but the review included 'before he gets his first grey hair, it is time for a new edition'.

Here it is, updated to 1993. As before it is strictly aimed at the practising clinician, including, wherever appropriate, a review reference for the resident or specialist who needs a lead into the details of that subject.

The past few years have seen a number of changes in the field of connective tissue disease — the worldwide recognition of the spectrum of the antiphospholipid syndrome, the dominance of methotrexate in the treatment of rheumatoid arthritis, the syndromes associated with silicone implants, the eosinophilic myalgic syndromes, the rapid increase in recognition (and numbers) of various vasculitic syndromes — notably limited forms of Wegener's granulomatosis. These changes are all highlighted and referenced in the fourth edition.

I am grateful to my colleagues in the lupus arthritis research unit at St Thomas' Hospital for their help and advice.

London 1993   *G.R.V. Hughes*

TO THE FIRST EDITION

The connective tissue diseases present some of the most taxing clinical problems in medicine. Although recent advances, particularly in immunology, have contributed to a finer definition of some of these diseases, their diagnosis and management rely heavily on clinical criteria.

The emphasis of this book is towards diagnosis, though current theories regarding aetiology are discussed and recent references are included.

The reputation of the Hammersmith Hospital as a referral centre for patients with connective tissue diseases has been largely due to the work of Professor E.G.L. Bywaters. His help and advice in the writing of this book have been invaluable. I am also grateful to Dr Charles Christian,

Cornell University, New York, for his advice, to Dr R. Travers for proof-reading and indexing, and to Mrs J. Andrews and Mrs O. Wong for typing the manuscript.

London 1977   *G.R.V. Hughes*

1: *Introduction*

Implicit in the term connective tissue disease is the assumption that members of the group have a common pathogenesis or aetiology. Although the generally accepted members of the group of diseases, systemic lupus erythematosus, rheumatoid arthritis, scleroderma, dermatomyositis and the various vasculitides, have enough features in common to ensure their acceptance as a clinical family they differ in many aspects and do not have any consistent pathological or immunological features. A negative common feature of the group is the lack of a proven aetiological agent. Rheumatic fever, known to be a hypersensitivity reaction to streptococci, is now excluded, though other members still included may have similar aetiological mechanisms. For similar reasons, the genetically determined connective tissue diseases such as Ehlers–Danlos syndrome — perhaps the only 'true' connective tissue diseases — are excluded.

Aetiology

Three headings appear repeatedly in the aetiology sections of this book — immunological, viral and genetic. All of the diseases discussed demonstrate immunological abnormalities, particularly the presence of humoral auto-antibodies. In some cases, such as the haemolytic anaemia of SLE, these autoantibodies clearly have a direct pathogenetic role. For the most part, however, they may merely be epiphenomena, reflecting a more basic defect of the immune system such as loss of T-cell suppressor activity. Considerable knowledge has accumulated of immune complex disease mechanisms, where pathological change, particularly in renal glomeruli and blood vessels, is brought about by complement-mediated inflammatory processes, secondary to the deposition of antigen–antibody complexes.

Immune complex tissue damage is a secondary phenomenon. The initiating factors leading to altered immunity in these diseases are unknown, though evidence for both infective and genetic mechanisms is strong. Perhaps most attention, in terms of aetiological factors, has been given to SLE, and for this, as well as other reasons, more space is devoted to SLE than to the other diseases.

A number of the diseases have clear inheritance patterns, and evidence from family and twin studies, as well as inferences made from animal models, suggests that genetic factors may play an important pathogenetic role. The concept that a disease pattern of response to an infection might be genetically determined has received impetus from the work on immune-response genes in mice, and the finding of strong associations of spondylitis and sacroiliitis with HLA-B27, including those examples following gastro-enteric infection. An increasing number of examples of genetic deficiencies of various complement components has been recognized. A significant number of these patients have subsequently developed one or other of the connective tissue diseases, in particular SLE. During the past decades, overwhelming evidence for an increased prevalence of a C4 null allele on the 6th chromosome in SLE has provided further support for a genetic hypothesis.

Diagnosis

In the majority of cases, a clear diagnosis of one or other connective tissue disease can be made. However, many examples of 'overlap' do occur. The finding of a serological marker for 'mixed connective tissue disease' demonstrated that the use of immunological tests may contribute further to 'splitting'. During the past two decades, the development of tests for studying 'extractable nuclear antigens' has played a useful role in the definition of subsets of lupus-like diseases. In many ways, it was the refusal to conform to 'classical' definitions which led to the discovery of the antiphospholipid syndrome.

To fall into the temptation of making the all-embracing diagnosis of 'connective tissue disease' or 'overlap syndrome' is to put the clock back on the development of this subject. It is salutary to remember that until relatively recently ankylosing spondylitis was considered by some to be a variant of rheumatoid arthritis — a view that could have delayed the discovery of its relationship to HLA antigen.

An intelligent approach to classification has been in the drawing up of criteria for classification. While these cannot be used for diagnosis, the use of statistical analysis must play a part in assessment of such complicated disease patterns and their prognosis.

Nevertheless, at the bedside, initial diagnosis is made largely on clinical grounds and the emphasis of this volume is directed towards clinical diagnosis, exemplified where possible by case reports.

It is becoming increasingly clear that a spectrum of severity is seen in each of these diseases. Thus what might appear to be rapidly progressive scleroderma might be benign eosinophilic fasciitis, or a young woman with SLE psychosis and DNA binding values of 100% may yet have a very good prognosis. Indeed with the development of serological tests, the concept of 'minimal lupus' might be extended to other members of the group, leading to a recognition of milder variants of these diseases, and offering, if nothing else, more hope to the patient.

2: *Systemic Lupus Erythematosus*

Systemic lupus erythematosus (SLE), because of its widespread clinical manifestations, and because of rapidly increasing knowledge concerning its pathogenetic mechanisms, has achieved an importance among the connective tissue diseases out of all proportion to its clinical frequency. During the past three decades, the prevalence of lupus appears to have increased — indeed in some countries in the Caribbean and in the Far East, it has overtaken rheumatoid arthritis in importance.

SLE is predominantly a disease of young women and, until relatively recently, was widely regarded as having an almost uniformly poor prognosis. The introduction of sensitive immunological tests, particularly antinuclear antibodies, antiDNA antibody and complement estimations, has led to the recognition of milder forms of the disease, which in turn has contributed to the apparent increase in prevalence.

SLE may affect any organ of the body, though for some reason the liver is rarely clinically affected (the confusing terminology of 'lupoid hepatitis' is now abandoned). The characteristic pattern of disease is one of exacerbation and remission. While it was once thought to lead to death in the majority of cases, it is now recognized that permanent remission may occur and indeed may be common in mild cases.

SLE characteristically affects the vasculature (leading to renal, cerebrovascular, pulmonary, and widespread organ involvement) as well as serosal surfaces (leading to pleurisy, pericarditis and peritonitis). In particular it is characterized by a profound and widespread disturbance of immune mechanisms, leading to the formation of autoantibodies and immune complexes. While renal, central nervous system (CNS) and cardiac lesions are prognostically most important, the most frequent manifestations of SLE are of skin and of joint disease, and in a proportion of patients the disease appears to be confined to these parts of the body. For a number of reviews of developments in SLE, the reader is referred to Hughes (1982b), Lahita (1993) and Wallace & Hahn (1993).

HISTORICAL

While SLE has probably been recognized for a number of centuries as one of the causes of facial 'lupus', it was not until the 19th century that

4

Cazenave, Hebra & Kaposi (1875) recognized the distinct systemic form of the disease, and separated it from discoid lupus. Kaposi associated the facial 'butterfly' eruption with 'more or less fever of an irregularly remittent type ... attended by general prostration and disturbed consciousness, resulting in coma or stupor or complicated with pleuro-pneumonia and ending in death'.

It is William Osler (1895) who deserves the credit, however, for describing the disease in the form in which we currently recognize it: '... polymorphic skin lesions ... arthritis occasionally, and a variable number of visceral manifestations, of which the most important are gastrointestinal crisis, endocarditis, pericarditis, acute nephritis and haemorrhage from the mucous surfaces. Recurrence is a special feature of the disease and attacks may come on month after month or even throughout a long period of years.'

Over the ensuing decades, various morbid anatomical and clinical features were described but in 1948, the next major advance came with the discovery of Hargraves, Richmond and Morton (1948) of the LE cell in bone marrow preparations of patients with SLE. This led to the recognition both of milder forms of lupus and of the widespread immunological disturbance present in the disease.

In 1969–70 the DNA-binding test and its clinical applications were described (Pincus *et al*. 1959) and in 1983, the antiphospholipid antibody syndrome was described (see Chapter 3).

PREVALENCE

SLE in the male is extremely rare, and most series agree on a female : male ratio of 9:1. The disease is commonest in the childbearing years, and especially in the later teenage years and early twenties.

Although it has been difficult to analyse ethnic prevalence differences, the disease does appear to be commoner in black populations, particularly in the USA and the West Indies. The author, during one year in Jamaica, saw 81 new cases of SLE, and the prevalence of the disease on this island may approach 1 in 250 women. In one 10-year study (Siegel, Holley & Lee 1970) the age-adjusted mortality prevalence rates were three times greater for black females than white females in New York City, and 4·3 times greater in Jefferson County, Alabama — a close agreement for such widely separated communities. Further difficulties have arisen because of differences in diagnostic interpretation in some studies, for example, inclusion of 'rheumatoid arthritis and LE'. The widespread use of diagnostic criteria such as those suggested by the American Rheumatism Association (see below) may lead to further classification, as will the development of more

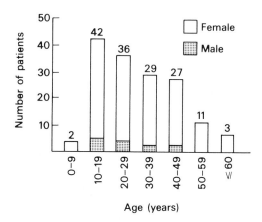

Fig. 2.1 The age distribution of patients at the onset of multisystem disease. The number at the top of each bar refers to the total number of patients in each decade. (From Estes & Christian 1971.)

specific diagnostic tests such as measurement of antiDNA antibodies.

The epidemiology of SLE was extensively reviewed in the 1970s by Siegel & Lee (1973). The highest incidence reported at that time was in New York: 14 new cases per 100 000 were reported in black females between the ages of 15 and 44 in 1960. The prevalence (i.e. number of people suffering from the disease at any one time) in this group on July 1st 1965 was 80·9 per 100 000 or just under 1 in 1000. Fessel (1974) in an extensive survey of residents of San Francisco noted a prevalence in women (aged 15−64 years) of 1 in 2000. The prevalence in black women rose to 1 in 245. Thus SLE is not a rare disease — indeed in parts of South East Asia, prevalence figures may exceed those of rheumatoid arthritis. In London, admittedly in a referral practice, there are now 1000 lupus patients listed in the St Thomas' lupus clinic.

PATHOLOGY

Table 2.1 summarizes the main pathological features. Despite the long list, surprisingly little diagnostic help in SLE is obtained from histology. The most striking histological feature is the so-called 'fibrinoid necrosis' which affects particularly the small arteries, arterioles and capillaries (as distinct from polyarteritis nodosa which affects predominantly medium-sized vessels such as the coronary and mesenteric arteries). Fibrinoid necrosis also affects the interstitial collagen and membranes such as the pleura and joint capsules. It occurs in a number of well-defined stages. First, increased

Table 2.1 Principal pathological changes in SLE

General
Fibrinoid necrosis
Haematoxylin bodies ('tissue LE cells')
Deposition of immune complexes along basement membranes

Skin
Discoid — follicular plugging and scarring
Systemic — immune complexes in dermal/epidermal junction

Kidneys
Immune complex deposition ('lumpy-bumpy' immunofluorescence)
Focal or diffuse glomerulonephritis
Fibrinoid necrosis of arterioles or arteries

CNS
Microinfarcts
Choroid plexus complexes

Heart
Pericarditis
Myocarditis
Libman—Sachs endocarditis

Blood vessels
Arteriolitis and capillaritis
Major arteries less frequent
Micro-thrombi

Spleen
'Onion-skin' thickening

Joints
Fibrinoid deposition

Lungs and pleura
Fibrinoid. Adhesions. Effusions
Interstitial pneumonitis
Recurrent atelectasis. Infections

amounts of mucopolysaccharide cause the swelling of collagen ground substance. The collagen fibres then swell and become fragmented, finally dissolving into a homogeneous hyaline or finely granular periodic acid—Schiff (PAS)-positive substance. Immunofluorescent studies have shown that this fibrinoid contains large amounts of gammaglobulin, with fibrin or ground substance, together with complement and fibrinogen.

The other feature highly suggestive of SLE is the haematoxylin body, the tissue counterpart of the LE cell, that represents the pyknosis of nuclei, with resultant coalescence or phagocytosis.

Kidney. There are no pathognomonic changes, though a number of features are regularly seen. The 'classical' change — the *wire loops*; eosinophilic thickening of the basement membrane of some capillary loops — is seen only in more advanced cases. Other light microscopic changes include a local or generalized focal glomerulitis — with or without crescent formation, capsular adhesions and glomerular fibrosis — haematoxylin bodies and interstitial infiltration by plasma cells and lymphocytes. In other (rare) patients, the predominant lesion is a diffuse membranous glomerulonephritis. Fibrinoid necrosis may develop, especially in afferent arterioles (Fig. 2.2).

Electron microscopy has revealed that the main lesion in lupus nephritis is the deposition of electron-dense material on the endothelial aspect of the membrane, either in linear or 'lumpy-bumpy' distribution. Immunofluorescent examination, which has now largely replaced light microscopy as an investigative tool in SLE, has shown this material to consist largely

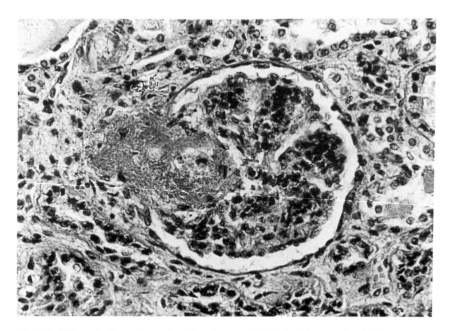

Fig. 2.2 SLE nephritis. Glomerulus showing marked fibrinoid necrosis of afferent arteriole. (H & E ×340. Dr Shirley Amin, University Hospital of the West Indies.)

of gammaglobulin (particularly IgG), complement and fibrinogen. The globulin has antinuclear activity, particularly against DNA. The distribution of complement is generally similar to that of immunoglobulin suggesting that both are deposited in the form of immune complexes. Demonstration of the antigen has proved far more difficult though DNA has been localized histochemically. The pathological features of lupus nephritis have been extensively reviewed by Lahita (1993) and Wallace & Hahn (1993).

Skin. The more benign discoid lupus has the more florid clinical and pathological changes, with hyperkeratosis, follicular plugging, vacuoliz-ation of basal cells, perivascular infiltrate with lymphocytes and plasma cells and fibrinoid necrosis in the dermis. Immunofluorescent studies of skin have proved diagnostically useful, especially in SLE, showing deposition of gammaglobulin and complement along the dermal–epidermal junction. This finding may be present in clinically uninvolved skin.

Central nervous system (Harris & Hughes 1985). Very little is known about the neuropathology of CNS lupus. In the study of Johnston & Richardson (1968) the predominant lesions related to small blood vessels where de-structive and proliferative changes were found, associated with scattered microinfarcts. In retrospect, perhaps the most striking finding of this 'classic' study was the notable *absence* of vasculitis — microthrombi being more a feature. Likewise, evidence that cerebral immune complex depo-sition (including choroid plexus immunoglobulin and lowered CSF C_4 levels), is a major cause of CNS lupus is scanty (reviewed by Hughes 1980), though the choroid plexus and glomerular basement membrane do have striking morphological and functional similarities, and share common antigenic determinants. IgG antigen and C_3 have been demonstrated in the choroid plexuses of animals with acute serum sickness (Koss, Chernack & Griswold 1973) and, in the New Zealand mouse (Lampert & Oldstone 1973).

An alternative mechanism of neuropsychiatric involvement is suggested by the observations that human brain shares antigens with lymphocyte membranes and cross-reacts with antilymphocyte antibodies (Bluestein & Zvaifler 1976). Cold-reactive antilymphocyte antibodies are found more frequently in those patients with neuropsychiatric disease (Fig. 2.3a) (Bresnihan *et al*. 1977). Furthermore, only those seen in the CNS group of patients are absorbable by the brain (Fig. 2.3b). Further studies have shown that a subgroup of antineuronal antibodies exists which are warm-reactive IgG and probably directed against the neuronal cell membrane (Bresnihan *et al*. 1979). Their presence correlates broadly with clinical CNS involvement.

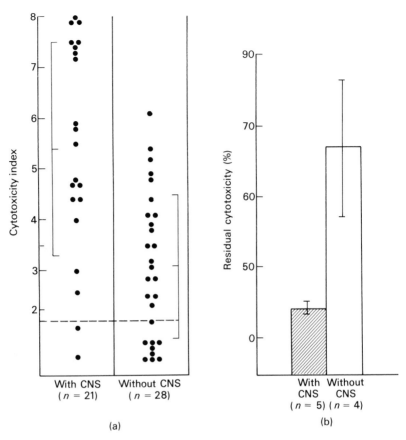

Fig. 2.3 (a) Maximal cytotoxicity index of SLE patients with and without CNS involvement. The titres of lymphocytotoxic antobodies were significantly higher ($P<0.001$) in those with CNS disease. (b) However, comparison of lymphocytotoxins from CNS and non-CNS patients showed that only those from the CNS group could be absorbed out by incubation with brain homogenates. (From Bresnihan *et al.* 1977.)

Perhaps one of the key changes of emphasis in the pathology of SLE has been the recognition of the importance of thrombotic mechanisms in the disease, particularly in many cases of CNS lupus, where the thrombotic tendency associated with antiphospholipid antibodies (see Chapter 3) is implicated not only with thrombotic strokes, but with other cerebral and ocular features including epilepsy, chorea and myelopathy (Montalban *et al.* 1991).

Other organs. The commonest cardiac lesion is fibrinoid deposition on the pericardium. Mild myocarditis, with focal fibrinoid change in the walls of small arteries and fibrinoid deposition in the septa and near blood vessels is the second most frequent finding. The well-known endocardial ('Libman–Sachs') vegetations (Fig. 2.4) — dry granules on either surface of any of the valves — are found only rarely, and in patients with severe generalized disease. The valvular lesion of SLE, in particular valvular thrombosis and Libman–Sachs endocarditis are now known to be strongly associated with antiphospholipid antibodies and their pro-thrombotic tendencies (Khamashita *et al.* 1991).

The spleen may show a very characteristic 'onion-skin' lesion, said to be one of the most pathognomonic histological findings in SLE, and due to marked perivascular fibrosis around the central and peripheral arteries (Fig. 2.5).

In the lungs, recurrent pleurisy and adhesions may lead to progressive elevation of the diaphragm and a restrictive lung pattern on respiratory function tests. An interstitial pneumonitis may be seen and wire-loop lesions of pulmonary capillaries have been described.

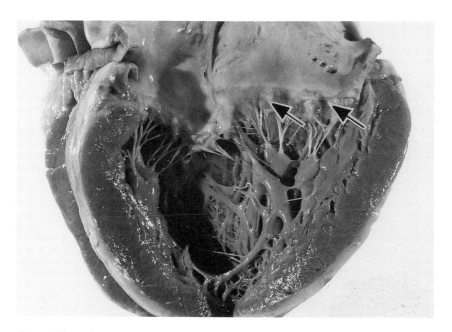

Fig. 2.4 Heart showing non-infective (Libman–Sachs) vegetations on and below the line of closure of the mitral valve.

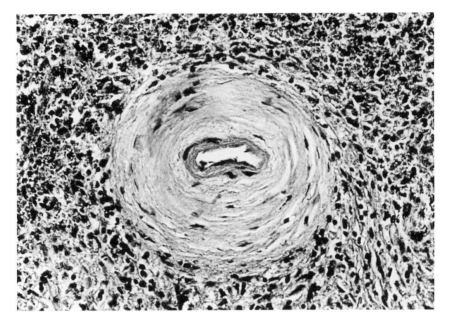

Fig. 2.5 Spleen in SLE, showing concentric 'onion-skin' periarterial fibrosis. (H & E ×340. Dr Shirley Amin, University Hospital of the West Indies.)

AETIOLOGY

Immunological changes

In no other disease are there more widespread immunological abnormalities. Particularly prominent are humoral antibodies of the non-organ specific group. The most specific finding appears to be the presence of antibodies against double-stranded DNA (p. 298) though antibodies are found against other nuclear constituents, as well as a wide variety of non-specific antigens. Less prominent are antibodies against organ-specific antigens such as thyroid and gastric parietal cells. The wide range of serological abnormalities has led to the suggestion that there might be a general defect of 'self tolerance' or in T-cell suppressor function (Alarcon-Segovia 1982; Searles & Williams 1982). While this is almost certainly the case in the New Zealand mouse (see later), the evidence for a defect in cell-mediated immunity in human SLE has been less clear-cut (reviewed by Hahn 1975) (Table 2.2). Other factors, such as a reduced level of thymic hormone (Bach, Dardenne & Bach 1973) may also contribute.

Some of the various theories of 'autoimmunity' have been reviewed by

Table 2.2 Evidence for reduced cell-mediated immune responses in SLE
(from Hahn 1975)

In humans	In New Zealand mice
Reduced delayed hypersensitivity*	Reduced *in vitro* lymphocyte transformation to allogeneic cells
Reduced *in vitro* lymphocyte transformation to specific antigens*	Reduced *in vitro* lymphocyte transformation to non-specific mitogens
Reduced *in vitro* lymphocyte response to non-specific mitogens*	Circulating antibodies against T cells present during active disease
Reduced cell-mediated immune response to DNA in face of enhanced antibody response	Reduced ability of lymphocytes to produce graft vs. host reactions
Reduced numbers of circulating T cells during active disease	Reduced ability to reject allografts
Circulating antibodies against T cells present during active disease	Resistant to induction of immune tolerance*
	Reduction of T-cell helper effects on antibody formation
	Reduction of T-cell suppressor effects on antibody formation
	Acceleration of autoantibody formation and nephritis by reduction of T-cell function

* Conflicting results are reported in the literature.

Rabin & Winkelstein (1975). Current views on the aetiology of SLE are reviewed in Hughes (1982b) and by Talal (1992).

Virus infection

In 1975, De Horatius and Messner published a paper in which they demonstrated lymphocytotoxins in 68% of close household contacts of SLE patients. This finding, provided support for the participation of a transmissible agent in the aetiology of human SLE. Nevertheless, direct attempts at virus isolation in SLE have failed.

Most of the evidence supporting a virus infection in SLE has come from observations on animal models (see below). The role of type-C virus in SLE has been reviewed by Pincus (1976) and in considerable detail in *Arthritis and Rheumatism* **21** (No. 5) (Suppl.) 1978.

Animal models (reviewed by Mountz & Edwards 1992)

The New Zealand mouse. Much of the research in SLE and indeed in other connective tissue diseases has been catalysed by observations made in the New Zealand B/W hybrid (NZB/W F1) mouse, which develops LE cells, antinuclear antibodies including those against DNA and RNA, autoimmune haemolytic anaemia and immune complex glomerulonephritis (reviewed by Whaley, Webb & Hughes 1976). These animals, whose disease expression can be modified by cross-breeding experiments, have a number of major immunological defects (Table 2.3). The relevance of these findings to human SLE is discussed by Talal (1975), Steinberg *et al.* (1978) and by Mountz & Edwards (1992).

A number of mouse models have been studied intensively, notably the MRL-lpr/lpr model, and these animal models have provided information on a number of aspects relevant to SLE, including macrophage defects, cytokine regulation, arthritis, renal and CNS disease, mechanisms of the antiphospholipid syndrome mechanisms in Sjøgren's disease, and even possible therapeutic regimens (reviewed by Mountz & Edwards 1992).

Canine lupus. A colony of dogs has been raised in which the clinical and laboratory features are strikingly similar to human SLE, with auto-immune haemolytic anaemia, purpura, polyarthritis, nephritis and anti-nuclear factors. Injection of cell-free filtrates from the spleens of these animals led to the development of ANA LE cells and, in some cases, antiDNA antibodies in the recipients (Lewis *et al.* 1973). A recent review is provided by Fournel *et al.* (1992).

Genetic factors

Epidemiological studies and the observations made on the New Zealand mouse hint strongly at genetic factors in SLE. Family studies have shown an increased incidence not only of SLE and other connective tissue diseases, but also of other immunological abnormalities in the relatives of SLE patients (reviewed by Walport *et al.* 1982 and Miles & Isenberg 1993).

Table 2.3 Immunological defects in NZB/W F1 mice

Genetic predisposition to autoallergic disease
Failure of T cells to maintain tolerance
Excessive B-cell activity
Loss of circulating T lymphocytes
Spontaneous production of lymphocytotoxic antibody

Cell-mediated immunity	Hypergammaglobulinaemia
↓	Circulating 'auto'antibodies
Persistence of viral infection	↓
Malignancy	Immune complex disease

Block *et al*. (1975) reviewed the literature on SLE and twins and collected an additional 12 twin pairs. They noticed a high concordance for ARA criteria (over 70%) and concluded that the evidence from the twin studies clearly suggested a strong genetic component in the pathogenesis of SLE.

Two situations have been defined in which a clear 'lupus diathesis' exists. The first is in patients with persistent false-positive serological tests for syphilis, of whom a significant number ultimately develop SLE or other connective tissue diseases (Dubois 1974). The second is the rapidly expanding number of patients identified with inherited complement deficiencies, and the marked propensity of these individuals to ultimately develop SLE or its variants (reviewed by Rynes 1982). In particular patients with deficiencies of the early components (Clr, Cls, C2 and C4) developing SLE have been described.

In the majority of HLA studies the association is with the haplotype A1 B8 DR3 (Black *et al*. 1982).

In 1983, our group published a study suggesting the association might be with C4 null alleles. (Fielder *et al*. 1983). The families of 29 patients with SLE and 42 normals were studied. Null (silent) alleles for C4A or C4B were found in 82% of patients. C4 null alleles were in close linkage disequilibrium with DR3 (Fielder *et al*. 1983). This study provides a possible link between the known complement deficiency associations, and the HLA association (Hughes & Batchelor 1983).

Since that time, it is clear that partial deficiency of C4 (especially C4A) is strongly associated with SLE. Partial C4A deficiency occurs in 10−20% of the population, but is found in up to 80% of SLE patients. There appears to be a gene dose-effect with a relative risk for SLE of 3 with one C4A-null allele, and 17 with 2 alleles (reviewed by Liszewski *et al*. 1989). For an up to date review, the reader is recommended to read that by Reveille (1992).

DNA as the antigen

Despite the almost invariable presence of DNA antibodies in active SLE, native DNA itself does not appear to be an immunogen. It is possible, however, that other factors such as UV light and drugs might modify the DNA, rendering it immunogenic.

Hormonal (see Talal 1982; Lahita 1990, 1992)

While all the current evidence points to an interaction of genetic and infective factors in the aetiology of SLE, any theory of causation must account for the fact that women sufferers outnumber males by 9 to 1, and that pregnancy and oestrogens affect the phenotypic expression of the disease. SLE in the male is an extremely rare disease (Miller *et al.* 1983), and it is of interest that Klinefelter's syndrome associated with SLE has been described. Lahita and his colleagues at the Rockefeller Institute have found that both males and females with SLE have abnormal metabolism of oestradiol. Furthermore, abnormal metabolism of testosterone has been reported (Jungers, Dougados & Pellisier 1982). Interesting data have emerged from studies of the New Zealand mouse where female NZB/W mice have an earlier onset and greater severity of immune complex nephritis than do male mice. The development of nephritis has been associated with a switch from predominantly IgM anti-DNA production to predominantly IgG anti-DNA antibody production and this switch can be delayed in female mice by androgen administration and accelerated in male mice by prepubertal castration (Roubinian *et al.* 1977).

During the past five years, the evidence pointing to an endocrine–immune disease link in SLE (for example, by invoking an increased aromatase action in patients with SLE) has become compulsive (Lahita 1992).

CLINICAL FEATURES

General

Table 2.4 gives the incidence of major clinical manifestations developing in 150 SLE patients studied by Estes & Christian (1971). While this shows that muscular, articular and cutaneous forms of the disease are commonest, neuropsychiatric manifestations occurred in nearly two-thirds of all cases. While almost any constellation of symptoms and signs may be seen in SLE, a number of disease patterns tend to recur in the same patient.

Perhaps the greatest change in diagnosis has come in the recognition

Table 2.4 Major clinical manifestations of SLE in 150 patients (from Estes & Christian 1971)

Manifestation	Percentage
Musculo-articular	95
Cutaneous	81
Fever	77
Neuropsychiatric	59
Renal	53
Pulmonary	48
Cardiac	38

of milder forms of SLE. With such recognition, it is apparent that seemingly 'non-specific' complaints can precede the onset of more recognizable features by as long as 20 years. General malaise is common during exacerbations of the disease, and may be contributed to by fever, synovitis and anaemia (most commonly normochromic, normocytic). Depression is sometimes marked and may be due to organic cerebral disease (see later).

Premenstrual exaggeration of symptoms, particularly headaches, is a common feature of SLE.

When fever is prominent, it may be difficult to be certain that the patient does not have septicaemia, or, in the patient on corticosteroid therapy, disseminated tuberculosis. The measurement of C-reactive protein, normally low in SLE, may help in this regard (Pepys, Lanham & De Beer 1982). Two problems are presented by the patient with fever. Firstly, infections, particularly urinary tract infections, may precipitate disease exacerbations of SLE, and secondly, their treatment, particularly with penicillin and sulphonamides may result in a disease flare. Such allergies (as distinct from drug-induced lupus) are frequent in SLE and some patients may give a history of allergy to several drugs or chemicals (Sequeira *et al.* 1993). One group of drugs which deserves consideration is the oral contraceptive agents which occasionally provoke a disease flare (Travers & Hughes 1978; Jungers *et al.* 1982a).

It is always difficult to pinpoint a single triggering factor in a disease which waxes and wanes as SLE but in some patients the circumstantial evidence is strong:

Case report. *A 20-year-old girl developed SLE with synovitis, skin rash, fever, pleurisy and raised antiDNA antibody titres 3 months after starting oral contraceptives for the first time. She stopped taking the contraceptive pill and was treated for a short period with prednisolone with an improvement in symptoms and signs. Eight months later, she decided to restart the 'pill'. After 10 weeks she again developed a similar flare of SLE. A year later the patient was clinically well and with normal antiDNA antibody titres. She again started taking an oral contraceptive, and within 3 weeks complained of arthralgias and was found to have a temperature of 99·5°F. DNA binding was 73%.*

An important precipitating factor in SLE is UV light. Some patients appear unduly sensitive to sunlight, with only brief exposure resulting in generalized disease activity.

Case report. *A 34-year-old woman journalist had suffered from discoid LE for 3 years. There were no systemic features. DNA binding activity was normal. She moved to Los Angeles and spent her free time sunbathing. Within a month she complained of arthralgia, headaches, limb girdle pain and vague visual disturbances. On her return to the UK 2 months later, she was noted to have widespread discoid lesions on the face, arms, chest and legs. There was patchy alopecia, and synovitis of several metacarpophalangeal joints. She was emotionally labile and was noted to have a rotatory tremor of the head and choreiform movements of the hands. The ESR was 65 mm/hr and serum DNA binding had risen to 70% (see Fig. 2.6). ASO titres were normal. With chloroquine and corticosteroid treatment, the symptoms and signs regressed rapidly.*

It has not proved possible to forecast the SLE patient who will prove UV sensitive, and it is possible that previous publications have overemphasized the frequency of this manifestation. In my own experience, approximately one-half of SLE patients show clear photosensitivity. Furthermore, the tendency to photosensitivity sometimes disappears when the disease goes into remission. The presence of anti-Ro antibodies is associated with photosensitivity.

Skin and mucous membranes (reviewed by Gilliam & Sontheimer 1982)

The most 'classical' feature of SLE is the 'butterfly' rash on the cheeks and

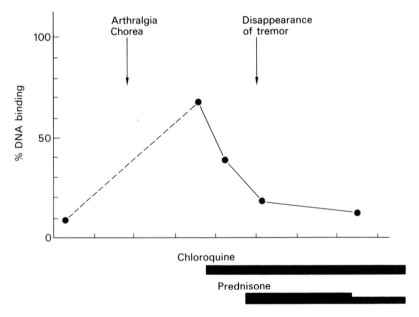

Fig. 2.6 Serial DNA-binding values in a patient with discoid LE, developing arthralgia and chorea following sun exposure.

bridge of the nose (Fig. 2.7). The incidence of this manifestation in more recent series is falling, as more sensitive diagnostic methods become more widely used. In Estes & Christian's series (1971) it was noted in 39% of patients. It may be transient, and especially in children, can be almost indistinguishable from a febrile malar flush. In some patients it appears only after sunshine exposure. A large variety of other skin manifestations can occur in SLE (Table 2.5). These include urticaria, palmar and plantar rashes (Fig. 2.8), digital vasculitis (Fig. 2.14A, B), subungal erythema, and pigmentation (Fig. 2.9). Always look at the elbows — a prominent place for the development of vasculitic lesions, varying from pigmentation to pinpoint blisters to ulceration.

A peculiar, and characteristic skin lesion is 'subacute cutaneous LE' — often circular or serpiginous, with a clear border, and prominent in exposed areas, particularly the upper chest. This highly photosensitive rash is often found in ANA-negative LE patients who demonstrate anti-Ro

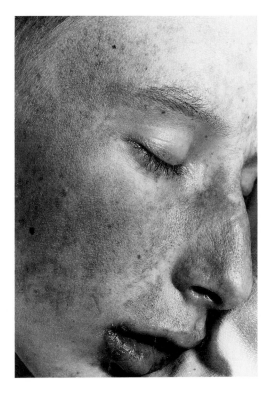

Fig. 2.7 'Butterfly' eruption in SLE. (Professor E.G.L. Bywaters, formerly Royal Postgraduate Medical School, Hammersmith Hospital.)

Chapter 2

Table 2.5 Mucocutaneous manifestations of SLE in 50 patients (from Grigor *et al.* 1978)

Manifestation	Percentage
Cutaneous vasculitis	70
Facial rash	68
Alopecia	64
Positive Shirmer's test	40
Mouth ulcers	34
Raynaud's phenomenon	32
Photosensitivity	28
Purpura	24
Subcutaneous nodules	22
Discoid lesions	20

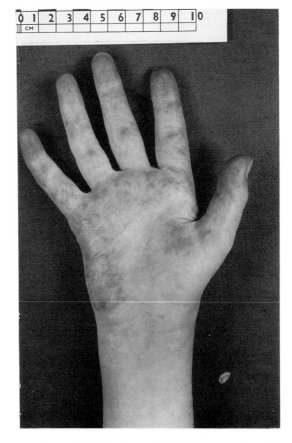

Fig. 2.8 Palmar vasculitis in SLE. (Professor E.G.L. Bywaters, formerly Royal Postgraduate Medical School, Hammersmith Hospital.)

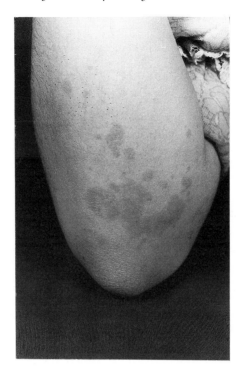

Fig. 2.9 Elbow pigmentation in SLE.

(reviewed by Gilliam & Sontheimer 1982). Discoid lesions may be found in some SLE patients.

Of all the mucocutaneous manifestations, perhaps the two most important are alopecia and livedo reticularis. Alopecia occurred in almost two-thirds of a series of SLE patients studied in an earlier series (Davis *et al.* 1973). It varied from mild non-scarring patchy alopecia, associated with the new growth of short hairs on the upper forehead, to total alopecia. Its pathogenesis is uncertain but it serves as a sensitive and useful guide to disease activity in SLE, occasionally paralleling rises in DNA antibody titres as the only clinical sign of activity. Alopecia also occurs in discoid LE (Fig. 2.10). Like other manifestations of lupus it may occur in advance of others.

Case report. *A 23-year-old girl with acute SLE recalled that 4 years earlier she had suffered from an acute 'viral' illness in which almost all her hair fell out and in which the 'joints were painful for several weeks'.*

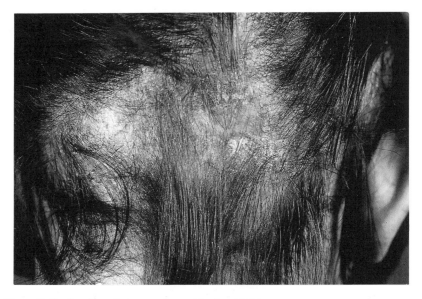

Fig. 2.10 Patchy alopecia in a patient with discoid LE.

Skin biopsy has become a widely used diagnostic tool in SLE. Immuno-fluorescent studies reveal the presence of deposits of gammaglobulin in affected skin, usually in the dermal−epidermal junction region, in up to 90% of SLE cases. These findings are noted in clinically unaffected skin in up to 50% of SLE cases and in virtually 100% of discoid lesions (reviewed by Gilliam & Sontheimer 1982).

In practice, we have tended to use skin biopsy less in recent years, largely because of the increasing information now obtained by serological tests. For example 'subacute cutaneous LE' (see Gilliam & Sontheimer 1982) is characterized by anti-Ro antibodies (Maddison 1982). See p. 306.

Livedo reticularis is an important though often subtle clinical finding in SLE. Its blotchy, patterned, bluish appearance may be seen in otherwise normal subjects but patients with SLE frequently learn to recognize its appearance. It is a distinct sign of vasculopathy and in our own experience has been associated in a number of patients with CNS involvement. The most striking clinical association of livedo is with the thrombotic tendency — especially the transient and not-so-transient cerebrovascular thrombosis, associated with antiphospholipid antibodies (Hughes 1984b) (see Chapter 3).

Other mucocutaneous manifestations in SLE are 'rheumatoid-like nodules' some of which have demonstrable haematoxylin bodies on biopsy, panniculitis (sometimes related to withdrawal of corticosteroid therapy) and leg ulcers. Nasal and oral ulceration is reported to be frequent in some series.

Skeletal system

Arthralgias occur in 90–100% of SLE patients, and may be marked, even in the absence of synovitis. Occasionally, the joint pain appears to be out of proportion to the degree of synovitis; in such patients, the effect of salicylates and even corticosteroids can be disappointing in the relief of symptoms.

While SLE is often considered an 'arthritic' condition, it is inflammation of the tendons which is most prominent — the patient often being unable to place her fingers and palms flat together. Tendon contractures also lead to an almost pathonogmonic thumb deformity in SLE (Fig. 2.11) — the 'hitch hiking' thumb. Interestingly, in our study of families with SLE, we noted a number of clinically normal relatives with the identical 'hitch hiking' thumb. Management of chronic tendon contractures in SLE has, to date, been one of our greatest therapeutic failures.

An important feature of SLE synovitis is the absence of erosions. Even where synovitis has been present for many years, erosions are rare. A small percentage develop a deforming but non-erosive arthritis. Superficially, such cases — so-called Jaccoud's arthritis (Fig. 2.11) — resemble chronic rheumatoid arthritis, with ulnar deviation, swan-neck deformities and joint subluxations. However, X-rays reveal that in most cases the cartilage and bone are not eroded (Fig. 2.12). These deformities are almost certainly due to tendon contractures. Similar deformities occasionally occur in the feet.

Of importance in SLE is aseptic necrosis of bone, usually of the hip. Almost invariably related to corticosteroid therapy, rather than to a local vasculitis, it should be considered as a differential diagnosis of pain in the hip or knee in SLE patients. The diagnosis has hitherto been based on the

Table 2.6 Musculoskeletal manifestations in 50 patients (from Grigor *et al.* 1978)

Manifestation	Percentage
Non-deforming arthritis or arthralgia	88
Deforming arthritis	10
Avascular necrosis	6
Erosions	6
Myalgia or myositis	32
Tendon contractures	12

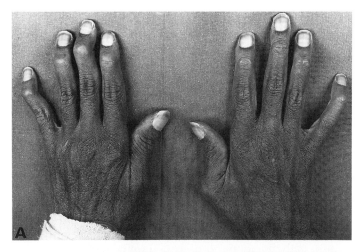

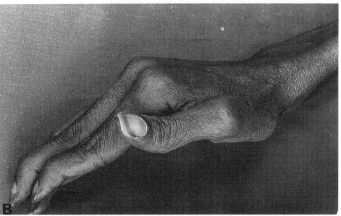

Fig. 2.11 A, B. Mild deforming arthritis in SLE.

X-ray appearances, with the distinctive demarcated area of 'ground glass' necrotic bone (Fig. 2.13). Bone scanning now provides a useful aid to diagnosis, changes being detectable before X-ray abnormalities appear.

It is almost certain that as a more conservative approach to management in SLE becomes accepted, the incidence of this complication will fall.

Nevertheless, there remains a strong clinical impression that individuals differ considerably in their propensity to develop avascular necrosis. It remains possible that underlying vascular pathology (e.g. the vasculopathy associated with anticardiolipin antibodies — see Chapter 3) may contribute to this complication of SLE.

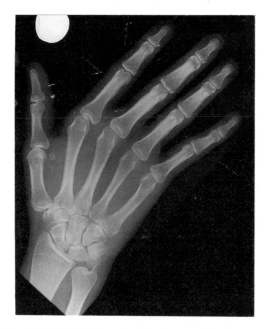

Fig. 2.12 'Jaccoud' arthritis in SLE, showing the absence of erosions.

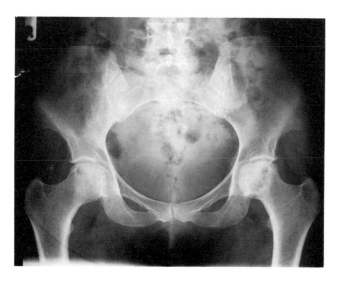

Fig. 2.13 Aseptic necrosis of both hips. The left hip in particular shows the well-demarcated area of necrotic femoral head.

Muscles

While many SLE patients on corticosteroids may have steroid-induced muscle changes, a true inflammatory myositis may occur (Estes & Christian 1971). A clinical clue to its presence may be provided by periorbital oedema, and there may be slight eyelid discoloration as in dermatomyositis. While such cases may be close to the 'borderland' of mixed connective tissue disease or other 'overlap' syndromes they deserve recognition, firstly because of the significant contribution of myositis to morbidity, and secondly because of the usually good clinical response to steroids in the majority of cases.

A rarer, though well-recognized, manifestation of SLE is myasthenia, and thymomas have been reported in association with SLE. In one such case, anti-acetylcholine receptor antibodies were detected (Valesini *et al.* 1983). The clinical relationships between lupus and thymomas can be difficult to interpret, as in the following unusual case.

Case report. *A 64-year-old woman developed acute polyarthritis and pleurisy. DNA binding was 100% and anticardiolipin antibodies were raised. Rheumatoid factor and ENA were negative. There was no past history of any clinical illness other than the removal of a thymoma 7 years earlier.*

Arteries

While SLE is one of the arteritides, clinical evidence of artery disease varies considerably from patient to patient.

The gross pattern of involvement is in medium-to-small vessels and the commonest manifestations are in the skin. Common sites of clinical vasculitis are at the elbow, on the knuckles, where there may be either purplish discoloration or erythema, and in the finger tips where periungal or subungal microinfarcts as well as livedo reticularis occur (Fig. 2.14).

Raynaud's phenomenon, although reported in up to 25% of cases is, in our experience, not a major feature of SLE (as distinct from systemic sclerosis and mixed connective tissue disease), and even when present it is quite frequently mild.

A separate, and possibly highly important, pathology in some cases may be endarterial thrombosis. Recently, this feature of SLE has been shown to be associated with the presence of antiphospholipid antibodies such as that responsible for the so-called 'lupus anticoagulant'. Patients with high titres of anticardiolipin antibodies are subject not only to venous thrombosis (including recurrent deep-vein thromboses) but may develop cerebral, limb and coronary artery thromboses (Asherson *et al.* 1985, 1986; Hughes, Harris & Gharavi 1986) (see Chapter 3).

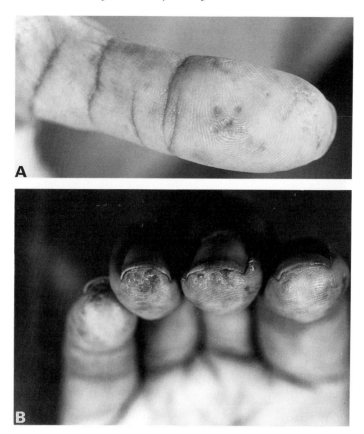

Fig. 2.14 Digital vasculitis (A) and finger tip infarction (B) in SLE.

Heart

The commonest cardiac lesion is pericarditis. In our patients, subclinical pericardial effusions, detectable by echocardiography, were seen in up to two-thirds of cases of active SLE (Davis *et al.* 1973). While pericarditis is most frequently transient and mild, it can be life threatening (Estes & Christian 1971; Chang 1982).

Case report. *An 18-year-old secretary had been attending the dermatology clinic with a 1-year history of disfiguring facial discoid LE. There had been no prior evidence of systemic disease. For 2 weeks prior to admission she had complained of joint pains, tiredness, and for 1 week of increasing dyspnoea. With the development of ankle swelling the dyspnoea worsened rapidly and she was admitted as an emergency, with central cyanosis and pericardial tamponade.*

Pericardial aspiration was considered, but she responded rapidly to high dose prednisone, and diuretics.

Fortunately, the majority of cases respond to corticosteroids, and aspiration is very rarely needed.

Cardiomyopathy due to SLE may also be more frequent than hitherto realized. Its only manifestation may be a persistent tachycardia, or relatively non-specific ECG changes.

Pulmonary hypertension is an occasional feature in SLE — possibly underdiagnosed. It may be an extension of the clotting syndrome associated with antiphospholipid antibodies (Asherson *et al.* 1983; Hughes 1993).

The classical endocarditis of SLE — the so-called Libman—Sachs endocarditis — is an autopsy diagnosis, and cannot be diagnosed with certainty in life. Murmurs in SLE patients are common and presumably related to anaemia, tachycardia or fever. However, aortic valvular lesions have been described and have led to aortic valve perforation. We have seen rapidly progressive mitral valve disease in association with peripheral vasculopathy and anticardiolipin antibodies (Khamashita *et al.* 1991). With increasing longevity in SLE, and prolonged use of steroids, ischaemic heart disease may well become a new risk factor — though again, we may discover in the next few years that anticardiolipin antibodies predispose to coronary artery thrombosis.

Pulmonary involvement

One of the commonest manifestations of SLE is serositis, in particular pleurisy. Almost half of the 150 patients of Estes & Christian (1971) had pulmonary complications and of these 60 had pleural effusions. In the multi-centre series of 245 patients collected by the American Rheumatism Association (Cohen *et al.* 1971) 60% had had pleurisy. The effusion is usually an exudate (protein exceeding 3 g/100 ml) and in contrast to rheumatoid arthritis the pleural fluid sugar is generally normal. As with other effusions of active SLE the pleural fluid complement level is low.

In some SLE patients, the pleurisy may be 'dry' and may be a cause of recurrent or persistent pain in a patient in otherwise total remission.

A variety of other pulmonary abnormalities may occur, including recurrent atelectasis and non-bacterial pneumonia (reviewed by Turner-Stokes & Turner-Warwick 1982). One of the more frequent chest X-ray findings in such patients is a gradual elevation of the diaphragms, with obliteration of the costophrenic angles leading to 'small lungs'. In some unfortunate patients, the lungs progressively 'shrink' despite all forms of therapy (Fig. 2.15).

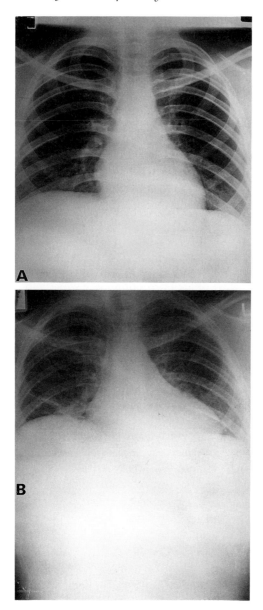

Fig. 2.15 A, B. Progressive elevation of the diaphragm over a 1-year period in a 19-year-old girl with SLE (despite antibiotics, prednisone and azathioprine).

Occasionally, diffuse interstitial lung disease occurs. Estes & Christian (1971) noted that 14 of their 150 patients had diffuse lung infiltrates and 9 had X-ray evidence of pulmonary fibrosis. In a detailed pulmonary function study, 30 consecutive SLE patients attending our lupus clinic were examined clinically, radiologically and physiologically in an attempt to detail the nature of the pulmonary involvement. Patients were studied regardless of whether or not respiratory symptoms were present. Functional abnormalities were found in 80% of these patients. Diffusing capacity was below normal in 80%, and a reduced total lung capacity in 43%. An interesting observation was that weakness of the respiratory muscles, in particular the diaphragm, may contribute to the reduction of lung volumes and may account for the elevated diaphragms seen radiographically in some patients with otherwise unexplained dyspnoea and orthopnoea (Gibson, Edmonds & Hughes 1977).

In the patient on steroids or immunosuppressive drugs, the acute development of widespread pulmonary shadows and pneumonitis may present diagnostic difficulties from pulmonary tuberculosis, pneumocystis or other pulmonary infection (Matthay *et al.* 1974).

Case report. *A 26-year-old West Indian woman with clinically active SLE (joint disease, skin rashes, alopecia and renal involvement) had been on azathioprine and prednisone for 2 years. She was admitted as an emergency with marked dyspnoea and widespread 'miliary' shadowing on both lung fields on chest X-ray (Fig. 2.16). A Mantoux test 2 years previously had been negative. Laboratory tests included Hb 10·6 g%, WBC 3500 (Neut. 35%, Lymph. 54%), complement (C3) 33% mg per cent, DNA binding 100%. The patient had a dry cough but no sputum was obtainable. Although a tentative diagnosis of miliary tuberculosis was made, the only immediate treatment given was an increase in prednisone to 80 mg daily. Within 24 hours the symptoms had dramatically improved and subsequent chest radiographs showed rapid disappearance of the lesions. No evidence of tuberculosis was obtained.*

Reticuloendothelial system

Occasionally patients present with massive lymphadenopathy at the onset of their disease, though the commoner picture is of slight 'rubbery' lymph node enlargement only. Lymphadenopathy occurs in 30% of cases, being twice as common as clinical splenomegaly (Table 2.7) (see also Chapter 7). Despite the T-cell disturbance in SLE, the thymus is small, or normal in size.

Recent studies have suggested that a significant number of patients with SLE may have a functional hyposplenism. Interestingly, in one of the

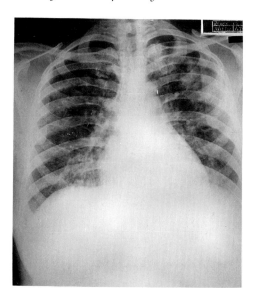

Fig. 2.16 Miliary shadowing in acute SLE. The lesions cleared rapidly on prednisone.

Table 2.7 Reticuloendothelial and haematological manifestations in 50 patients (from Grigor *et al.* 1978)

Manifestations	Percentage
Lymphadenopathy	30
Splenomegaly	16
Anaemia	52
Haemolytic anaemia	12
Leucopenia	46
Lymphopenia	82
Thrombocytopenia	26

first of these studies, 2 of 4 patients with SLE and evidence of hyposplenism developed salmonella septicaemia (Lovy *et al.* 1981) suggesting a parallel with sickle cell disease.

Blood (Table 2.7) (reviewed by Budman & Steinberg 1977)

Red cells. A normochromic, normocytic anaemia is the commonest haematological manifestation of SLE, occurring in one-half to three-quarters of all patients. In the multi-centre ARA survey (Cohen *et al.* 1971) haemolytic anaemia was detected in 16% of cases. A similar figure was noted in our

Chapter 2

series (Grigor *et al.* 1978) and in Estes & Christian's series with a positive direct Coombs test demonstrable in 38 of 150 patients, 18 of whom had evidence of haemolysis. In 3 additional patients, acute haemolytic episodes, with sudden drops in haematocrit, rises in serum bilirubin, reticulocytosis or absent serum haptoglobins, occurred in the absence of a positive direct Coombs test. Bohner *et al.* (1968) looked at the causes of positive direct Coombs reactions seen in a university hospital. The largest single group was SLE which accounted for 18%.

White cells. Leucopenia (WBC $< 4500/mm^3$) occurs in up to two-thirds of SLE patients. In particular, an absolute lymphopenia is common, even in the presence of a normal total WBC. Leucopenia, while rarely of clear pathogenetic significance in SLE is of fundamental diagnostic importance in the differentiation from other vasculitides, the majority of which demonstrate a leucocytosis or a normal WBC. The increased tendency to infection in SLE may be contributed to not only by quantitative leucopenia, but reduced phagocytosis of the leukocytes as shown by reduction of nitroblue tetrazolium dye reduction (Wenger & Bole 1973).

Using the lymphocyte toxicity test, cytotoxic antibodies to lymphocytes have been detected in three-quarters of SLE sera (Mittal *et al.* 1970). Lymphocytotoxins are complement dependent, and may be 7S or 19S. Their presence is broadly related to disease activity in SLE, particularly to fever, skin, haematological and CNS involvement (Butler *et al.* 1972; Bluestein & Zvaifler 1976; Bresnihan *et al.* 1977).

Platelets. While mild thrombocytopenia is common, severe degrees ($10-30 000$ platelets/mm^3) are unusual, occurring in less than 5% of cases. The overlap between idiopathic thrombocytopenic purpura (ITP) and SLE is strong and ITP may antedate the development of SLE by many years. Studies of antiphospholipid antibodies has thrown light on to the pathogenesis of thrombocytopenia in SLE. A significant number of patients with antiphospholipid antibodies develop thrombocytopenia. In our studies, there was a strong statistical correlation between elevated IgG anticardiolipin antibody levels and thrombocytopenia ($P > 0.001$) and of the 20 patients with the highest IgG anticardiolipin levels, 16 had thrombocytopenia (Harris *et al.* 1985a). Preliminary studies have shown that these are primarily directed against negatively charged phospholipids — those sited mainly on the inner layer of the bilipid platelet membrane. Possibly in those patients with severe episodes of thrombocytopenia, additional factors are operative in exposing this inner membrane.

As might be expected, a significant number of patients with *idiopathic* thrombocytopenic purpura have antiphospholipid antibodies. Time will tell whether this subset of patients develop other features of SLE (Harris *et al.* 1985a).

In view of such findings, one wonders whether splenectomy is, in the long term, advisable in SLE, though the short-term results are good – 9 out of 16 in the series of Breckenridge, Moore & Ratnoff (1967) improving.

Clotting factors. Clotting defects have been recognized in SLE since 1952, when Conley and Hartmann described two SLE patients with prolonged whole blood clotting and prothrombin times.

A wide variety of clotting abnormalities have been described (reviewed by Byron 1982). These include the finding of antithrombin III in some patients (Loizou *et al.* 1984). Clinical bleeding problems are rare. The important lupus anticoagulant, and its association with arterial and venous thrombosis, are discussed in Chapter 3.

Kidney

While earlier studies of SLE gave the incidence of renal involvement as 50%, it is now recognized that subclinical involvement is more frequent, with fluctuation and reversibility of lesions probably being common during the earlier stages of the disease.

Based on light microscopy, three broad categories are defined: focal, diffuse proliferative and membranous. While different series give different percentages some generalizations can be made. Focal nephritis (Fig. 2.17, A) is the commonest lesion, especially with recognition of milder SLE cases. This lesion carries the best prognosis and may be reversible. The second type, the diffuse proliferative lesion (Fig. 2.17, B), carries the worst prognosis. The third (membranous) type is the least common and usually presents with the nephrotic syndrome (though the other varieties of lesions may also do so) and, somewhat surprisingly, carries a reasonably good prognosis, probably irrespective of steroid administration (reviewed by Adu & Cameron 1982; Gladman 1992; Ginzler & Antoniadis 1992).

While the majority of patients remain 'true to type' within these broad categories, overlap does occur. No renal biopsy can be said to be pathognomonic of SLE — for example, wire-loop lesions can be seen in other vasculitides. Despite these limitations, renal biopsy is still used in SLE in order to provide an approximate prognostic assessment, especially in active, early disease with persistent hypocomplementaemia (Baldwin *et al.* 1977).

The kidney has a limited number of clinical responses to insult, and the renal manifestations of SLE — nephrotic syndrome, haematuria, acute

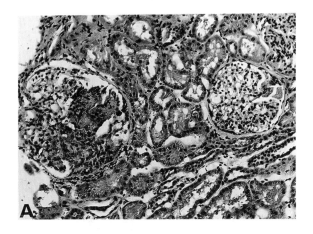

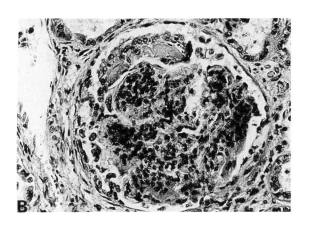

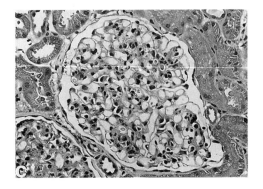

renal failure, hypertension — do not reflect closely the pathological picture. The 'end-stage' kidney in SLE is no different pathologically from that in other diseases (Fig. 2.18).

Immunofluorescence has proved most useful in assessment of renal lupus. In focal lupus nephritis, immunofluorescence shows that the granular deposits of IgG and C3 are found in *all* glomeruli, predominantly in mesangial regions (Fig. 2.19, A). In diffuse proliferative disease, the deposits are seen in all sites, in severe cases (more than 30% of glomeruli involved) granular staining for IgG and C3 is heavy (Fig. 2.19, B) and fibrin deposits may be seen in, and adjacent to, crescents.

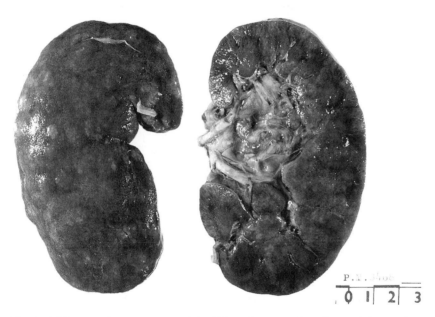

Fig. 2.18 Macroscopic appearances of the kidney from a patient dying of chronic SLE nephritis, showing coarse granularity of the surface and cortical thinning. (Dr Shirley Amin, University Hospital of the West Indies.)

Fig. 2.17 (*facing page*) A, Kidney (×160). Focal proliferative glomerulonephritis with necrosis. Exudation of polymorphs and local crescent formation in one glomerulus. The second glomerulus shows a small area of fibrinoid change. (Dr Shirley Amin, University Hospital of the West Indies.) B, Kidney (×350). Diffuse proliferative nephritis, with basement membrane thickening. Also demonstrates fibrin in Bowman's space, giving rise to crescent formation. (Dr Shirley Amin, University Hospital of the West Indies.) C, Kidney (×350). Mild mesangial thickening only. (Dr Shirley Amin, University Hospital of the West Indies.)

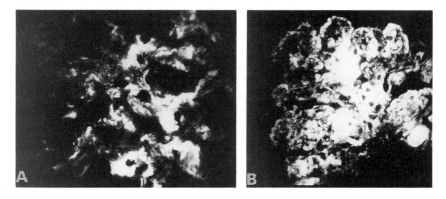

Fig. 2.19 Patterns of immunofluorescence in the SLE kidney (×340) using conjugated anti-C3 antiserum. A, Mesangial staining. B, Lumpy and granular deposits along basement membrane and in the mesangium. (Dr Shirley Amin, University Hospital of the West Indies.)

A further guide to assessment of severity and prognosis is provided by electron microscopy, where electron-dense deposits suggest a poorer outlook (Fig. 2.20, A). More recent studies have concentrated on the presence of glomerular thrombi and extensive sub-endothelial deposits, these two features being predictive of an increase in glomerular sclerosis in a subsequent second renal biopsy (Kim *et al.* 1988).

It has become rather traditional to regard high anti-DNA antibody levels as a harbinger of renal disease. This is wrong. Many, many patients in clinics throughout the world remain free from any clinical renal disease, despite high DNA levels. Other measurements will also have to be taken into account, for example C3 levels (Houssiau *et al.* 1991), anti-DNA complexes (Sasaki *et al.* 1991), rheumatoid factor (Howard *et al.* 1991, Houssiau *et al.* 1991), anti-endothelial cell antibodies (D'Cruz *et al.* 1991), thrombomodulin (Takaya 1991), antiphospholipid antibodies (D'Cruz *et al.* 1991, Frampton 1991).

It is apparent that 'subclinical' renal involvement may be present for years prior to the development of proteinuria or hypertension and it is not uncommon to find immunofluorescent evidence of immune complex deposition in renal biopsies performed on patients whose sole clinical evidence of renal involvement was a lowered serum complement level.

Urinalysis in SLE reveals abnormalities in approximately one-third to one-half of SLE (Table 2.8).

Other urinary findings may be those of disturbed tubular function, such as renal tubular acidosis (Tu & Shearn 1967). Renal vein thrombosis is a rare but serious manifestation of SLE (Appel *et al.* 1976). We described

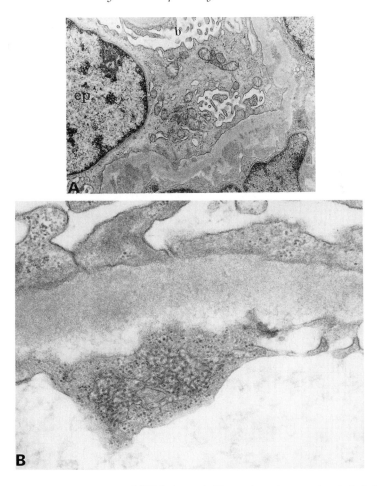

Fig. 2.20 Electron microscopy of SLE kidney. A, Dense deposits on subendothelial aspects of the basement membrane (ep = epithelial cell; b = Bowman's space.). B (EM ×57 600). Microtubular structure in endoplasmic reticulum of endothelial cell. (Dr J. Audrecht, University Hospital of the West Indies.)

Table 2.8 Renal manifestations in 50 patients (from Grigor *et al.* 1978)

Manifestation	Percentage
Proteinuria (>1 g/24 h)	26
Abnormal urine sediment	30
Raised serum creatinine	10
Abnormal histology	34

four cases in whom a clotting tendency, as well as the lupus anticoagulant, was present (Asherson *et al.* 1984).

Nervous system (Khamashta, Cervera & Hughes 1991)

One of the major clinical trends in SLE during the past decade has been the appreciation of the frequency of CNS involvement in SLE, in particular the incidence of psychosis and more subtle neuropsychiatric presentations. Indeed it might even be proposed that SLE be redefined as a primarily neurological disease. While it is possible that immune complex deposition in the cerebral vasculature accounts for some of the neuropathology, it has proved difficult to obtain proof of immune complex deposition in the majority of cases. In our own hands, the majority of cases have had normal CSF complement levels (C4 in the CSF represents about 1/200−1/300 of that in serum, and more sensitive estimation techniques may increase the clinical usefulness of CSF complement levels.)

Kaposi, in his original description of SLE, noted recurrent delirium in 2 out of 11 patients. In the 150 patients studied by Estes & Christian (1971) CNS involvement was noted in no less than 59% of patients and was second only to renal involvement as a cause of death.

The spectrum of CNS involvement is wide and encompasses almost the whole range of neurological disease (reviewed by Harris & Hughes 1985; Khamashta, Cervera & Hughes 1991). By far the most frequent manifestations are depression and psychosis, and SLE patients have been diagnosed as schizophrenic before the real nature of the disease was recognized. The mental changes vary from mild depressive states (which may mistakenly be attributed to a general reaction to the disease or to corticosteroid therapy) through to a rapidly developing profound dementia.

Case report. *A 53-year-old Jamaican woman was initially seen as an outpatient with mild labile hypertension and depression. Four years later she was noted to have active synovitis in the small joints of the hands and ankles. In addition, she was severely depressed, had marked muscle weakness, and a pericardial friction rub. Investigations included ESR 98 mm/h, WBC 4600 with an absolute lymphopenia, a positive WR with negative* Treponema pallidum *immobilization test, positive LE cell and ANA tests and DNA binding activity of 78%. Evidence of myositis was obtained by EMG and muscle enzyme abnormalities. Over the course of her first week in hospital, she became progressively more withdrawn and uncommunicative. She developed paranoid ideas about other patients and became frankly schizophrenic. Ten days after admission her level of consciousness deteriorated rapidly. No focal neurological signs were found. The spinal fluid was normal, but EEG showed marked*

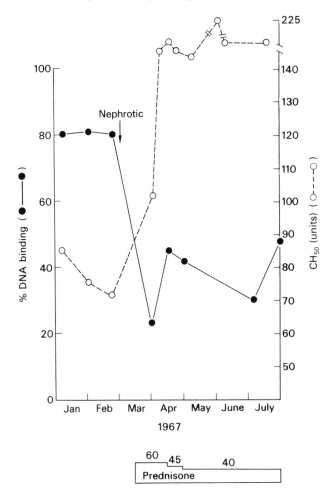

Fig. 2.21 Serial study in SLE nephritis. The DNA binding of 80% (continuous line) and low CH_{50} result (normal > 150 units) preceded the development of proteinuria.

Table 2.9 Principal CNS involvement in SLE

Depression	Cerebellar ataxia
Psychosis	Chorea
Seizures	Myelitis
Hemiplegia	Meningitis
Paraplegia	Peripheral neuropathy
Cranial nerve lesions	

generalized abnormalities. She was started on high-dose corticosteroid therapy.
Within 24 hours there was noticeable improvement in her level of consciousness.
Three days later a normal sleep pattern was restored and she was fully orientated
and feeding herself. During the 12 months follow-up period, in which the
prednisone was gradually discontinued, there was no active synovitis or recur-
rence of depression. The DNA binding activity was less than 20%. She was a
highly intelligent woman with considerable insight who could recount in detail
what went on when she was in a state of apparent stupor.

Milder forms of neuropsychiatric disturbance may be commoner than hitherto realized, and SLE may well come to be recognized as a relatively important 'medical' cause of neuropsychiatric disease in young women.

Baker (1973) in a review of the psychopathology of SLE noted that psychiatric symptoms had been noted in up to 52% of SLE patients. In his own study, 17 patients with SLE were evaluated psychiatrically. Serious psychiatric syndromes were observed in 41% of the patients. Of 11 episodes observed, a mixed syndrome (characterized by a combination of organic symptoms and either affective or schizophreniform symptoms) was the most common type of psychopathology and occurred in 45% of the episodes. It was concluded that:

1 Psychiatric episodes do not represent an intensification of psychopathology present before the onset of SLE in most cases.
2 SLE is not merely acting as a non-specific stress to predisposed individuals.
3 There is considerable variability.
4 The episodes are totally reversible in the majority of cases.
5 Somatic treatment may alleviate the psychiatric disturbances.

The diagnosis of this group of patients has proved particularly difficult. All too often the depression in a young SLE patient has been ascribed to the presence of chronic disease or to steroid therapy. That even the most subtle behavioural changes may be due to organic disease is hinted at by the usually highly abnormal electroencephalograms seen in such patients.

Unfortunately, serological testing, conventional brain scanning and even computed tomography have limited diagnostic value. Preliminary data have suggested that MRI scanning may have some value in CNS lupus (Bernstein 1983), though only where focal lesions are expected, for example in association with antiphospholipid antibodies (Montalban *et al.* 1991).

Scanning using inhaled oxygen-15 has been found to show marked abnormalities both of cerebral flow and metabolism in a variety of patients with cerebrovascular disease. In a study of 47 patients with SLE, abnormalities in regional distribution of oxygen utilization and blood flow were seen in 23 out of 24 patients with definite CNS involvement (Pinching *et al*. 1978). Even in patients with subtle psychiatric changes, gross defects were often seen (Fig. 2.22).

The previously mentioned association between lymphocytotoxic antibodies and cerebral disease has suggested that, in future, serological assays for antineuronal antibodies may have clinical potential (Bresnihan & Hughes 1979).

Epilepsy. Epilepsy has been reported in 17−50% of patients with CNS lupus (Bennett *et al*. 1972) all types having been noted. It is not uncommon to see SLE patients diagnosed at, say, 20 years, who have had epilepsy since being teenagers or even in childhood.

Case report. *A 25-year-old patient developed vasculitis, arthritis, fever and a rash 2 weeks after the delivery of her first child.*

She had suffered from mild epilepsy since the age of 13. At the age of 14 she was alleged to have had an attack of 'rheumatic fever'.

In a study of our own patients, the incidence of 'premorbid' epilepsy was eight times the national 'background' figure (Mackworth-Young & Hughes 1985). Epilepsy is also an important clinical feature in some patients with antiphospholipid antibodies.

Migraine. Migraine attacks are a well-known feature of SLE and were prominent in our patients (Grigor *et al*. 1978). While they are generally related to disease activity, they are not consistently responsive to steroid therapy. The subject has been reviewed by Brandt & Lusell (1978). Our own clinical experience also shows migraine to be an important clinical component of the antiphospholipid syndrome (see Chapter 3).

One of the commonest antecedent histories obtained in SLE patients is of teenage migraine. With increasing awareness of mild SLE, it is commonplace to see young girls in clinic whose only manifestations of disease are premenstrual migrainous headaches and a high DNA-binding activity.

Transient ischaemic attacks. These may be difficult to differentiate from migraine. Nevertheless, they are of great significance, and are not uncommon. Clinical features include partial loss of vision, transient unilateral blindness, transient hemiphagia and, sometimes, not so transient effects:

Case report. *A 15-year-old schoolgirl had complained for 1 year of intermittent abdominal pains and episodic arthralgia. Twenty-four hours before admission she had experienced a sharp pain above the eyes, associated with nausea,*

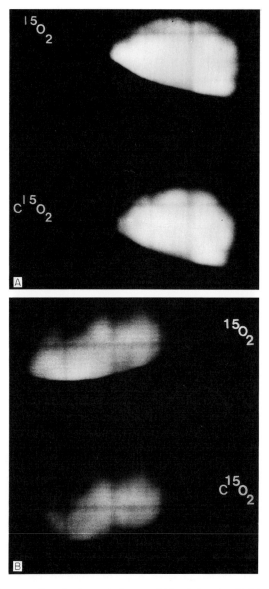

Fig. 2.22 Disturbances of cerebral metabolism and blood flow in CNS lupus. A, Normal oxygen-15 (cerebral metabolism) and $^{15}CO_2$ (cerebral blood flow). B, Scans in a 21-year-old girl with SLE in whom the only CNS abnormality was of mild behavioural disturbance and depression. This technique is now being adapted for computed tomography (Dr T. Jones, Hammersmith Hospital).

followed by a sensation of multicoloured flickering lights in both visual fields. Within 24 hours these had become lateralized to the left homonomous temporal fields and 12 hours later she was found to have a complete left-sided homonomous hemianopia. In addition she had a facial 'butterfly' rash, subungal splinter haemorrhages, and livedo reticularis over the forearm and dorsum of the right hand. Brain scan and lumbar puncture were normal. The EEG showed frequent irregular low-to-medium voltage delta waves in the right posterior quadrant. The DNA binding activity was 81% and complement levels were normal. With the exception of the homonomous hemianopia she responded rapidly to steroid therapy and has remained well, asymptomatic and at work for the past 3 years.

This case — first described in 1972 (Bennett *et al.* 1972) — deserves updating.

Case report. She remained well throughout her teenage years, though the hemanopia was permanent. In 1982 she married. Her first pregnancy in 1982 was complicated by livedo reticularis. Two days following delivery of a normal infant, she developed thrombocytopenia (platelets 5000/mm³). Over the ensuing year, on reducing doses of prednisolone, the platelets returned to 150000/mm³. During this episode, the serum contained high titres of anticardiolipin antibodies.

In 1993, high levels of anticardiolipin persist and the platelet count fluctuates (on no treatment) in the 60000 region. The patient remains otherwise well.

Perhaps in this patient it is even more important to ask why the pregnancy did not end in miscarriage.

Hemiplegia. Of 15 patients developing cerebrovascular attacks in our SLE series, 13% had moderate or high titres of anticardiolipin antibodies (Harris *et al.* 1984). This association was also seen in patients with normal DNA-binding values and otherwise relatively quiescent disease.

Although hemiplegia in SLE was recognized by Osler in 1895 (he described it in a young doctor), it is only recently that the significance of transient and permanent cerebral ischaemia has been emphasized. This major subject, with implications for stroke patients far beyond the clinical limits of SLE, will be discussed in Chapter 3.

Cranial nerve lesions

These are relatively uncommon (Bennett *et al.* 1972), though facial pain (and occasionally trigeminal neuralgia) may be prominent.

Unilateral ptosis (the pathogenesis of which is obscure) is a recurrent feature in a number of patients we have studied.

Myelopathy. Myelopathy is a rare though important manifestation of SLE (Penn & Rowan 1968; Morgan *et al*. 1986). In such cases, the CSF protein may be high and the CSF complement level reduced. In a review of 26 patients with transverse myelopathy associated with SLE, the diagnosis of SLE was made in only 60% before the onset of the myelopathy. Thirteen patients died, 9 had permanent neurological defects and only 4 recovered nearly normal function (Andrianakos *et al*. 1975).

A multiple sclerosis-like clinical picture is occasionally seen in SLE, and an interesting group of six patients has been described in whom chronic false-positive tests for syphilis and a clinical picture resembling multiple sclerosis was associated with laboratory findings suggestive of SLE. The commonest neurological finding was spastic paraplegia. The patients all had chronic biological false-positive tests for syphilis (Fulford *et al*. 1972). It was this study that led us to look at 'Jamaican neuropathy' — a clinically similar condition — and set out on our studies of antiphospholipid antibodies. Myelopathy in SLE is probably one of the stronger associations of antiphospholipid antibodies (see Chapter 3).

Disorders of movement. Chorea has been the most widely reported disorder of movement of SLE. It may be subtle, and, especially in children with chorea, SLE is an important differential diagnosis from rheumatic fever. In a review by Donaldson & Espiner (1971) the mean age of onset was 18 years, somewhat older than that in rheumatic fever. In 8 of the 2 cases, chorea was the initial manifestation of the disease. In 12 cases other neurological abnormalities were present. The development of chorea in the postpartum period should suggest the possibility of lupus (Donaldson & Espiner 1971). Chorea has been associated, in our studies, with anti-cardiolipin antibodies (see Chapter 3).

Cerebellar ataxia is occasionally seen. Dubois (1974) reports one patient in whom cerebellar ataxia recurred each time the prednisolone dose was reduced below 15 mg daily.

Peripheral neuropathy. This is uncommon in SLE, a point of differentiation from polyarteritis nodosa and rheumatoid arthritis. It is usually of the mixed, symmetrical type, though a mononeuritis multiplex has been described. Also described is an exclusive motor loss with raised levels of spinal fluid protein without a pleocytosis, as in the Guillain–Barré syndrome (Lewis 1965). We have described a patient with SLE, thrombocytopenia and Guillain–Barré syndrome in whom antiphospholipid antibodies appeared to cross-react with sphingomyelin (Harris *et al*. 1983).

Retinopathy. Although SLE not infrequently causes retinopathy, visual impairment is uncommon. The clinically observed retinal lesions include cotton-wool exudates and haemorrhages. Rarely, perivascular sheathing and fibrosis may occur. Retinal exudates in the absence of other pre-disposing causes (hypertension, diabetes, severe anaemia) are called 'cytoid bodies' and may develop acutely.

Less florid forms may be picked up by fluorescein dye retinal angio-graphy (Santos *et al.* 1975) though this technique has not yet been widely assessed as an investigative aid in cerebral vasculitis. Our own experience using routine fluorescein angiography was disappointing (Lanham *et al.* 1982). Although leakage was seen, the changes did not closely parallel the clinical features. It is likely that the incidence of cytoid bodies reported in older series is high, representing a more severely ill group of patients.

INFECTION IN SLE

Infection has been a major cause of morbidity and mortality in SLE, both in the pre-steroid and post-steroid eras. Clearly, a number of factors such as corticosteroids, immunosuppressives and uraemia may themselves heighten any tendency to develop infection (Table 2.10).

It still is doubtful, however, whether asymptomatic SLE patients, or those in total remission, have an increased propensity to infection. Having said this, salmonella infection (possibly associated with functional hypo-splenism in lupus — Lovy *et al.* 1981) is common.

Some light was shed on the problem in a survey where data from 223 SLE patients were analysed by computer. The frequency of infections increased progressively with increased steroid dosage, reaching an eight-

Table 2.10 Possible factors leading to increased infection in SLE

Lowered complement levels
Defective phagocytosis
Decreased leukocyte chemotaxis
Circulating lymphocytotoxins
Impaired delayed hypersensitivity
Selective defects of cellular immunity
Antibody to circulating granulocytes
Reduced nitroblue tetrazolium dye reduction
Lowered antibody response (especially IgM) to certain antigens
Functional hyposplenism

Also:
Corticosteroids
Immunosuppressives
Uraemia
Nephrotic syndrome

fold increase in patients receiving 40 mg prednisone daily or over (Ginzler
et al. 1978).

The review by Watanabe-Duffy and Gladman (1991) is recommended.

SLE AND PREGNANCY

Provided that renal and cardiac function are not impaired, pregnancy is
not contraindicated in SLE (Grigor *et al.* 1977; Jungers, Dougados & Pelissier
1982a). Fertility and sterility rates are normal in SLE patients (Fraga *et al.*
1974) but abortion rates are significantly higher than normal, both before
and after the onset of SLE. Exacerbations of SLE may occur at any time
during pregnancy though the immediate postpartum period is critical,
and close medical supervision is required during the 8 weeks following
delivery (Lockshin 1993).

With the exception of the rare but interesting association with congenital
heart block (Scott *et al.* 1983), the fetus does not appear to be at risk of
congenital abnormalities in SLE. Thus the reason(s) for the increased
abortion rate remain unclear. Immunological mechanisms have been
suggested. Lymphocytotoxic antibodies (normally absent in healthy SLE
pregnancies) many cross-react with trophoblast antigens and serve as
'blocking' antibodies (Bresnihan *et al.* 1977). Anticardiolipin antibodies
have been clearly associated wtih thrombosis and abortion in SLE (Hughes
1983; Harris *et al.* 1983). In a study of SLE pregnancies ending in abortion,
most were associated with anticardiolipin antibodies. In those placentae
available for histology, placental vessel thrombosis was prominent (Derue
et al. 1985).

As lupus affects mainly women of childbearing age, there have been
worldwide studies of lupus in pregnancy — indeed most major institutions
now run lupus-in-pregnancy clinics. Lupus itself is not a contraindication,
but hypertension, renal disease, and antiphospholipid associated miscarriage (see Chapter 3) are problems for particular groups of patients.

DISCOID LUPUS

Discoid lupus characteristically produces inflammatory plaques on the
face, arms and trunk (Fig. 2.23). The characteristic pathological lesion in
chronic discoid LE are erythema, hyperkeratosis and scaling, follicular
plugging, telangiectasia and atrophy of skin appendages. Positive immunofluorescent 'band' tests are obtained on involved skin.

As well as the face and exposed areas of skin, scalp and mucocutaneous
lesions are frequent.

The lesions vary from localized and minimal, to widespread and severely

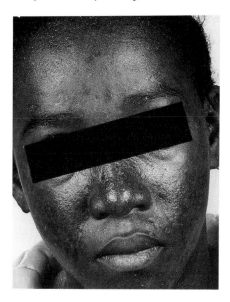

Fig. 2.23 Chronic discoid LE.

disfiguring. In approximately one-half of patients, there is a history of photo-sensitivity, and in occasional cases local skin trauma is considered to be an exacerbating factor.

A wider age group is affected than with SLE, patients of 70 years and older being reported.

Although SLE patients may develop discoid lesions, in the main there is a relatively small risk of patients with chronic discoid LE subsequently developing systemic LE. The figure usually quoted is 5%, though detailed studies of individual discoid LE patients sometimes reveal subtle systemic abnormalities such as abnormal EEGs or pulmonary function abnormalities. When chronic discoid LE patients *do* develop systemic features, these are often transient, as in the case described earlier and in the following case.

Case report. *A 49-year-old woman had had discoid lesions of the face, upper arms and scalp for 4 years. Following prolonged sun exposure on holiday, there was worsening of the skin lesions, together with the development of mild widespread synovitis, which lasted for 2 months before resolving.*

As knowledge of lupus grows, so the recognition of clinical subjects widens. There are, for example, three clinical groups of discoid LE patients in whom 'systemic features' may occur — late onset arthritis (sometimes resembling rheumatoid arthritis), neurological disease, notably depression, and the antiphospholipid antibody syndrome (Chapter 3) which may appear with devastating consequences such as stroke in discoid lupus patients who have hitherto showed no features of 'systemic' lupus erythematosus.

DRUG-INDUCED LUPUS

Clinical (reviewed by Harmon & Portonova 1982; Mongey & Hess 1989)

Although drugs have been suggested as one of the causes of the apparent increase in the prevalence of lupus, drug-induced lupus is distinctly rare — possibly ten times less common than SLE (Lee, Rivero & Siegel 1966). Some of the drugs more frequently implicated are listed in Table 2.11 (adapted from Alarcon-Segovia 1975).

In general, the development of lupus on the first group of drugs is dose related, while those in the second group may have an 'allergic' mechanism. In addition, positive ANA tests were more frequent in patients receiving the former group of drugs, the incidence of positive ANA tests being

Table 2.11 Drugs implicated in drug-induced LE

Frequent
Hydralazine
Procainamide
Anticonvulsants (phenytoin, hydantoins, primidone)
Isoniazid
Chlorpromazine
Oral contraceptives (may exacerbate pre-existing SLE)
Rare
Aminosalicylic acid
D-Penicillamine
L-Dopa
Methylthiouracil
Propylthiouracil
Phenylbutazone
Beta-blockers
Quinidine
Reserpine
Sulphonamides ⎱ may exacerbate pre-existing SLE
Penicillin ⎰

many times higher than the incidence of clinical SLE induced by these agents. (Reviewed by Hughes 1982a, and Hess 1982.)

The main features of drug-induced LE are listed in Table 2.12.

The clinical features closely resemble those of SLE proper (though pulmonary involvement may be commoner in drug-induced LE and may be life-threatening. Remission following withdrawal of the drug may take several months (or even years in the case of hydralazine) but a conservative therapeutic approach is required.

Case report. A 30-year-old male solicitor had suffered from intermittent epilepsy since the age of 6 years; treated intermittently with anticonvulsants. At the age of 28 years, whilst on diphenylhydantoin, which had had been receiving for 2 years, he developed athralgias, facial rash and pleurisy. LE cell tests were positive. The anticonvulsant was changed and he was started on ACTH 40 units, alternate days, on which he remained until his referral. During the previous 6 months he had complained of bilateral knee and hip joint pains and it was felt that the lupus was again becoming active. He was found to have marked Cushing's syndrome and bilateral aseptic necrosis of the hips, but no evidence of lupus activity. DNA binding, complement and renal function tests were normal.

In general, there has been, if anything, a tendency to overplay the significance of positive ANA tests in patients taking drugs. Only rarely are they followed by the development of clinical symptoms. Furthermore, clinical symptoms generally become prominent only if undiagnosed.

Case report. A 54-year-old receiving a beta-blocker for mild hypertension was found on serological testing (by a study group monitoring ANAs in patients

Table 2.12 Features in drug-induced LE

Polyarthritis and arthralgia
Skin eruptions
Polyserositis
Hepatomegaly
Lymphadenopathy
Pulmonary infiltrates
Renal and CNS involvement rare
Hypergammaglobulinaemia, leucopenia, ANA, LE cells
DNA antibodies (double stranded) negative
Complement normal
Resolves on withdrawal of the offending drugs

*receiving these drugs) to have an ANA of >1 in 2000. On checking, the patient
had recently suffered increasing arthralgias for which her practitioner had
started ibuprofen. The pains resolved on changing the antihypertensive therapy
and the ANA reverted to normal.*

Serological tests in drug-induced LE

ANA tests are almost invariably positive in patients with drug-induced
LE and LE cells are plentiful. (Some of the best teaching preparations of
LE cells are from cases of drug-induced LE). DNA antibodies are usually
absent or in low titre (Hughes 1971; Winfield & Davis 1974) (reviewed by
Hughes *et al.* 1981 and Hess 1982).

Tan and his colleagues have demonstrated that the antinuclear antibody
is largely directed against nuclear histone. The antibodies are non-
complement fixing, which may in part explain the low incidence of renal
involvement (Fritzler & Tan 1978; Hess 1982).

Aetiology of drug-induced LE

It is currently believed that at least some of the drugs act as immunogens
or haptens leading to disease in genetically predisposed individuals.
Acetylation in the liver is, for isoniazid as for hydralazine, a major metabolic
pathway and it is likely that slower acetylators are more likely than
fast acetylators to develop isoniazid-induced LE (Perry *et al.* 1970). Some
evidence for a genetically determined predisposition comes from studies
of the past histories and family histories of patients with drug-induced
lupus (Alarcon-Segovia 1969).

A study from our group of patients taking hydralazine confirmed the
slow-acetyletor link, showed a female predominance, and, more significantly, suggested an HLA DR$_4$ association (Mansilla-Tinoco *et al.* 1982).

LABORATORY INVESTIGATIONS IN SLE

Table 2.13 lists some of the principal immunological abnormalities in SLE.

Antinuclear antibodies, DNA antibodies and the LE cell phenomenon
are discussed in the Appendix.

Antiphospholipid antibodies (Harris *et al.* 1983, 1985). These are discussed in
Chapter 3.

Rheumatoid factor. Rheumatoid factor is found in up to 40% of SLE patients. It
appears to have little pathogenic significance in SLE, and while it might
theoretically facilitate the phagocytosis of circulating immune complexes

Table 2.13 Principal immunological abnormalities in SLE

Antinuclear antibodies ⎱ see Appendix
Anticytoplasmic antibodies ⎰
Rheumatoid factors
Cryoproteins
False-positive tests for syphilis
Circulating anticoagulants
Antiviral antibodies
Lymphocytotoxins

its presence does not appear to exert either a beneficial or harmful effect on the course of the renal disease.

False-positive tests for syphilis. Patients with chronic biologically false-positive (BFP) reactions develop a high incidence of autoimmune diseases, especially SLE, Sjøgren's syndrome, autoimmune haemolytic anaemia, Hashimoto's thyroiditis and rheumatoid arthritis. In a 16-year survey by Catterall (1973), 134 patients attending a venereal disease clinic were found to have a persistent BFP reaction. Of these, 10 developed SLE and 4 discoid LE. A BFP reaction is found in up to 10% of patients with SLE. The association between false-positive serological tests for syphilis, the lupus anticoagulant and the tendency to thrombosis and abortion is discussed in Chapter 3.

In addition to 'false'-positive serology, the occasional unfortunate SLE patient may demonstrate a positive FTA test. In this situation, where the patient may be falsely diagnosed as having syphilis, the pattern of immunofluorescence in the FTA may be helpful, showing a 'beaded' appearance (thought to result from antinuclear antibody attaching to the test treponeme), rather than the usual homogeneous pattern (Kraus, Haserick & Lantz 1970).

Lymphocytotoxic antibodies (Winfield 1985). Up to 80% of SLE sera contain antibodies which react with sites on the surface of lymphocytes. Although both IgG and IgM classes are recognized, the cold-reactive IgM antibodies have received most attention because of their ease of measurement by complement-dependent microcytotoxicity assays. The IgM antibodies are broadly reactive with both B- and T-cell subpopulations. IgG antibodies react equally well at 4°C and 37°C.

Their role in the pathogenesis of SLE is not yet clear. However, important possibilities include an effect on lymphocyte subpopulations, a marker for virus infection and secondary pathogenetic effects on brain (Bresnihan *et al.* 1977) and placenta (Bresnihan *et al.* 1977).

Immunoglobulins. Polyclonal hyperglobulinaemia is found in up to 75% of SLE patients (Estes & Christian 1971; Dubois *et al.* 1974). Occasional cases of IgA deficiency in SLE are seen (Bach, Pillay & Kark 1971). In addition to raised IgG levels, turnover rates for IgG are twice as fast as in normals (Levy *et al.* 1970).

Sedimentation rate. While the ESR is elevated in 90% of patients with active SLE, it is not a particularly useful guide to disease activity or to therapy. Normal values are occasionally seen in patients with florid (especially CNS) lupus, and persistent elevations are seen in some patients otherwise in remission.

C-reactive protein

C-reactive protein (CRP) has emerged from the doldrums to become a major investigation in the connective tissue diseases. Put at its simplest, the SLE patient has an ESR of 100 and a CRP of zero. It is a regular and striking finding that SLE patients fail to mount a significant CRP response (Becker *et al.* 1980). Even in the presence of infection, the rise is rarely striking (Honig, Gorevic & Weissman 1977). So regular is this finding in SLE that we have proposed it as a candidate consideration amongst the ARA criteria (Perreira da Silva *et al.* 1980). The subject of CRP in general has been reviewed by Pepys *et al.* (1982).

Serum amyloid A

Similarly, SLE patients fail to achieve a high serum amyloid A level (De Beer *et al.* 1982), perhaps a clue to the apparently low incidence of amyloid in SLE.

DIFFERENTIAL DIAGNOSIS

The development of antiDNA antibody estimations has simplified the diagnosis of SLE. However, other antigens play a part in the immune complex pathogenesis of this disease, and cases of active SLE are sometimes seen in whom antiDNA antibodies are absent (reviewed by Hughes 1984a). Conversely, rare patients are seen with diseases other than SLE in whom antinative DNA antibodies are detectable. As always, it is the diseases in which differential diagnosis is most difficult — Sjøgren's syndrome and chronic active hepatitis — for example, where the occasional raised antiDNA antibody titre has been demonstrated. It should be stressed that high titres (e.g. over 50% DNA binding) of DNA antibodies are almost exclusive to SLE.

Because of the wide variety of presentations (listed in Table 2.14) and features (Fig. 2.24) not only diagnosis but classification become difficult, and a number of earlier reviews of SLE may well have included cases of mixed connective tissue disease, or rheumatoid arthritis plus Sjøgren's syndrome.

The American Rheumatism Association publish criteria for the classification of SLE (Table 2.15).

It has been stressed that such criteria should be reserved for classification

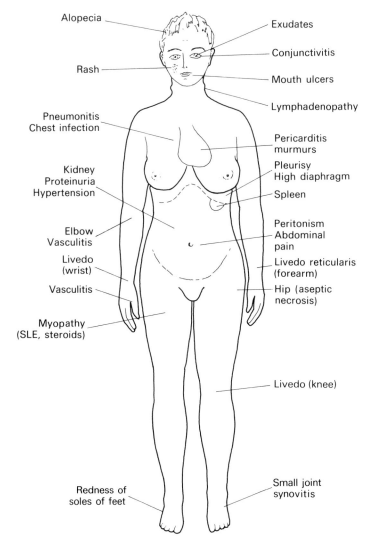

Fig. 2.24 More frequent physical findings in SLE.

Table 2.14 Initial manifestation of SLE in 150 patients (from Estes & Christian 1971)

Manifestation		Patients (%)
Arthritis or arthralgia		53
Cutaneous		
Discoid lesions	9 ⎫	
Malar rash	9 ⎬	19
Other	1 ⎭	
Nephritis		6
Fever		5
Epileptiform seizures		3
Raynaud's phenomenon		3
Pleurisy		3
Pericarditis		2
Anaemia		2
Thrombocytopenic purpura		2
Biologically false-positive Wassermann reaction		1
Jaundice		1

Table 2.15 The 1982 revised ARA criteria for the classification of SLE (Tan *et al.* 1982)

1 Butterfly rash
2 Discoid lupus
3 Photosensitivity
4 Oral ulcers
5 Arthritis
6 Serositis
7 Kidney disease (proteinuria >0.5 g/day, cellular casts)
8 Neurologic disorder (seizures or psychosis)
9 Blood disorder
  (a) Haemolytic anaemia
  (b) WBC <4000 on 2 or more occasions
  (c) Lymphopenia <1500 on 2 or more occasions
  (d) Thrombocytopenia <100 000
10 Immunologic disorder (LE cells, antiDNA, antiSm, false-positive STS)
11 Antinuclear antibody

purposes and not for diagnosis. They have been criticized as being too 'classical', and probably exclude many milder cases of SLE.

One of the diagnostic difficulties in SLE concerns the patient with mild renal disease. Again the DNA binding test may prove of value in this situation. For example, in a study of group of 64 children with different renal diseases, including hypocomplementaemic nephritis carried out with Dr T. Pincus, we observed titres only in the SLE group (Fig. 2.25) (Pincus

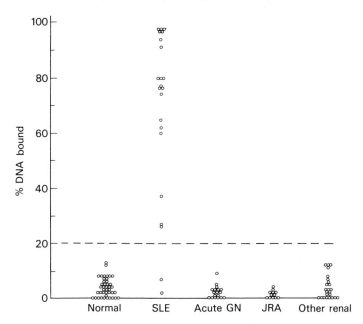

Fig. 2.25 DNA binding values in a series of children with SLE, other acute glomerulonephritides, juvenile rheumatoid arthritis and a variety of other renal diseases. (From Pincus *et al.* 1971.)

et al. 1971). In these children the SLE had previously been diagnosed by other criteria, but the implication is that mild renal disease with a strongly positive ANA test and, more specifically, a positive DNA-binding test should be suspected as being due to SLE. In such cases, the finding of a low complement value might weigh in favour of a renal biopsy.

Joint pain is the commonest manifestation of SLE, and the differentiation from rheumatoid arthritis in its early stages may be difficult. The two pointers to SLE which have already been mentioned include the generally milder nature of the synovitis, and the lack of erosions. Table 2.16 lists the more important distinguishing features between rheumatoid arthritis and SLE.

While a number of cases of 'overlap' have been described, in particular cases of rheumatoid arthritis progressing to SLE, a number of these have, in the past, reflected the lack of diagnostic aids or precision. It is becoming clear that SLE in minor form may masquerade for many years as other diseases before diagnosis. This aspect is discussed further in the section on management, but the following case illustrates the point.

Table 2.16 Rheumatoid arthritis versus SLE — distinguishing features

Feature	RA	SLE
Usual age	>40	Under 40
Sex (F : M) ratio	3 : 1	9 : 1
Synovitis	++	+/−
Stiffness	++	+−
Erosions (1 year)	+	−
Alopecia	−	+
Skin rashes	−	+
Renal disease	−	+
Fever	Acute onset only	+
Rheumatoid factor	80%	30−40%
ANA	10−20%	100%
DNA antibodies	0%	80−100%
Complement	N or raised	Lowered or N
CRP	High	Low
Serum amyloid A	Raised	Low

Case report. *A 53-year-old woman had suffered from arthritis for 22 years. This had largely consisted of intermittent synovitis of the finger and toe joints, though large joints were occasionally involved. Her health had otherwise been good. During the episodes of synovitis, which lasted for several weeks at a time, she took prednisone tablets, and generally took a holiday until the arthritis improved. She had been diagnosed by one practitioner as palindromic rheumatism. She was found to have 3 g proteinuria daily, in addition to minimal synovitis. There were no radiographic joint erosions. The only other significant feature in the past history was of two episodes of pleurisy several years earlier. Investigation included a negative latex test, positive ANA, DNA binding of 100% and a C3 level of 50% of normal. A renal biopsy showed focal proliferative nephritis. Skin biopsy gave a positive 'band' test.*

One of the most difficult diagnostic problems is the patient with exclusively neuropsychiatric or neurological problems. Cases of SLE may attend psychiatric or neurological institutions long before the diagnosis is clear; diagnosis in such cases rests more on the awarenees of the physician than on any individual laboratory investigation. Furthermore, an increasing number of patients with diffuse cerebral vasculitis, in whom no other clinical evidence of SLE exists are being seen in lupus and neurological centres.

In summary, the 'classical' criteria for a diagnosis of SLE are of limited value in diagnosis. The physician who diagnoses SLE only in the presence of renal disease, 'butterfly' face rash and LE cells will miss the vast majority of cases.

Table 2.17 contains a list of features which, though not diagnostic, provides useful clues to the early or atypical case of SLE. A 'screening' ANA should be a standard investigation in all cases where these features are seen.

MANAGEMENT OF SLE
(reviewed by Miller 1992)

General measures

The most important thing in the management of SLE is to make the diagnosis. In the light of the improved prognosis, it follows that treatment should be tailored as conservatively as the clinical situation allows (Hughes 1982c).

While not all SLE patients are UV light sensitive, it is wise to advise against excess sun exposure, and probably worthwhile using UV light barrier creams. Advice regarding avoidance of other antigenic stimuli is not always clear cut. Vaccination is best avoided during episodes of disease activity, and penicillin and sulphonamides — well-known poten-

Table 2.17 Diagnosis of SLE — useful pointers

Female
Black > White
Age under 40 years
No joint erosions after $\geqslant 2$ years arthritis
Lymphopenia
History of drug allergies
History of 'epilepsy' in childhood
History of 'growing pains' in childhood
Alopecia
Neuropsychiatric disturbances
Recurrent abortions
Livedo reticularis
Elbow vasculitis
False-positive serological tests for syphilis
Positive immunofluorescent test on skin biopsy
High DNA binding
Low serum complement
Low CRP–high ESR
Positive ENA

tiating factors in patients with SLE — should be used only under close supervision.

That antigenic stimuli do lead to exacerbations of SLE is shown in the following bizarre case history.

Case report. A 21-year-old Oxford undergraduate had had recurrent haemolytic anaemia, arthralgias, alopecia and episodes of emotional disturbance. A diagnosis of SLE had been made and supported by the finding of LE cells and raised DNA binding. During a period of relative quiescence, she had been advised by a practitioner to undergo a course of therapy in a clinical specializing in the injection of extracts of embryo tissues. Within a few weeks she developed skin rashes, marked arthralgias, haemolytic anaemia and florid psychiatric disturbances. On her return she was noted for the first time to have proteinuria. No cryoglobulins were detected, but the complement level had fallen below normal and DNA binding had risen to 100%.

Salicylates

The incidence with which salicylate-induced liver function abnormalities occur in SLE is not known, but our own experience (Travers & Hughes 1978) suggests that it may be high. During an 18-month period, six patients were seen in whom marked rises in liver enzymes (particularly SGOT) were seen, reverting to normal on stopping the drug. In other studies, rechallenging with aspirin resulted in a return of the abnormalities.

In four patients (Fig. 2.26) aspirin was changed to diflunisal, an aspirin derivative without the ortho-acetyl group. Over a two-month follow-up period on 500 mg twice daily, adequate analgesia was obtained and no patient showed a rise on SGOT or other enzymes.

These data suggest that the hepatotoxicity of salicylates in SLE may be associated with the ortho-acetyl moiety, and that diflunisal might be a useful alternative anti-inflammatory agent in this disease.

Antimalarials

These drugs, championed by Dubois (1978), have re-emerged as major therapeutic agents in the management of SLE (Lanham & Hughes 1982). (Reviewed in *Lupus* 1992, Suppl 1: 1–200.)

Their mode of action is not yet elucidated in SLE, though they have a long list of pharmacological properties. Their therapeutic effect in SLE may well extend beyond their well-known use in the skin and joint manifestations of SLE, though evidence for this remains anecdotal.

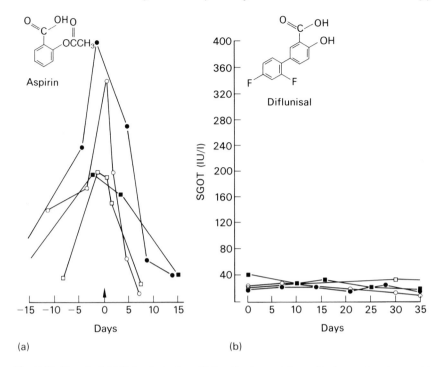

Fig. 2.26 Rises in SGOT levels in four SLE patients receiving salicylates, showing rapid return to normal levels on withdrawal of the drug (day 0). The right-hand chart shows the lack of change in SGOT levels in the same four patients challenged with diflunisal.

Case report. *During a double-blind trial of hydroxychloroquine versus placebo tablets, a patient with mild SLE developed nephrotic syndrome. On breaking the dosage code, this disease flare occurred soon after the switching from active ingredient to placebo.*

Dosage regimes of less than 6 mg/kg/day have been recommended by Mackenzie & Scherbel (1980). The loading dose of 400 mg often leads to mild diplopia and fears in the patient about ocular toxicity. Higher doses are sometimes required for short periods, especially in resistant discoid lupus. Eye checks, though possibly over-cautious at the lower dosage regimes, are still recommended. We have recently completed a five-year prospective study of the retinal effects of hydroxychloroquine and have detected no adverse ocular effects on doses of 200 mg daily or less. For resistant cases the addition of mepacrine 50 mg daily (100 mg leads to excessive pigmentation) may be valuable. The successful use of thalidomide in severe, crippling discoid lupus has been reported (Krop *et al.* 1983).

Corticosteroids

SLE differs from some of the other vasculitides described in this book in its generally favourable response to moderate doses (10–30 mg daily) of prednisone. Some features, especially the fever, pleurisy, pericarditis and haemolytic anaemia respond regularly to steroid therapy. Others, particularly CNS manifestations, are particularly difficult to manage. Dubois (1974) pioneered the use of massive steroid dosage in CNS lupus patients. However, while heroic treatment may be briefly tried in patients with widespread organic brain disease, in those with pure psychosis, the side effects have, in our experience, far outweighed the benefits. Sergent *et al.* (1975) have analysed the results of corticosteroid therapy in their own cases of CNS lupus. Of the deaths in the series, two were due to probable active SLE involving the CNS, while in five, death was attributable to complications of therapy. Furthermore, detailed analysis has shown that corticosteroid therapy, above all else, is associated with the tendency to infection seen in SLE (Ginzler *et al.* 1978). More and more it is becoming realized that once the acute or life-threatening episode is over, the steroid dose may be fairly rapidly reduced and, as frequently as not, either totally stopped or maintained on dosages of 10 mg daily or less. The positive aspects of such an approach are shown by one report (Grigor *et al.* 1978) where the mean prednisolone dose, over a period of 1433 patient-months, was 7·5 mg daily. The estimated mean five-year survival was 98% and no new cases of aseptic necrosis were seen.

Pulse methylprednisolone

Experience with the use of large 'pulse' intravenous doses of methylprednisolone has become widespread, especially in the management of renal graft rejection. In fulminating SLE, the initial and anecdotal experience is good. The commonly used dosage — 1 g i.v. on three successive days — has proved surprisingly free from major complications, though its efficacy may be short lived (Mackworth-Young, Walport & Hughes 1984).

Immunosuppressives

Felson and Anderson (1984) pooled data from all previously published clinical trials in which patients had been randomly assigned to receive either prednisone alone or prednisone plus immunosuppressive. They

showed that in the patients (with lupus nephritis) there was significantly less deterioration with the latter group. Both cyclophosphamide
and azathioprine were associated with a 40% reduction in rates of adverse
renal outcomes. They concluded that immunosuppressive drugs and steroids together are more effective and that previously published trials reached
false conclusions because of small sample sizes (see Gladman 1992).

Pulse cyclophosphamide

Another lesson learnt from the oncologists is the use of intermittent
(usually intravenous) cyclophosphamide. Tolerance is excellent, and the
short-term side effects minimal.

So favourable has been our impression of this drug that it has taken
over as a first-line treatment (together with steroids) in SLE patients with
active vasculitis or nephritis. Dosage regimens vary but at present we use
between 500 and 1000 mg given i.v. (usually with an anti-emetic). Our
own ('St Thomas') regimen is to give 3 × 500 mg pulses at weekly intervals.
To avoid cystitis, MESNA is added and a high fluid intake is maintained. The
subsequent treatment is generally for monthly 500 mg cyclophosphamide
pulses or for conversion to azathioprine.

The most favourable indications for pulse cyclophosphamide in SLE
are not yet clear, but may be surprisingly diverse, as in the case we
reported (Walport & Hughes 1982), where aplastic anaemia in a girl with
active SLE was reversed with 'pulse' cyclophosphamide.

Other forms of therapy

A number of forms of therapy, many untried, have theoretical application
in SLE.
1 Thoracic duct cannulation — a small number of patients have undergone
this procedure without convincing evidence of improvement.
2 Plasmapheresis. A number of centres, including our own, have tried
this method in advanced SLE (Fig. 2.27) (reviewed by Kimberley 1982).
This treatment not only affects circulating immune complex levels, but
also has an effect of reticuloendothelial function (Fig. 2.28) (Lockwood
et al. 1979). It still, nearly two decades on, does not stand up to close
scientific scouting (Wallace 1993).
3 Sex hormone modulation. For theoretical reasons discussed earlier, and
from observations on experimental animals, sex hormone modulation might
be considered.

To date, the practicalities have proved too much, though we have
reported the successful use of danazol (a drug with mild androgen effects)

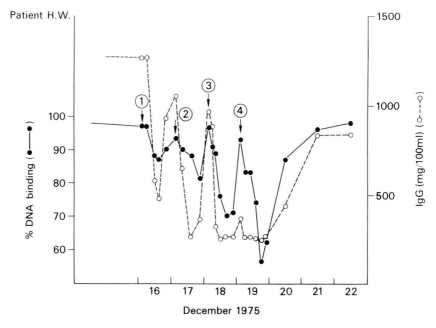

Fig. 2.27 Plasma exchange. Change in IgG (dash line) and DNA binding values in a patient undergoing four 4-litre plasma exchanges (arrowed). The temporary nature of the serological improvement is seen. (In collaboration with Dr Keith Peters.)

in 2 patients with marked premenstrual flares of their lupus (Morley *et al.* 1982). Unfortunately, subsequent use of this agent in SLE has, in our hands, been associated with a high incidence of rashes.

4 Renal transplantation — SLE is not *per se* a contraindication to trans- plantation. Indeed there is now widespread and successful experience in transplantation in SLE patients. Fortunately, by the time this end stage has been reached, the lupus itself rarely provides management problems (Coplon *et al.* 1983; Mejia *et al.* 1983; Miller 1992).

5 Antibiotics. Infection is still one of the major causes of death in SLE, and increasingly common is the problem of infection with atypical pathogens, such as *Cryptococcus* and *Mycoplasma*. Sieving, Kauffman & Watanakunakorn (1975) surveyed 33 cases of deep fungal infection in SLE. All were receiving corticosteroid therapy. With the possible exception of sulphonamides no antibiotic is contraindicated in SLE provided there is no specific history of sensitivity.

6 General drug therapy. While drugs such as methyldopa, hydralazine and anticonvulsants may cause drug-induced lupus, their use is not contraindicated in SLE proper.

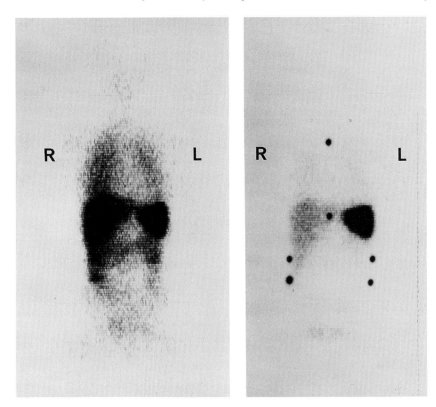

Fig. 2.28 Scans in a patient with SLE using chromium-labelled, heat-damaged red blood cells. The patient presented with marked dyspnoea and had abnormal lung function tests. The left-hand scan shows widespread uptake including marked uptake in the lungs. Following four 4-litre plasma exchanges (and no other therapy) there was improvement not only in the pulmonary function but also in immune complex titres. The repeat scan (right-hand) scan showed alteration in uptake of the heat-damaged red blood cells with a return to predominantly splenic uptake. (Dr D.M. Lockwood, Hammersmith Hospital.)

USE OF LABORATORY TESTS IN THE MONITORING OF SLE

Apart from routine blood counts and urinalysis, three tests — DNA antibodies, anticardiolipin antibodies and serum complement estimations — are of considerable value in the month-to-month management of SLE patients.

In the majority of SLE patients, rapidly rising antiDNA titres predict a flare of disease activity (Lightfoot & Hughes 1976). Equally important is the knowledge that serological abnormalities may also spontaneously revert to normal without treatment. This recognition of 'subclinical' flares of SLE, or of 'minimal' disease has implications for the management of the disease and presents a strong argument for therapeutic conservatism wherever possible as illustrated in these two cases.

Case report. A 38-year-old nurse had been diagnosed as having SLE 8 years previously, with synovitis, proteinuria, pericarditis, alopecia and a skin rash. Three years previously she had gone into clinical remission and had remained well and active as a theatre sister since that time. Over the period 1972–3 her DNA-binding values had begun to rise, reaching a level of 62%. The complement (C3) remained normal and apart from minimal synovitis there were no new clinical abnormalities. No treatment was given and the DNA binding returned to normal, the synovitis disappearing.

Case report. A 23-year-old woman with SLE in remission became pregnant. During the first trimester and again during the puerperium, the DNA binding values rose to over 60%, on both occasions without clinical exacerbations.

The benefits of this approach have been seen in the decreased infection rate and the strikingly low incidence of avascular bone necrosis.

Furthermore, it is clear that high DNA-binding values may persist for months or even years in the absence of clinical disease activity — indeed one patient described here may qualify for the *Guinness Book of Records*!

Case report. A 45-year-old operating room sister had had SLE for 12 years; for the past 6 years she has remained clinically well and off all therapy. Her DNA-binding value over that period has never fallen below 60%.

Obviously, as with the experimental animal, some patients produce more antibody than others (it is a 'clinical impression' that children with SLE produce higher titres than adults, for example). Nevertheless, present evidence suggests that high titre DNA-binding values do not, *per se*, constitute grounds for treatment (Hughes 1971, 1975).

What about lowered serum complement levels? Although it has often been stated that low complement levels may point towards renal involvement, this need not be the case. Thus, in a series of SLE patients studied in Jamaica (Wilson & Hughes 1979) hypocomplementaemia occurred with equal frequency in the 'renal' and 'non-renal' groups. Some of the more active 'non-renal' SLE patients may have profound hypocomplementaemia, with marked activation of the classical pathway.

For these reasons, in the individual patient, neither hypocomplementaemia nor high titres of complexes *per se* should be regarded as indications for more aggressive therapy.

More than ever, and despite all the new tests, the management of SLE is still based mainly on clinical criteria.

PROGNOSIS (reviewed by Gladman 1992)

The prognosis of SLE continues to improve with the recognition of milder forms of the disease. Renal disease still carries the gravest prognosis, though CNS disease comes a close second (Fig. 2.29). Of the patients with renal disease, diffuse proliferative nephritis carried a poorer prognosis than focal proliferative or membranous. The prognosis of renal disease has also improved. Even pregnancy is not now totally contraindicated in the presence of renal disease. The reason for the improved prognosis are clear, and are summarised well by Gladman (1992).

With improving prognosis the case for a conservative therapeutic approach not only in the use of immunosuppressive but also with long-term steroids is strengthened — it has been reported, for example, that coronary artherosclerosis might be accelerated in SLE patients on corticosteroids

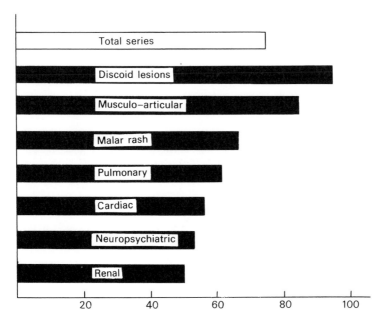

Fig. 2.29 Estimated five-year percentage survival for seven manifestations of SLE. (From Estes & Christian 1971.)

(Bulkley & Roberts 1975), though other factors such as the arteriopathy associated with anticardiolipin antibodies may also be relevant here.

Obviously, this widespread improvement both in adult (Grigor *et al.* 1978) and childhood (Caeiro *et al.* 1981) lupus has been largely due to earlier diagnosis. In communities where milder disease may not reach hospital, the figures remain somewhat less optimistic (Feng & Boey 1982; Gladman 1992).

REFERENCES

Adu D. & Cameron J.S. (1982) Lupus nephritis. In: *Clinics in Rheumatic Diseases*, Vol. 8, pp. 153–182, Ed: G.R.V. Hughes. Saunders, Philadelphia.

Alarcon-Segovia D. (1969) Drug induced lupus syndromes. *Mayo Clinic Proceedings*, **44**, 664.

Alarcon-Segovia D. (1975) Drug induced lupus erythematosus and related syndromes. In: *Clinics in Rheumatic Diseases*, Vol. 1, p. 573, Ed: N. Rothfield. Saunders, Philadelphia.

Alarcon-Segovia D. (1982) Cellular immunity of its regulation in SLE. In: *Clinics in Rheumatic Diseases*, Vol. 8, pp. 63–76, Ed: G.R.V. Hughes. Saunders, Philadelphia.

Andrianakos A.A., Duffy J., Suzuki M. & Sharp J.T. (1975) Transverse myelopathy in systemic lupus erythematosus. *Annals of Internal Medicine*, **83**, 616.

Appel G.B., Williams G.S., Meltzer J.I. & Pirani C.L. (1976) Renal vein thrombosis, nephrotic syndrome and systemic lupus erythematosus. *Annals of Internal Medicine*, **85**, 310.

Asherson R.A., Lanam J., Hull R.G., Boey M.L., Gharavi A.G. & Hughes G.R.V. (1984) Renal vein thrombosis in SLE: association with the lupus anticoagulant. *Clinical and Experimental Rheumatology*, **2**, 75–79.

Asherson R.A., Mackworth-Young C.G., Boey M.L., Gharavi A.E. & Hughes G.R.V. (1983) Pulmonary hypertension in SLE. *British Medical Journal*, **287**, 1024–1025.

Asherson R.A., Mackworth-Young C.G., Harris E.N., Gharavi A.E. & Hughes G.R.V. (1985) Multiple venous and arterial thromboses associated with the lupus anticoagulant and antibodies to cardiolipin in the absence of SLE. *Rheumatology International*, **5**, 91–93.

Asherson R.A., Morgan S.H., Harris E.N., Gharavi A.E., Krausz T. & Hughes G.R.V. (1986) Arterial occlusion causing large bowel infarction — a reflection of clotting diathesis in SLE. *Clinical Rheumatology*, **5**, 102–106.

Bach G.L., Pillay V.K.G. & Kark R.M. (1971) Immunoglobulin (IgA) deficiency in systemic lupus erythematosus. *Acta Rheumatologica Scandinavica*, **17**, 63.

Bach J.F., Dardenne M. & Bach M. (1973) Demonstration of a circulating thymic hormone in mouse and man. *Transplantation Proceedings*, **5**, 99.

Baker M. (1973) Psychopathology in systemic lupus erythematosus: I. Psychiatric observations. *Seminars in Arthritis and Rheumatism*, **3**, 95.

Baldwin D.S., Gluck M.C., Lowenstein J. & Gallo G.R. (1977) Lupus nephritis. Clinical course as related to morphologic forms and their transitions. *American Journal of Medicine*, **62**, 12.

Becker G.J., Waldburger M., Hughes G.R.V. & Pepys M.B. (1980) Investigation of fever in SLE. Value of C-reactive protein measurement. *Annals of the Rheumatic Diseases*, **39**, 50–52.

De Beer F.C., Mallya R.K., Fagan E.A., Lanham J.G., Hughes G.R.V. & Pepys M.B. (1982)

Serum amyloid-A protein concentration in inflammatory diseases and its relationship to the incidence of reactive systemic amyloidosis. *Lancet*, **11**, 231–234.

Bennett R.M., Hughes G.R.V., Bywaters E.G.L. & Holt P.J.L. (1972) Neuropsychiatric problems in systemic lupus erythematosus. *British Medical Journal*, **4**, 342.

Bernstein R. (1983) Nuclear magnetic resonance (NMR) imaging of the brain in SLE. *Journal of Computer Assisted Tomography*, **7**, 461–467.

Block S.R., Winfield J.B., Lockshin M.D., D'Angelo W.A. & Christian C.L. (1975) Studies of twins in systemic lupus erythematosus. A review of the literature and presentation of 12 additional sets. *American Journal of Medicine*, **59**, 533.

Bluestein H.G. & Zvaifler N.J. (1976) Brain-reactive lymphocytotoxic antibodies in the serum of patients with systemic lupus erythematosus. *Journal of Clinical Investigation*, **57**, 509.

Bohner R.F., Ultmann J.C., Gorman J.G., Farhangi M. & Scudder J. (1968) The direct Coombs' test: its clinical significance. Study in a large university hospital. *Annals of Internal Medicine*, **68**, 19.

Brandt K.D. & Lusell S. (1978) Migrainous phenomena in SLE. *Arthritis and Rheumatism*, **21**, 7.

Breckenridge R.T., Moore R.D. & Ratnoff O.D. (1967) A study of thrombocytopenia. New histologic criteria for the differentiation of idiopathic thrombocytopenia associated with disseminated lupus erythematosus. *Blood*, **30**, 39.

Bresnihan B. (1982) CNS lupus. In: *Clinics in Rheumatic Diseases*, Vol. 8, pp. 183–196, Ed: G.R.V. Hughes. Saunders, Philadelphia.

Bresnihan B., Oliver M., Grigor R. & Hughes G.R.V. (1977) Brain reactivity of lymphocytotoxic antibodies in systemic lupus erythematosus with and without cerebral involvement. *Clinical and Experimental Immunology*, **30**, 333.

Bresnihan B., Oliver M., Williams B. & Hughes G.R.V. (1979) An anti-neuronal antibody cross-reacting with erythrocytes and lymphocytes in SLE. *Arthritis and Rheumatism*, **22**, 313–320.

Bresnihan B., Grigor R., Oliver M., Lewkonia R. & Hughes G.R.V. (1977) Immunological mechanism for spontaneous abortion in SLE. *Lancet*, **ii**, 1205.

Bresnihan B. & Hughes G.R.V. (1979) An anti-neuronal antibody in SLE. *Arthritis and Rheumatism*, **2**, 313–320.

Budman D.R. & Steinberg A.D. (1977) Hematologic aspects of systemic lupus erythematosus. *Annals of Internal Medicine*, **86**, 220.

Bulkley B.H. & Roberts W.C. (1975) The heart in SLE and the changes induced by corticosteroid therapy. *American Journal of Medicine*, **58**, 243.

Butler W.T., Sharp J.T., Rossen R.D., Lidsky M.D., Mittal K.K. & Gard D.A. (1972) Relationship of the clinical course of SLE to the presence of circulating lymphocytotoxic antibodies. *Arthritis and Rheumatism*, **15**, 231.

Byron M.A. (1982) The clotting defect in SLE. In: *Clinics in Rheumatic Diseases*, Vol. 8, pp. 137–152, Ed: G.R.V. Hughes. Saunders, Philadelphia.

Caeiro F., Michielson F.M.C., Bernstein R.M., Hughes G.R.V. & Ansell B.M. (1981) SLE in childhood. *Annals of Rheumatic Diseases*, **40**, 325–331.

Catterall R.D. (1973) Biological false negative positive reactions and systemic disease. In: *Ninth Symposium on Advanced Medicine*, p. 97, Ed: G. Walker. Pitman, London.

Cazenave, Hebra F. & Kaposi M. (1875) *On Diseases of the Skin, Including the Exanthemata*, Vol. 4. Translated and edited by W. Tay. The New Sydenham Society, London.

Chang R.W. (1982) Cardiac manifestations of SLE. In: *Clinics in Rheumatic Diseases*, Vol. 8, pp. 197–206, Ed: G.R.V. Hughes. Saunders, Philadelphia.

Cohen A.S., Reynolds W.E., Franklin E.C., Kulka J.P., Ropes M.W., Shulman L.E. &

Wallace S.L. (1971) Preliminary criteria for the classification of systemic lupus erythematosus. *Bulletin of the Rheumatic Diseases*, **21**, 643.

Conley C.L. & Hartmann R.C. (1952) A haemorrhagic disorder caused by circulating anticoagulant in patients with disseminated lupus erythematosus. *Journal of Clinical Investigation*, **31**, 621.

Coplon N.S., Diskin C.J., Peterson J. & Swenson R.S. (1983) The long term clinical course of systemic lupus erythematosus in end stage renal disease. *New England Journal of Medicine*, **308**, 186–190.

Davis P., Atkins B., Josse R.G. & Hughes G.R.V. (1973) Criteria for classification of SLE. *British Medical Journal*, **3**, 88.

D'Cruz D., Houssain F., Ramirez, G. *et al.* (1991) Antibodies to endothelial cells in SLE: a potential marker for nephritis and vasculitis. *Clinical and Experimental Immunology*, **85**, 254–261.

De Horatius R.J. & Messner R.P. (1975) Lymphocytotoxic antibodies in family members of patients with systemic lupus erythematosus. *Journal of Clinical Investigation*, **55**, 1254.

Derue G.J., Englert H.J., Harris E.N., Hawkins D., Elder M. & Hughes G.R.V. (1985) Intra-uterine death in SLE; association with anticardiolipin antibodies. *Journal of Obstetrics and Gynaecology*, **5**, 207–208.

Donaldson I.M. & Espiner E.A. (1971) Disseminated lupus erythematosus presenting as chorea gravidarum. *Archives of Neurology*, **24**, 240.

Dubois E.L. (1974) *Lupus Erythematosus*. University of Southern California Press.

Dubois E.L. (1978) Antimalarials in the management of discoid and systemic lupus erythematosus. *Seminars in Arthritis and Rheumatism*, **8**, 33.

Dubois E.L., Wierzchowiecki M., Cox M.B. & Weiner J.M. (1974) Duration and death in SLE: an analysis of 249 cases. *Journal of the American Medical Association*, **223**, 1399.

Estes D. & Christian C.L. (1971) The natural history of systemic lupus erythematosus by prospective analysis. *Medicine*, **50**, 85.

Felson D.T. & Anderson J. (1984) Evidence for the superiority of immunosuppressive drugs and prednisone over prednisone alone in lupus nephritis. *New England Journal of Medicine*, **311**, 1528–1533.

Feng P.H. & Boey M.L. (1982) Systemic lupus erythematosus in Chinese: the Singapore experience. *Rheumatology International*, **2**, 151–154.

Fessel W.J. (1974) Systemic lupus erythematosus in the community. *Archives of Internal Medicine*, **134**, 1027.

Fielder A.H.L., Walport M.J., Batchelor J.R., Dodi I.A. & Hughes G.R.V. (1983) Family study of the major histocompatibility complex in patients with SLE: importance of null alleles of C4A and C4B in determining disease susceptibility. *British Medical Journal*, **286**, 425–429.

Fournel C., Chabane L., Caux C. *et al.* (1992) Canine SLE. A study of 75 cases. *Lupus*, **1** (3), 133–140.

Fraga A., Mintz G., Orozco J. & Orozco J.H. (1974) Sterility and fertility rates, fetal wastage and maternal morbidity in systemic lupus erythematosus. *Journal of Rheumatology*, **1**, 293.

Frampton G. (1991) Significance of antiphospholipid antibodies in patients with lupus nephritis. *Kidney International*, **39**, 1225–1231.

Fritzler M.J. & Tan E.M. (1978) Antibodies to histone in patients with drug-induced and idiopathic lupus erythematosus. *Arthritis and Rheumatism*, **21**, 556 (abstr.).

Fulford K.W.M., Catterall R.D., Delhanty J.J., Doniach D. & Kremer M. (1972) A collagen disorder of the nervous system presenting as multiple sclerosis. *Brain*, **95**, 373.

Gibson G.J., Edmonds J.P. & Hughes G.R.V. (1977) Diaphragm function and lung involvement in systemic lupus erythematosus. *American Journal of Medicine*, **63**, 926.

Gilliam J.N. & Sontheimer R.D. (1982) Skin manifestations of SLE. In: *Clinics in Rheumatic Diseases*, Vol. 8, pp. 207–218, Ed: G.R.V. Hughes. Saunders, Philadelphia.

Ginzler E.M. & Antoniadis I. (1992) Clinical manifestations of SLE, measures of disease activity and longterm complications. *Current Opinion in Rheumatology*, **4**, 672–680.

Ginzler E., Diamond H., Kaplan D., Weiner M., Schlesinger M. & Seleznick M. (1978) Computer analysis of factors influencing the frequency of infection in SLE. *Arthritis and Rheumatism*, **21**, 37.

Gladman D. (1992) Prognosis of SLE and factors that affect it. *Current Opinion in Rheumatology*, **4**, 681–687.

Grigor R., Edmonds J., Lewkonia R., Bresnihan B. & Hughes G.R.V. (1978) Systemic lupus erythematosus. A prospective analysis. *Annals of the Rheumatic Diseases*, **37**, 121.

Grigor R.R., Shervington P.C., Hughes G.R.V. & Hawkins D.F. (1977) Outcome of pregnancy in systemic lupus erythematosus. *Proceedings of the Royal Society of Medicine*, **70**, 99.

Hahn B.H. (1975) Cell mediated immunity in systemic lupus erythematosus. In: *Clinics in Rheumatic Diseases*, Vol. 1, p. 497, Ed: N. Rothfield. Saunders, Philadelphia.

Harmon C.E. & Portanova J.P. (1982) Drug-induced lupus: clinical serological studies. In: *Clinics in Rheumatic Diseases*, Vol. 8, pp. 121–136, Ed: G.R.V. Hughes. Saunders, Philadelphia.

Harris E.N. & Hughes G.R.V. (1985) Cerebral disease in SLE. *Springer Seminars in Immunopathology*, **8**, 251–266.

Harris E.N., Asherson R.A., Gharavi A.E. & Hughes G.R.V. (1985a) Thrombocytopenia in SLE and related autoimmune disorders: association with anticardiolipin antibodies. *British Journal of Haematology*, **59**, 227–230.

Harris E.N., Englert H., Derue G., Hughes G.R.V. & Gharavi A. (1983) Antiphospholipid antibodies in acute Guillain–Barré syndrome. *Lancet*, **ii**, 1361–1362.

Harris E.N., Gharavi A.E., Hegde U. & Hughes G.R.V. (1985b) Anticardiolipin antibodies in autoimmune thrombocytopenic purpura. *British Journal of Haematology*, **59**, 231–234.

Harris E.N., Gharavi A.E., Asherson R.A., Boey M.L. & Hughes G.R.V. (1984) Cerebral infarction in systemic lupus: association with anticardiolipin antibodies. *Clinical and Experimental Rheumatology*, **2**, 47–51.

Harris E.N., Gharavi A.E., Boey M.L. *et al.* (1983) Anticardiolipin antibodies: detection by radioimmunoassay and association with thrombosis in SLE. *Lancet*, **ii**, 1211–1213.

Harris E.N., Gharavi A.E. & Hughes G.R.V. (1985c) Antiphospholipid antibodies. In: *Clinics in Rheumatic Diseases*, Vol. 11, pp. 591–610, Ed: R.C. Williams. Saunders, Philadelphia.

Harris E.N. & Hughes G.R.V. (1985) Cerebral disease in systemic lupus erythematosus. *Springer Seminar on Immunopathology*, **8**, 251–266.

Hess E.V. (1982) Role of drugs and environmental agents in lupus syndromes. *Current Opinion in Rheumatology*, **4**, 688–692.

Honig S., Gorevic P. & Weissman G. (1977) C-Reactive protein in systemic lupus erythematosus. *Arthritis and Rheumatism*, **20**, 1065.

Houssain F., D'Cruz D., Vianna J. & Hughes G.R.V. (1991) Lupus nephritis: the significance of serological tests at the time of biopsy. *Clinical and Experimental Rheumatology*, **9**, 345–349.

Hughes G.R.V. (1975) Frequency of antiDNA antibodies in SLE, RA and other diseases.

Scandinavian Journal of Rheumatology, Supplement 11, p. 42.

Hughes G.R.V. (1971) The significance of anti-DNA antibodies in SLE. *Lancet*, **2**, 861.

Hughes G.R.V. (1980) CNS lupus: diagnosis and treatment. *Journal of Rheumatology*, **7**, 405−411.

Hughes G.R.V. (1982a) Hypotensive agents, beta-blockers and drug induced lupus. *British Medical Journal*, **284**, 1358−1359.

Hughes G.R.V. (ed.) (1982b) Systemic lupus erythematosus. *Clinics in Rheumatic Diseases*, Vol. 8. Saunders, Philadelphia.

Hughes G.R.V. (ed.) (1982c) The treatment of SLE: the case for conservative management. In: *Clinics in Rheumatic Diseases*, Vol. 8, 299−314. Saunders, Philadelphia.

Hughes G.R.V. (1983) Thrombosis, abortion, cerebral disease, and the lupus anticoagulant. *British Medical Journal*, **287**, 1088−1089.

Hughes G.R.V. (1984a) Autoantibodies in lupus and its variants: experience in 1000 patients. *British Medical Journal*, **289**, 339−342.

Hughes G.R.V. (1984b) Connective tissue disease and the skin (The 1983 Prosser−White oration). *Clinical and Experimental Dermatology*, **9**, 535−544.

Hughes G.R.V. (1993) The antiphospholipid syndrome − ten years on. *Lancet*, **342**, 341−344.

Hughes G.R.V. & Batchelor J.R. (1983) Genetics of systemic lupus erythematosus. *British Medical Journal*, **286**, 416−417.

Hughes G.R.V., Harris E.N. & Gharavi A.E. (1986) The anticardiolipin syndrome. *Journal of Rheumatology*, **13**, 486−489.

Hughes G.R.V., Rynes R.I., Gharavi A. *et al.* (1981) The heterogeneity of serologic findings and predisposing host factors in drug-induced lupus erythematosus. *Arthritis and Rheumatism*, **24**, 1070−1073.

Johnson R.T. & Richardson E.P. (1968) The neurological manifestations of systemic lupus erythematosus. A clinical pathological study of 24 cases and review of the literature. *Medicine*, **47**, 337.

Jungers P., Dougados M., Pelissier C. *et al.* (1982) Influence of oral contraceptive therapy on the activity of SLE. *Arthritis and Rheumatism*, **25**, 618−623.

Khamashta M.A., Cervera R., Asherson R. *et al.* (1990) Association of antibodies against phospholipids with heart valve disease in SLE. *Lancet*, **335**, 1541−1544.

Khamashta M.A., Cervera R. & Hughes G.R.V. (1991) The central nervous system in SLE. *Rheumatology International*, **11**, 117−119.

Kimberley R.P. (1982) Plasmapheresis in SLE. In: *Clinics in Rheumatic Diseases*, Vol. 8, pp. 243−260, Ed: G.R.V. Hughes. Saunders, Philadelphia.

Koss M.N., Chernack W.J. & Griswold W.R. (1973) The choroid plexus in acute serum sickness. *Archives of Pathology*, **96**, 331.

Kraus S.J., Haserick J.R. & Lantz M.A. (1970) Fluorescent treponemal antibody-absorption test reactions in lupus erythematosus. *New England Journal of Medicine*, **282**, 1287.

Krop J., Bonsmann G., Happle R. *et al.* (1983) Thalidomide in the treatment of 60 cases of chronic discoid LE. *British Journal of Dermatology*, **108**, 461−466.

Lahita R.G. (1990) Sex hormones and the immune system. In: *Ballieres Clinical Rheumatology*, Vol. 4, pp. 1−12, Ed: A. Parke. Balliere Tindall, London.

Lahita R.G. (1992) Sex steroids and SLE: metabolism of androgens to estrogens. *Lupus*, **1**, 125−127.

Lahita R.G. (1993) *Systemic Lupus Erythematosus*, 2nd edn. Wiley Medical, New York.

Lahita R.G., Kunkel H.G. & Bradlow H.L. (1983) Increased oxidation of testosterone in SLE. *Arthritis and Rheumatism*, **26**, 1517−1521.

Lampert P.W. & Oldstone M.B.A. (1973) Host immunoglobulin G and complement deposits in the choroid plexus during spontaneous immune complex disease. *Science*, **180**, 408.

Landry M. (1977) Phagocytic function and cell-mediated immunity in systemic lupus erythematosus. *Archives of Dermatology*, **31**, 1477.

Lanham J.G., Barne T., Kohner E.M. & Hughes G.R.V. (1982) SLE retinopathy: evaluation by fluorescein angiography. *Annals of Rheumatic Diseases*, **41**, 473–478.

Lanham J.G. & Hughes G.R.V. (1982) Antimalarial therapy in SLE. In: *Clinics in Rheumatic Diseases*, Vol. 8, pp. 279–298, Ed: G.R.V. Hughes. Saunders, Philadelphia.

Lee S.L., Rivero I. & Siegel M. (1966) Activation of systemic lupus erythematosus by drugs. *Archives of Internal Medicine*, **117**, 620.

Levy J., Barnett E.V., MacDonald N.S., Klinenberg J.R. (1970) Altered immunoglobulin metabolism in SLE and RA. *Journal of Clinical Investigation*, **49**, 708.

Lewis D.C. (1965) Systemic lupus and polyneuropathy. *Archives of Internal Medicine*, **116**, 518.

Lewis R.M., Andre-Schwartz J., Harris C.S., Hirsch M.S., Black P.H. & Schwartz R.S. (1973) Canine systemic lupus erythematosus. Transmission of serological abnormalities by cell free filtrates. *Journal of Clinical Investigation*, **52**, 1893.

Lightfoot R.W. & Hughes G.R.V. (1976) The significance of persisting serological abnormalities in SLE. *Arthritis and Rheumatism*, **19**, 837.

Liszewski M.K., Kahl L.E. & Atkinson J.P. (1989) The functional role of complement genes in SLE and Sjøgrens syndrome. *Current Opinion in Rheumatology*, **1**(3), 347–352.

Lockshin M.D. (1993) Does lupus flare during pregnancy? *Lupus*, **2**(1), 1–2.

Lockwood C.M., Worrledge S., Nicholas A., Cotton C. & Peters D.K. (1979) Reversal of impaired splenic function in patients with nephritis or vasculitis (or both) by plasma exchange. *New England Journal of Medicine*, **300**, 524–530.

Loizou S. *et al.* (1984) Antithrombin III in SLE. *Clinical and Experimental Rheumatology*, **2**, 53–56.

Lovy M. *et al.* (1981) Concurrent SLE and salmonellosis. *Journal of Rheumatology*, **8**, 605–612.

Mackenzie A.H. & Scherbel A.L. (1980) Chloroquine and hydroxychloroquine in rheumatological therapy. *Clinics in Rheumatic Diseases*, Vol. 6, pp. 545–566. Saunders, Philadelphia.

Mackworth-Young C., Walport M.J. & Hughes G.R.V. (1984) Thrombocytopenia in a case of SLE: repeated administration of 'pulse' methyl prednisolone. *British Journal of Rheumatology*, **23**, 4, 298–300.

Mackworth-Young C. & Hughes G.R.V. (1985) Epilepsy — an early symptom of SLE. *Journal of Neurology, Neurosurgery, Psychology*, **48**, 185–192.

Maddison P.J. (1982) ANA-negative SLE. In: *Clinics in Rheumatic Diseases*, Vol. 8, pp. 105–120, Ed: G.R.V. Hughes. Saunders, Philadelphia.

Mansilla-Tinoco R., Harland S.J., Ryan P.J. *et al.* (1982) Hydralazine, antinuclear antibodies and the lupus anticoagulant. *British Medical Journal*, **284**, 936–939.

Matthay R.A., Schwartz M.I., Petty T.L., Stanford R.E., Gupta R.C., Sahn S.A. & Steigerwald J.C. (1974) Pulmonary manifestations of systemic lupus erythematosus. *Medicine*, **54**, 397.

Mejia G., Zimmerman S.W., Glass N.R., Miller D.T., Sollinger H.W. & Belzer F.O. (1983) Renal transplantation in patients with SLE. *Archives of Internal Medicine*, **143**, 2089–2092.

Miles S. & Isenberg D. (1993) A review of serological abnormalities in relatives of SLE patients. *Lupus*, 2(3), 145–150.

Miller M.H., Urowitz M.B., Gladman D.D. & Killinger D.W. (1983) SLE in males. *Medicine*, 62, 327–334.

Miller M.L. (1992) Treatment of SLE. *Current Opinion in Rheumatology*, 4, 693–699.

Mittal K.K., Rossen R.D., Sharp J.T., Lidsky M.D. & Butler W.T. (1970) Lymphocyte cytotoxic antibodies in SLE. *Nature*, 225, 1255.

Mongrey A.B. & Hess E.V. (1989) Drug-related lupus. *Current Opinion in Rheumatology*, 1, 353–359.

Montalban J., Codina A., Ordi J., Vilardell M., Khamashta M.A. & Hughes G.R.V. (1991) Antiphospholipid antibodies in cerebral ischaemia. *Stroke*, 22, 750–753.

Morgan S.H., Kennett R.P., Dudley C., Mackworth-Young C., Hull R. & Hughes G.R.V. (1986) Acute polyradiculo-neuropathy complicating systemic lupus erythematosus. *Postgraduate Medical Journal*, 62, 291–294.

Mountz J.D. & Edwards C.K. (1992) Murine modes of autoimmune disease. *Current Opinion in Rheumatology*, 4, 621–629.

Osler W. (1895) On the visceral complications of erythema exudativum multiforme. *American Journal of the Medical Sciences*, 110, 629.

Penn A.S. & Rowan A.J. (1968) Myelopathy in SLE. *Archives of Neurology*, 18, 337.

Pepys M.B., Lanham J. & De Beer F. (1982) C-Reactive protein in SLE. In: *Clinics in Rheumatic Diseases*, Vol. 8, pp. 91–104, Ed: G.R.V. Hughes. Saunders, Philadelphia.

Perreira Da Silva J.A., Elkon K., Hughes G.R.V., Dyck R.F. & Pepys M.B. (1980) CRP levels in systemic lupus erythematosus — a classification criteria. *Arthritis and Rheumatism*, 23, 770–771.

Perry H.M., Jr, Tan E.M., Carmody S. & Sakamoto A. (1970) Relationship of acetyl transferase activity to antinuclear antibodies and toxic symptoms in hypertensive patients treated with hydralazine. *Journal of Laboratory and Clinical Medicine*, 76, 114.

Pinching A.J., Travers R.L. & Hughes G.R.V. *et al.* (1978) Oxygen-15 brain scanning for detection of cerebral involvement in systemic lupus erythematosus. *Lancet*, i, 898.

Pincus T. (1976) Complex host viral interactions: principles from the study of type C viruses which might be applicable to rheumatic diseases. In: *Modern Topics in Rheumatology*, Ed: G.R.V. Hughes. Heinemann, London.

Pincus T., Hughes G.R.V., Pincus D., Tina L.U. & Bellanti J.A. (1971) Antibodies to DNA in childhood SLE. *Journal of Paediatrics*, 78, 981.

Reveille J.D. (1992) The molecular genetics of SLE and Sjøgrens syndrome. *Current Opinion in Rheumatology*, 4, 644–656.

Roubinian R., Papoian R. & Talal N. (1977) Androgenic hormones modulate autoantibody responses and improve survival in murine lupus. *Journal of Clinical Investigation*, 59, 1066.

Rynes R.I. (1982) Inherited complement deficiency states in SLE. In: *Clinics in Rheumatic Diseases*, Vol. 8, pp. 29–48, Ed: G.R.V. Hughes. Saunders, Philadelphia.

Santos R., Barojas E., Alarcon-Segovia D. & Ibanez G. (1975) Retinal microangiography in systemic lupus erythematosus. *American Journal of Ophthalmology*, 80, 249.

Scott J.S., Maddison P.J., Taylor P.V., Esscher E., Scott O. & Skinner R.P. (1983) Connective tissue disease, antibodies to ribo-nucleoprotein and congenital heart block. *New England Journal of Medicine*, 309, 209–212.

Searles R.P. & Williams R.C. Jr (1982) Lymphocyte-reactive antibodies in SLE. In: *Clinics in Rheumatic Diseases*, Vol. 8, pp. 77–90, Ed: G.R.V. Hughes. Saunders, Philadelphia.

Sequeira J., Cesic D., Keser G. *et al.* (1993) Allergic disorders in systemic lupus erythematosus. *Lupus*, **2**(3), 187–192.

Sergent J.S., Lockshin M.D., Klempner M.S., Lipsky B.A. (1975) Central nervous system disease in systemic lupus erythematosus. *American Journal of Medicine*, **58**, 644.

Siegel M., Holley H.L. & Lee S.L. (1970) Epidemiologic studies on systemic lupus erythematosus, comparative data for New York City and Jefferson County, Alabama. 1956–1965. *Arthritis and Rheumatism*, **13**, 802.

Siegel M. & Lee S.L. (1973) The epidemiology of systemic lupus erythematosus. *Seminars in Arthritis and Rheumatism*, **3**, 1.

Sieving R.R., Kauffman C.A., Watanakunakorn C. (1975) Deep fungal infection in SLE – 3 cases reported, literature reviewed. *Journal of Rheumatology*, **2**, 61.

Steinberg A.D., Klassen L.W., Ravecha E.S. *et al.* (1978) Study of the multiple factors in the pathogenesis of autoimmunity in New Zealand mice. *Arthritis and Rheumatism*, **21**, S.190.

Takaya M. (1991) Serum thrombomodulin and anticardiolipin antibodies in patients with SLE. *Clinical and Experimental Rheumatology*, **9**, 495–499.

Talal N. (1975) Animal models for systemic lupus erythematosus. In: *Clinics in Rheumatic Diseases*, Vol. 1, p. 485, Ed: N. Rothfield. Saunders, Philadelphia.

Talal N. (1982) Sex hormones and modulation of immune response in SLE. In: *Clinics in Rheumatic Diseases*, Vol. 8, pp. 23–26, Ed: G.R.V. Hughes. Saunders, Philadelphia.

Talal N. (1992) SLE and Sjøgren's syndrome. Editorial overview (and subsequent articles). *Current Opinion in Rheumatology*, **4**, 609–611.

Tan E.M., Cohen A.S., Fries J.F. *et al.* (1982) 1982 revised criteria for the classification of systemic lupus erythematosus. *Arthritis and Rheumatism*, **25**, 1271–1277.

Travers R. & Hughes G.R.V. (1978) Salicylate hepatotoxicity in systemic lupus erythematosus. A common occurrence? *British Medical Journal*, **2**, 1532.

Turner-Stokes L. & Turner-Warwick M. (1982) Intra-thoracic manifestations of SLE. In: *Clinics in Rheumatic Diseases*, Vol. 8, pp. 229–242, Ed: G.R.V. Hughes. Saunders, Philadelphia.

Tu W.H. & Shearn M.A. (1967) SLE and latent renal tubular dysfunction. *Annals of Internal Medicine*, **67**, 100.

Valesini G., Pastore R., De Berardinis P.G. *et al.* (1983) Appearance of anti-acetylcholine receptor antibodies coincident with onset of myasthenic weakness in patient with SLE. *Lancet*, **i**, 831.

Wallace D.J. (1993) Plasmapheresis in lupus. *Lupus*, **2**(3), 141–144.

Wallace D.J. & Hahn B. (Eds) (1993) *Dubois' Lupus Erythematosus*, 4th edn. Lea & Febiger, New York.

Walport M.J., Black C.M. & Batchelor J.R. (1982) The immunogenetics of SLE. In: *Clinics in Rheumatic Diseases*, Vol. 8, pp. 3–22, Ed: G.R.V. Hughes. Saunders, Philadelphia.

Walport M. & Hughes G.R.V. (1982) Reversal of aplastic anaemia secondary to SLE by high dose intravenous cyclophosphamide. *British Medical Journal*, **285**, 769–770.

Watanabe-Duffy K.N. & Gladman D.D. (1991) Infection and disease activity in SLE: a review of hospitalized patients. *Journal of Rheumatology*, **18**, 1180–1184.

Wenger M.E. & Bole G.G. (1973) Nitroblue tetrazolium (NBT) dye reduction by peripheral leucocytes from patients with RA and SLE. *Journal of Laboratory and Clinical Medicine*, **82**, 513.

Whaley K., Webb J. & Hughes G.R.V. (1976) Human and animal SLE. In: *Recent Advances in Rheumatology*, Eds: W.C. Dick & W.W. Buchanan. Academic Press, London.

Wilson W.A. & Hughes G.R.V. (1979) Rheumatic diseases in Jamaica. A 3 year study.

Annals of Rheumatic Diseases, **38**, 320.

Winfield J.B. (1985) Anti-lymphocyte antibodies in SLE. In: *Clinics in Rheumatic Diseases*, Vol. 11, pp. 523–550, Ed: R.C. Williams. Saunders, Philadelphia.

Winfield J.B. & Davis J.S. (1974) AntiDNA antibody in procainamide induced lupus erythematosus. *Arthritis and Rheumatism*, **17**, 97.

3: *The Antiphospholipid Syndrome*

In the early 1980s we published a series of paper describing a syndrome, consisting of multiple thrombosis, multiple abortions, thrombocytopenia and neurological disease. Other features include livedo reticularis and labile hypertension (Hughes 1983, 1984, 1985, 1991; Hughes, Gharavi & Harris, 1986).

Although these features have long been recognized in SLE, it is now clear that they may, and often do, exist as a syndrome in ANA-negative patients, or in ANA-positive, DNA-binding negative patients (Table 3.1).

In our studies (Boey *et al.* 1983) of 31 patients with the lupus anticoagulant (LA), 18 had a history of venous or arterial thrombosis. Nine women had one or more abortions. Of seven patients with SLE and pulmonary hypertension, five had lupus anticoagulant activity, suggesting that intrapulmonary arterial coagulopathy may be an aetiological factor (Asherson *et al.* 1983). The other test showing increased positivity in this group of patients is the VDRL (antibody against cardiolipin).

Clinically, LA and VDRL tests have severe technical limitations. Figure 3.1 demonstrates that these antibodies are, in fact, directed against phospholipids.

Harris *et al.* (1983) described a sensitive radioimmunoassay for the detection of anticardiolipin antibodies. This test, up to 400 times more sensitive than VDRL testing, has opened up new avenues in research not only in SLE but in other diseases where thrombosis and/or thrombocytopenia are prominent features. (*See:* First World Symposium on Antiphospholipid Antibodies, *European Journal of Rheumatology and Inflammation*, 1984, **7**, No. 1.).

In the paper by Harris *et al.*, patients with lupus or lupus-like diseases were selected. In this group of patients (including some with discoid LE and ANA-negative lupus) there was a striking association with high titres of anticardiolipin antibodies and a tendency to thrombotic disease (Table 3.1).

Table 3.1 The antiphospholipid syndrome (after Hughes 1985)

Arterial thrombosis
Strokes
Ocular occlusions
Myocardial infarction
Peripheral vascular occlusion
etc.

Venous thrombosis
Recurrent venous thrombosis
Deep vein thrombosis
Pulmonary emboli (later pulmonary hypertension)
Adrenal vein (Addison's)
Renal vein
Liver vein (Budd–Chiari, etc.)
Leg ulcers
etc.

Recurrent abortion
Placental infarction

Immunological and blood
Thrombocytopenic (occasional)
Coombs' positive haemolytic anaemia
Microsomal antibodies
Thyroid antibodies
ANA
VDRL in a few

Other associations
Heart valve thrombosis
Libman–Sachs endocarditis
Splinter haemorrhages and clubbing
Chorea
Epilepsy
Livedo reticularis
Migraine
Amaurosis fugax
Hip avascular necrosis
Skin necrosis and gangrene
Myelopathy

Rare associations
Acute 'catastrophic' antiphospholipid syndrome
DIC
Adult respiratory distress syndrome
Thrombotic thrombocythaemia syndrome

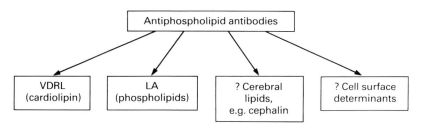

Fig. 3.1 Cross-reactivity of antiphospholipid antibodies.

PREVALENCE

At present, the prevalence of this syndrome both within the SLE spectrum, or outside it, is unknown. It seems likely that a wide range of clinical syndromes in which vasculopathy or thrombosis are implicated may come to be studied for evidence of such antibody-mediated mechanisms.

PATHOGENESIS (reviewed in Harris *et al.*, 1992)

Immunology

The antiphospholipid antibodies are of all immunoglobulin classes.

In general, IgG anticardiolipin antibodies are more often associated with clinical disease. Anticardiolipin antibodies have not, so far, been found in significant titres in normal population studies.

Pathogenesis of thrombosis

The strong association between antiphospholipid antibodies and thrombosis suggests a cause-and-effect relationship. The mechanisms are unknown. Carreras & Vermylen (1982) suggested an effect on endothelial membrane.

Alternatively, a direct effect on platelet membrane phospholipids might be of significance. Harris and colleagues showed that anticardiolipin antibodies reacted best with negatively charged phospholipids such as phosphatidylinositol. These phospholipids are predominantly on the inner platelet membrane, and it was possible to absorb anticardiolipin antibodies in these studies by sonicating platelets (Fig. 3.2) (Harris *et al.*, 1985). It is possible therefore that additional factors are required to initiate the platelet damage prior to thrombocytopenia or thrombosis (reviewed by Khamashta, Asherson & Hughes 1989).

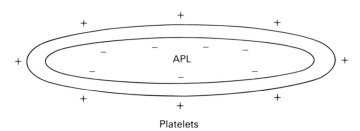

Platelets

Fig. 3.2 Antiphospholipid antibodies and thrombocytopenia — possible mechanism. Anticardiolipin reacts preferably with negatively charged phospholipids. Absorbed by sonicated platelets, in which the inner membrane (negatively charged phospholipid) is exposed.

CLINICAL FEATURES

General (Hughes 1984, 1991, 1993; Sugai 1992)

To date, the selection of patients has been influenced by the known predisposition of SLE patients to develop this syndrome. Thus the majority of patients are young and female, though an older age-group (40–60-year olds) may be equally at risk — notably some patients whose previously 'classical' SLE had apparently gone into remission.

Livedo reticularis is often prominent, especially over the knees and wrists. Some patients develop labile hypertension — in the absence of overt renal disease — and this may be due to a renovascular mechanism.

The constellation of neurological, thrombotic and thrombocytopenic features may occur simultaneously or over many years.

Thrombosis

Venous. In view of the known previous association between the lupus anticoagulant and venous thrombosis, it was no surprise to find a strong association between anticardiolipin antibodies and recurrent venous thrombosis. Some of these patients give a past history of multiple venous thromboses, including deep venous thromboses, axillary vein thrombosis and even subclavian thrombosis. In general, the thromboses do not occur when the patient is anticoagulated. The syndrome also occurs in patients without obvious SLE:

Case report. *A 27-year-old female had had three previous deep vein thromboses. Anticoagulant was discontinued 2 years after the third episode. Two years later she became pregnant. At 27 weeks the fetus died. Placental vessels showed numerous thromboses. The patient had anticardiolipin antibodies in titres of >20 S.D. No other antibodies or serological abnormalities were detected.*

Other thromboses have included renal vein thrombosis (Asherson *et al.* 1983) and retinal vein thrombosis.

Other non-SLE conditions in which the presence of venous thrombosis and anticardiolipin antibodies have been associated are Behçet's syndrome (Hull *et al.*, 1984), Degos' disease (Englert *et al.* 1984), Budd–Chiari syndrome (Hughes *et al.* 1984; Mackworth-Young *et al.* 1985), adrenal infarction and Addison's disease (Asherson & Hughes 1991).

Perhaps one of the most striking findings during these studies was the possible association of antiphospholipid antibodies, demonstrated indirectly in early studies by the lupus anticoagulant test, with pulmonary hypertension (Asherson *et al.* 1983) suggesting a possible mechanism for this condition.

Arterial. More sinister, however, is the association with arterial disease. In a study of SLE patients with cerebral infarction (Harris *et al.* 1984), 13 out of 15 had anticardiolipin antibodies.

These observations make us take very much more seriously the common transient ischaemic attacks seen in some of our SLE patients.

Case report. A 33-year-old patient had presented 5 years previously with post-partum epilepsy and retinal vein thrombosis. She made a gradual recovery with partial return of vision. Over the ensuing 5 years she remained well, with one episode of joint pains and parotid swelling. Serological studies revealed antiRo and anticardiolipin antibodies. In association with a rising titre of the latter, she developed transient loss of vision, each episode lasting some 10–15 months. On separate occasions, she developed transient speech disturbances. There were no clinical abnormalities apart from underlying sicca syndrome. She was treated with anticoagulants and the episodes ceased.

The arterial lesions have been widespread and often dramatic and have included occlusions of the femoral, renal, mesenteric and cerebral arteries (Asherson *et al.* 1985b, 1986b; Asherson, Mackay & Harris 1986a) as well as an aortic arch syndrome (Asherson *et al.* 1985c). It is tempting to speculate that this might be the cause of some of the 'early' deaths from coronary artery disease reported in some SLE studies.

Multiple abortions

A tendency to multiple abortions has been recognized as a feature of SLE patients for some years (see Chapter 2). Early studies of the lupus anti-coagulant (and false-positive serological tests for syphilis) showed that these antibodies were associated with this tendency. We studied the association between anticardiolipin antibodies and noted a strong corre-lation between these antibodies and the tendency to intrauterine deaths. Indeed, 19 out of 28 patients with raised antibody titres developed spon-taneous abortion or intrauterine deaths. Placental histology showed throm-bosis (Derue *et al.* 1985). Lubbe *et al.* (1983) studied women with the lupus anticoagulant and multiple abortions and investigated whether treatment aimed at reducing anticardiolipin antibody titres improved their prognosis. By treating his patients with corticosteroids and suppressing antibody activity, six patients produced live healthy babies. During the past decade, management of these patients has, in general, moved away from steroids towards various form of anticoagulation, such as aspirin and heparin (Cowchock 1991).

Neurological disease

Cerebral thrombosis is clearly associated. However, it is tempting to suggest that some of these antibodies may cross-react directly with cerebral phospholipids.

Epilepsy and chorea have been prominent features in some of our patients. Some years ago, the author, during a year in Jamaica, studied a number of patients with 'Jamaican neuropathy', a meningomyelitis of unknown aetiology affecting young women. Of interest was the finding that many of the patients had false-positive STS (Wilson & Hughes 1975). The syndrome resembled a myelopathy described by Fulford *et al.* (1972) which was discovered in a small number of patients followed over some years because of false-positive STS. Atypical 'multiple sclerosis', myelopathy and Guillain–Barré syndrome are now well-recognized features of the syndrome (Asherson 1991).

Thrombocytopenia

A recurring problem in some patients with anticardiolipin antibodies is thrombocytopenia. This problem, as it relates to SLE, is discussed in Chapter 2. In a recent study, anticardiolipin antibodies were seen in 30% of patients with idiopathic thrombocytic purpura and no other features of SLE (Harris *et al.* 1985b).

Platelet counts in these patients often run at around 100 000 units/mm^3, sometimes falling precipitously (Asherson 1991).

TREATMENT

The effect of prednisolone and immunosuppressives on the antibodies, as well as on the syndrome itself are variable. In some patients, doses of 10–15 mg prednisolone appear to abort the symptoms. In others, doses over 40 mg daily appear to have little effect. The short-term effect of anticoagulants in those patients with thromboses is effective. Long-term dosage schedules are unclear, through recurring thrombosis has occurred in patients with anticardiolipin antibodies whose anticoagulants have been stopped (Asherson *et al*. 1985a).

PROGNOSIS

The prognosis of this syndrome remains uncertain. Its description has opened a new set of clinical problems for patients with SLE and lupus-like syndromes. The patient who at the age of 40 has otherwise gone into remission may yet be in danger of an acute vascular episode. Clearly, it is impossible at present to predict the wider ramifications of these findings, especially the long-term risk factor for vascular disease.

It is now a decade since our initial descriptions of the antiphospholipid syndrome. During that time, it has become clear that for some patients at least, the syndrome is severe and sinister. There must be, in hospitals throughout the world, thousands of patients with strokes, myocardial infarction, peripheral vascular disease, epilepsy, recurrent abortions, etc. in whom the underlying mechanism can now, with some precision, be identified.

REFERENCES

Asherson R.A. (1991) The 'primary' anti-phospholipid syndrome. In: *Phospholipid-Binding Antibodies*. pp. 377–386. Eds: E.N. Harris *et al*. CRC Press, Boca Ratan, Florida.

Asherson R.A. & Hughes G.R.V. (1991) Hypoadrenalism, Addison's disease and anti-phospholipid antibodies. *Journal of Rheumatology*, **18**, 1–3.

Asherson R.A., Chan J.K.H., Harris E.N., Gharavi A.E. & Hughes G.R.V. (1985a) Anti-cardiolipin antibody, recurrent thrombosis and warfarin withdrawal. *Annals of Rheumatic Diseases*, **44**, 823–825.

Asherson R.A., Harris E.N., Gharavi A.E., Derksen R.H., Kater L., Lendrum R., Bird G. & Hughes G.R.V. (1985b) Arterial occlusions associated with antibodies to cardiolipin. *Arthritis and Rheumatism (Supplement)*, **28**, 589.

Asherson R.A., Mackay I.R. & Harris E.N. (1986a) Myocardial infarction in a young male with SLE, deep vein thrombosis and antiphospholipid antibodies. *British Heart Journal*, **56**, 190–193.

Asherson R.A., Mackworth-Young C.G., Boey M.L., Hull R.G., Saunders A., Gharavi

A.E. & Hughes G.R.V. (1983) Pulmonary hypertension in SLE. *British Medical Journal*, **287**, 1024–1026.

Asherson R.A., Mackworth-Young C.G., Harris E.N., Gharavi A.E. & Hughes G.R.V. (1985c) Multiple venous and arterial thromboses associated with the lupus anti-coagulant and antibodies to cardiolipin in the absence of SLE. *Rheumatology International*, **5**, 91–93.

Asherson R.A., Morgan S.H., Harris E.N., Gharavi A.E., Kransz T. & Hughes G.R.V. (1986b) Arterial occlusion causing large bowel infarction — a reflection of clotting diathesis in SLE. *Clinical Rheumatology*, **5**, 102–106.

Boey M.L., Colaco C.B., Gharavi A.E., Elkon K.B., Loizou S. & Hughes G.R.V. (1983) Thrombosis in SLE: striking association with the presence of circulating lupus anticoagulant. *British Medical Journal*, **287**, 1021–1023.

Carreras L.O. & Vermylen J.G. (1982) Lupus anticoagulant and thrombosis — possible role of inhibition of prostacyclin formation. *Thrombosis and Haemostasis*, **48**, 38.

Cowchock S. (1991) Alternative approaches to treatment of women with anti-phospholipid antibodies and fetal loss. In: *Phospholipid-Binding Antibodies*. pp. 347–354. Eds: E.N. Harris *et al.* CRC Press, Boca Ratan, Florida.

Derue G.J., Englert H.J., Harris E.N., Gharavi A.E., Morgan S.H., Hull R.G., Elder M.G., Hawkins D.F. & Hughes G.R.V. (1985) Fetal loss in systemic lupus: association with anticardiolipin antibodies. *Journal of Obstetrics and Gynaecology*, **5**, 207–209.

Englert H.J., Hawkes C.H., Boey M.L., Derue G.M., Loizou S., Harris E.N., Gharavi A.E., Hull R. & Hughes G.R.V. (1984) Degos' disease: association with anticardiolipin antibodies. *British Medical Journal*, **285**, 576–577.

Fulford K.W., Catterall R.D., Delhanty J.J. *et al.* (1972) A collagen disorder of the nervous system presenting as multiple sclerosis. *Brain*, **95**, 373–386.

Harris E.N., Asherson R.A., Gharavi A.E., Morgan S.H., Derue G.J. & Hughes G.R.V. (1985b) Thrombocytopenia in SLE and related autoimmune disorders: association with anticardiolipin antibodies. *British Journal of Haematology*, **59**, 227–230.

Harris E.N., Exner J., Hughes G.R.V. & Asherson R. (Eds) (1992) *Phospholipid-Binding Antibodies*. CRC Press, Boca Ratan, Florida.

Harris E.N., Gharavi A.E., Asherson R. & Hughes G.R.V. (1984) Cerebral infarction in systemic lupus: association with anticardiolipin antibodies. *Clinical and Experimental Rheumatology*, **2**, 47–56.

Harris E.N., Gharavi A.E., Boey M.L., Patel B.M., Mackworth-Young C.G., Loizou S. & Hughes G.R.V. (1983) Anticardiolipin antibodies: detection by radioimmunoassay and association with thrombosis in SLE. *Lancet*, **ii**, 1211–1213.

Harris E.N., Gharavi A.E. & Hughes G.R.V. (1985a) Anti-phospholipid antibodies. In: *Clinics in Rheumatic Diseases*, Vol. II, pp. 591–609, Ed: R.C. Williams. Saunders, Philadelphia.

Hughes G.R.V. (1991) The antiphospholipid antibody syndrome. *Seminars in Clinical Immunology*, **1**, 5–9.

Hughes G.R.V. (1983) Thrombosis, abortion, cerebral disease and the lupus anticoagulant. *British Medical Journal*, **287**, 1088–1089.

Hughes G.R.V. (1984) Connective tissue disease and the skin. *Clinical and Experimental Dermatology*, **9**, 535–544.

Hughes G.R.V. (1985) The anticardiolipin syndrome. *Clinical and Experimental Rheumatology*, **3**, 285–286.

Hughes G.R.V. (1993) The antiphospholipid syndrome — 10 years on. *Lancet*, **342**, 341–344.

Hughes G.R.V., Gharavi A.E. & Harris E.N. (1986) The anti-cardiolipin syndrome. *Journal of Rheumatology*, **13**, 486–489.

Hughes G.R.V., Mackworth-Young C., Harris E.N. & Gharavi A.E. (1984) Veno-occlusive disease in SLE: possible association with anticardiolipin antibodies. *Arthritis and Rheumatism*, **27** (9), 1071–1072.

Hull R.G., Gharavi A.E., Tincani A., Asherson R.A., Denman M., Froude G. & Hughes G.R.V. (1984) Anticardiolipin antibodies: occurrence in Behçet's syndrome. *Annals of Rheumatic Diseases*, **43**, 746–748.

Khamashta M., Asherson R.A. & Hughes G.R.V. (1989) Possible mechanisms of action of the antiphospholipid binding antibodies. *Clinical and Experimental Rheumatology*, **7**, Suppl 1, 1.

Lubbe W.F., Butler W.S., Palmer S.J. *et al.* (1983) Fetal survival after prednisolone suppression of maternal lupus anticoagulant. *Lancet*, **i**, 1361–1363.

Mackworth-Young C.G., Gharavi A.E., Boey M.L. & Hughes G.R.V. (1985) Portal and pulmonary hypertension in a case of systemic lupus erythematosus: possible relationship with a clotting abnormality. *European Journal of Rheumatology*, **7**, 1–5.

Sugai S. (1992) Antiphospholipid antibody and antiphospholipid antibody syndrome. *Current Opinion in Rheumatology*, **4**, 666–671.

Wilson W.A. & Hughes G.R.V. (1975) Aetiology of Jamaican neuropathy. *Lancet*, **i**, 240.

4: *Sjøgren's Syndrome*

Sjøgren's syndrome occupies a central position amongst the 'autoimmune' diseases, and deserves detailed consideration. Its recognition, together with an appreciation of its widespread clinical and immunological ramifications, simplifies the diagnosis of many of these diseases.

For reviews of primary Sjøgren's syndrome, the reader is referred to Fox *et al.* (1984) and Moutsopoulos & Talal (1989).

DEFINITION

The full triad of Sjøgren's syndrome consists of keratoconjunctivitis sicca (dry eyes), xerostomia (dry mouth) and a connective tissue disorder — usually rheumatoid arthritis (Table 4.1). The term 'sicca syndrome' is reserved for cases in which only the first two features are present. The dryness frequently extends to other epithelial surfaces, such as the nasal cavity, pharynx, trachea, bronchi, oesophagus, skin and vagina.

Hypergammaglobulinaemia may be marked, and there is a high incidence of non-organ specific autoantibodies, particularly antiglobulins and antibodies against nuclear and cytoplasmic antigens (notably the ENA Ro).

HISTORICAL

While arthritis associated with keratitis filamentosa had been described as long ago as 1889, it was Henrick Sjøgren, a Swedish ophthalmologist who in 1933 and in a number of subsequent studies, drew attention to the widespread changes seen in this disorder. Of the 19 females reported in his monograph on keratoconjunctivitis sicca, 13 had arthritis. It gradually became clear that in the majority of cases, the arthritis associated with the syndrome was rheumatoid arthritis. Modern knowledge of the clinical associations of Sjøgren's syndrome is due in large part of the studies of Bloch and Bunim and their colleagues at the NIH, Bethesda, USA (1965). It was from these studies that the complication of lymphoma development in this condition was recognized, providing a link between these connective tissue disorders and malignancy of the lymphoreticular system (Anderson & Talal 1972).

Table 4.1 Sjøgren's syndrome triad

Dry eyes $\rbrace$ sicca syndrome
Dry mouth
Connective tissue disease

EPIDEMIOLOGY

As in SLE, the female:male ratio is 9:1 (Bloch *et al.* 1965; Shearn 1971). The frequency in the general population is, however, unknown, and available figures depend largely on methods of diagnosis. Seifert and Geiler (1957) studied the parotid glands at 900 consecutive autopsies and showed that 0·44% had histological changes compatible with a diagnosis of Sjøgren's syndrome. Up to a third of all patients with rheumatoid arthritis may have Sjøgren's syndrome (see later). The features of sicca syndrome are commoner in elderly populations (Whaley *et al.* 1972a).

PATHOLOGY

One characteristic change in the salivary glands is a diffuse lymphocytic infiltration (Fig. 4.1). This in turn may be associated with destruction and

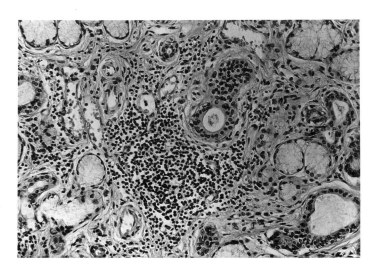

Fig. 4.1 Labial salivary gland biopsy showing a periductal focus of lymphocytes together with moderate diffuse lymphocytic infiltration (×210). (Dr D.M. Chisholm, Glasgow Dental Hospital.)

loss of salivary secretory tissues. In more severe cases, lymphoid follicles, complete with germinal centres, may be seen. In the most florid cases, total replacement of the gland occurs, and the differentiation from lymphomatous infiltration may be difficult. In general, however, the lobular architecture of the gland is preserved even in the presence of massive lymphocytic infiltration (Mason & Chisholm 1975).

Proliferation of the myoepithelial cells lining the ducts may lead to the so-called epimyoepithelial islands (Morgan−Castleman islands) though these are not confined to Sjøgren's syndrome.

Similar lymphoid infiltration may be seen in the lacrimal glands, the mucus secreting glands of the conjunctivae, the nasal cavity, pharynx, larynx, trachea, and bronchi, leading to secondary atrophy of these glands.

IMMUNOPATHOLOGY

The use of monoclonal antibodies has shown that the predominant cell is a T helper (Fox *et al*. 1984). B cells make up approximately 20% of the total infiltrate. Macrophages are poorly represented. More recently, the renal infiltrate has also been shown to be mainly T-helper cells.

'Mikulicz's syndrome'

In 1888 Mikulicz described a 42-year-old farmer who had massive lacrimal, parotid, buccal, palatal and submaxillary gland enlargement. Since that time considerable confusion has arisen regarding the relationship between Mikulicz's syndrome and Sjøgren's syndrome. Mikulicz's syndrome has come to be regarded as a heterogeneous group of conditions resulting in salivary or lacrimal gland enlargement (Table 4.2). In the majority of cases, Mikulicz's syndrome is synonymous with Sjøgren's syndrome. The additional eponymous term serves little useful purpose and will not be used again in the text.

Table 4.2 Causes of Mikulicz's syndrome

Sjøgren's syndrome
Leukaemia and lymphoma
(Sarcoidosis uveo-parotid fever)
Tuberculosis
Iodine and lead poisoning
(Mumps)

PATHOGENESIS

Autoimmunity

Labial gland biopsies of patients with rheumatoid arthritis in whom there is no clinical evidence of keratoconjunctivitis sicca reveal changes suggestive of early Sjøgren's syndrome in up to 25% of cases. This perhaps argues for a spectrum of salivary changes in rheumatoid arthritis, of which the full-blown sicca syndrome represents an extreme. The borderline between focal and diffuse histological lesions may be indistinct; Waterhouse and Doniach (1966) in a pathological study of salivary glands in a series of 525 necropsies, found focal lymphocytic lesions in over half of the women studied and in a quarter of the men. A raised prevalence and severity of adenitis in the salivary and lacrimal glands was found in subjects with rheumatoid arthritis. They pointed out the analogy with autoimmune thyroiditis, in which non-progressive focal lesions are far more prevalent than diffuse primary myxoedema.

Evidence of cell-mediated immune destruction of the salivary and lacrimal glands comes from studies showing cellular sensitization to salivary antigens in patients with rheumatoid arthritis as well as those with primary autoimmune liver disease and sicca complex. It is of interest that salivary and biliary ducts share antigenic determinants (McFarlane *et al.* 1976).

Natural killer cells, thought to be important in immune surveillance are reduced in patients with Sjøgren's (Miyasaka *et al.* 1983). This reduction may well be functional, as it can be restored by interleukin II (Pedersen *et al.* 1986).

Virus-like particles

As in most of the connective tissue diseases, tubulo-reticular structures have been observed in Sjøgren's syndrome — in the endothelium of glomeruli (Shearn 1971) as well as in the major and minor salivary glands (Daniels *et al.* 1974). As in the case of SLE, they may represent a host cell response to virus infection.

Animal models

The F_1 hybrid of the NZB/NZW mouse develops a lupus-like syndrome. These mice also develop lymphoid infiltrates in their salivary glands and have proved useful animal models for study. Immunofluorescent studies have shown that the first cells present in the lesions are B cells (Greenspan *et al.* 1974) though the recruiting stimulus for these cells is unknown. In the human predominant cell type in the lymphoid infiltrate has not been conclusively defined (Talal *et al.* 1974; Chused *et al.* 1974).

Genetic

In most series there is a strong association with the HLA haplotype A1, B8, DR3 (reviewed by Kassan & Gardy 1978). This highlights further the central role of Sjøgren's syndrome amongst the autoimmune diseases, as well as the association in rheumatoid arthritis between gold toxicity, HLA DR3 and Sjøgren's syndrome. During our family studies of SLE (Fielder *et al.* 1983), we noted clinical sicca syndrome, as well as antiRo antibodies in a number of the patients (unpublished). The HLA haplotype was taken further by the finding of a C_4 null allele in some of Sjøgren's patients (unpublished).

Exceptions to the HLA-DR3 primary Sjøgren's association were noted in certain ethnic groups — DR5 (Greeks) and DRw53 (Japanese) (reviewed by Moutsopoulos & Talal 1989).

CLINICAL FEATURES

The widespread clinical manifestations of Sjøgren's syndrome are shown in Table 4.3. It can be seen that many of the symptoms, while causing considerable suffering, are not dramatic, and may pass undetected by the physician, or alternatively, not be associated with the disease in question.

While the list is long, it must be stressed that in the majority of patients, the predominant complaints refer to the eyes and mouth.

General

Sjøgren's is possibly one of the most underdiagnosed conditions in both younger and older age groups. Often, the only symptoms are of tiredness and myalgia, and a number of my patients have been previously diagnosed as 'ME' (mylagic encephalitis). The value of the Schirmer's test (p. 102) — one of the most important bedside tests in medicine — cannot be exaggerated in this situation.

Case report. *A 59-year-old medical receptionist had complained of several years' fatigue and muscle aches. Previous investigation had been negative apart from one previously raised ESR. Various unsuccessful treatments had included antidepressives.*

On examination the Schirmer's tear test was completely dry. Investigation includes a positive latex, antiRo antibodies and moderate hypergamma globu-

Table 4.3 Clinical features of Sjøgren's syndrome

Eyes	*Nervous system*
Keratoconjunctivitis sicca	Cranial nerve lesions
Conjunctivitis	Peripheral neuropathy
Corneal vascularization	Neuropsychiatric features
Lacrimal gland enlargement	
	Respiratory system
Mouth	Tracheitis
Xerostomia	Bronchitis
Dental caries	Pneumonitis
Parotid gland enlargement	Atelectasis
Recurrent parotitis	Pleural effusions
	Diffuse interstitial pulmonary fibrosis
ENT	
Epistaxis	*Blood vessels*
Nasal septal perforation	Raynaud's phenomenon
Sinusitis	Hypergammaglobulinaemic purpura
Serous otitis media	
	Blood
GI tract	Anaemia
Dysphagia	Thrombocytopenia, leukopenia
Oesophageal web	Hyperglobulinaemia
Atrophic gastritis	Autoantibodies
Pancreatic disease	
	General
Genitourinary tract	Drug hypersensitivity
Renal tubular defects	Lymphoma development
Interstitial nephritis	
Vaginitis sicca	
Recurrent UTIs	

linaemia. She was treated with low-dose antimalarials (hydroxychloroquine) with improvement in the joint symptoms.

In younger (20–50-year-old) patients there is often a long history of intermittent parotid swelling, or lower limb purpura after exercise.

Keratoconjunctivitis sicca

The commonest complaint is not of dryness but of 'grittiness' or 'burning' in the eyes (Henderson 1950). Early in the course of the disease, the patient may actually complain of excessive lacrimation. Other symptoms include difficulty in opening the eyes in the morning, conjunctival discharge and occasionally photophobia.

Chapter 4

On examination, pericorneal injection, dullness of the conjunctiva, and superficial conjunctival scarring may be seen. Later there is punctate keratitis and keratitis filamentosa, with formation of threads and filaments (Fig. 4.2). Severe cases occasionally result in corneal vascularization.

Lacrimal gland enlargement is uncommon. The symptoms and signs of keratoconjunctivitis sicca are not specific for the condition, and the diagnosis must be confirmed by demonstrating diminished lacrimation, as shown by the Schirmer tear test (see p. 102) or by finding keratitis on slit-lamp examination of the cornea after the installation of dye into the conjunctival sac.

Patients with keratoconjunctivitis sicca frequently carry *Staphylococcus aureus* in the conjunctival sac, and although the incidence of infection is reduced by artificial tears, it remains an important risk (Williamson *et al.* 1970).

Xerostomia

In severe cases of xerostomia, there is atrophy of the oral mucosa, and a dry red furrowed tongue. Superinfection with *Candida* may complicate the picture, though this fortunately is rare. Even when there is severe damage to the major salivary glands, there is sufficient saliva for the inside of the mouth to appear moist. Clinical suspicion should be aroused by the absence of a normal pool of saliva around the base of the lingual frenulum.

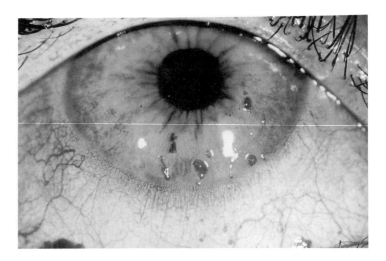

Fig. 4.2 Corneal vascularization and keratitis filamentosa in severe Sjøgren's syndrome. (Mr Peter Wright, Moorfield's Hospital.)

The frequent sipping of water required to facilitate swallowing may result in a spurious form of diabetes insipidus, as in the following patient:

Case report. *A 50-year-old nurse had complained of mild polyarthritis for several years. Rheumatoid factor was strongly positive, but there were no joint deformities or erosions. For 1 year she had complained of dryness at the back of the mouth and had resorted to frequent sipping of fluid. She took large jugs of water to bed at night, and woke at almost hourly intervals for micturition. Serum electrolytes and pituitary function were normal, and she was found to have Sjøgren's syndrome; despite the lack of ocular symptoms, there was less than 3 mm of tear secretion in 5 minutes.*

Such cases must be distinguished from occasional cases of nephrogenic diabetes insipidus seen in this condition (see later) and from sarcoidosis involving the basal meninges, joints and salivary glands.

Another sequel to the lack of saliva is dental caries, which may be severe and progressive. Painstaking dental care is required in such cases, especially in the fitting of dentures. Fortunately, problems in the wearing of well-fitted dentures in these patients are rare.

Salivary gland swelling

The majority of cases of Sjøgren's syndrome associated with rheumatoid arthritis do not have noticeable salivary gland enlargement. However, salivary (especially parotid) swelling may be marked, especially in cases of predominant sicca syndrome with minimal or no evidence of accompanying connective tissue disease.

Case report. *A 35-year-old dancer had noted intermittent parotid swelling for 10–15 years. The swelling became more prominent following 'allergic' reaction, especially to cheese. Sjøgren revealed hyperglobulinaemia and antiRo.*

During two episodes of active synovitis at the age of 31 and 34 years, the patient received short causes of prednisolone (7·5 mg daily). During each of these courses, the parotid swelling disappeared.

In long-standing Sjøgren's syndrome, sialectasis is almost the rule, and sudden enlargement in such cases may be due to a calculus or superinfection. These remains, nevertheless, a significant group of patients in whom the onset of Sjøgren's syndrome appears to be acute, in whom the sudden onset of salivary swelling is mistaken for mumps.

Ear, nose and throat

The dryness found in the salivary glands extends to the mucus-secreting tissues of the ear, nose, throat, alimentary and respiratory tracts. It is not surprising therefore that symptoms referable to the upper respiratory tract are common. Table 4.4 shows some of the data (in percentage) obtained in a series of patients studied in Glasgow (Doig *et al.* 1971). The last column represents a 'control' group of patients with rheumatoid arthritis in whom there was no evidence of Sjøgren's syndrome.

In addition to dryness of the throat, dysphagia and epistaxis, nasal crusting and atrophy, commonly cause nose bleeding and may (rarely) lead to perforation of the nasal septum and a suspected diagnosis of Wegener's or midline granuloma.

Gastrointestinal tract

Dysphagia may, in severe cases, be associated with postcricoid narrowing. Oesophageal webs, similar to those seen in iron deficiency, have been described (Doig *et al.* 1971). These are probably not premalignant.

Chronic atrophic gastritis is known to be associated with Sjøgren's syndrome. Buchanan (1966) found gastric parietal cell antibodies, histamine fast achlorhydria and gastritis in 3 of 6 Sjøgren's patients studied.

In a large series of patients studied in Glasgow (Whaley *et al.* 1972b) 28% of patients with Sjøgren's syndrome were found to have gastric parietal cell antibody as compared with 15% in a matched group of control patients.

The lymphocyte infiltration seen in the gastric mucosa in Sjøgren's syndrome is similar (using OKT markers) to that seen in the salivary glands (Kilpi *et al.* 1983).

While achlorhydria is found in Sjøgren's syndrome, the strength of any association with pernicious anaemia is uncertain. In a series of 171 patients with Sjøgren's syndrome, 6 were found to have pernicious anaemia,

Table 4.4 ENT symptoms in a Glasgow series

Symptom	Sicca syndrome (%)	Rheumatoid arthritis and sicca syndrome (%)	Rheumatoid arthritis alone (%)
Epistaxis	32	35	9
Soreness and dryness of throat	81	64	19
Nasal crusting	54	58	14

suggesting an association between the two conditions (Whaley *et al.* 1972a). Patients with pernicious anaemia, on the other hand, do not have an increased prevalence of keratoconjunctivitis sicca (Williamson *et al.* 1970).

Pancreatitis is (perhaps surprisingly) rare. Sporadic case reports of acute and of chronic pancreatitis have appeared, such as the case reported by Whaley *et al.* (1972b).

Case report. *A 64-year-old lady who had rheumatoid arthritis for 3 years, was diagnosed as having pernicious anaemia 1 year prior to being seen, on the basis of a macrocytic anaemia, megaloblastic bone marrow, histamine fast achlorhydria, gastric parietal cell antibody and response to cyanocobalamin therapy. In addition she complained of xerostomia, grittiness of the eyes, weight loss and diarrhoea. She was found to have typical rheumatoid arthritis, xerostomia and keratoconjunctivitis sicca. Laboratory values included a serum calcium of $8.6\,mg/100\,ml$, and phosphorus of $2.3\,mg/100\,ml$. The alkaline phosphatase was raised ($20.2\,KA\,units/ml$). Faecal fat excretion was $10.2\,g/day$ and radiological examination revealed osteomalacia. Xylose absorption was normal but a glucose tolerance curve was diabetic. Intestinal biopsy revealed a normal jejunal mucosa with normal maltose, sucrose and lactose concentrations. An X-ray of the abdomen showed pancreatic calcification.*

Subclinical evidence of pancreatitis as shown by secretin and pancreozymin tests, may be more common (Bloch *et al.* 1965; Hradsky, Bartos & Keller 1967).

Liver disease

The association of autoimmune liver disease and Sjøgren's syndrome is now well recognized. Mitochondrial antibody, a serological marker for autoimmune liver disease, is detectable in 10% of patients with sicca syndrome (without rheumatoid arthritis) compared with 0.7% of patients with rheumatoid arthritis alone (Whaley *et al.* 1972b). All but one of the positive group in this series had clinical or biochemical evidence of liver disease, the diagnoses including primary biliary cirrhosis and chronic active hepatitis. Of the 80 patients studied by Shearn (1971) 5 had either primary biliary cirrhosis or chronic active hepatitis. Sixty-three patients were investigated by Golding *et al.* (1970). The sicca syndrome was diagnosed in 42% of patients with chronic active hepatitis, 72% with primary biliary cirrhosis and 38% with cryptogenic cirrhosis. The overall incidence of sicca syndrome in these three 'autoimmune' liver diseases was 51%.

Chapter 4

Genito-urinary system

Vaginitis sicca may be a troublesome feature of the syndrome. In one of our patients recurrent severe vaginal moniliasis was an added problem.

It is a clinical impression that urinary tract infections are commonplace in Sjøgren's (as well as in SLE). Perhaps this relates to local mucosal abnormalities.

A variety of renal abnormalities have been described (Table 4.5). The most important association is with defects in renal tubular function, rather than primary glomerular disease, which is rare. In particular, renal tubular acidosis, or the failure to acidify urine normally, is seen in approximately a quarter of all patients with Sjøgren's syndrome (Shearn & Tu 1965, 1968; Talal, Zisman & Schur 1968; Shioji *et al.* 1970; Shearn 1971; Whaley *et al.* 1972b). Other tubular defects have included diabetes insipidus, renal tubular acidosis, generalized aminoaciduria, diminished renal tubular reabsorption of uric acid, and phosphaturia. A true Fanconi syndrome is, however, rare (Mason *et al.* 1970). A form of nephrogenic diabetes insipidus not reversible by pitressin has been described (Shearn & Tu 1965).

The aetiology of these defects is still under discussion. While interstitial nephritis and chronic pyelonephritis (Shearn 1971) may be the underlying factor in some of the tubular defects this seems unlikely to be the whole explanation. More important may be the effect of hyperglobulinaemia *per se*. Other diseases characterized by hyperglobulinaemia such as chronic active hepatitis, hyperglobulinaemic purpura, cryoglobulinaemia, sarcoid and SLE, are occasionally complicated by renal tubular acidosis (Morris, Johnson & Fudenberg 1964).

While glomerulonephritis and renal arteritis are unusual problems in Sjøgren's syndrome, a small series of patients with rheumatoid arthritis and features suggestive of Sjøgren's syndrome were described in whom

Table 4.5 Renal abnormalities in Sjøgren's syndrome

Physiological
Renal tubular acidosis
Other renal tubular defects
Nephrogenic diabetes insipidus
Renal failure

Pathological
Lymphocyte and plasma cell infiltrates
Interstitial pyelonephritis
Glomerular basal membrane thickening and glomerulonephritis
Necrotizing vasculitis

---

reduced C3 levels and glomerulonephritis were found. Immunofluorescence revealed glomerular deposition of IgM and C3 (Talal, Zisman & Schur 1968). In such patients the differentiation from SLE may be difficult. Glomerulonephritis may also be observed in patients with cryoglobulinaemia and Sjøgren's syndrome (Meltzer & Franklin 1968). Occasional patients with sicca syndrome have been noted to develop immune complex nephritis (Moutsopoulos *et al.* 1978).

Nervous system

Unlike SLE, central nervous system disease in Sjøgren's syndrome is rare. Isolated cranial nerve palsies are occasionally seen as well as cases of multiple cranial neuropathies (Kaltreider & Talal 1969). Peripheral neuropathy is more frequent, though whether it is related to the associated connective tissue disease or relates primarily to Sjøgren's syndrome is not clear.

Case report. *A 48-year-old solicitor was admitted with acute mononeuritis multiplex. These were small vasculitic lesions on the elbows and fingers, but otherwise the only abnormal clinical finding was of sicca syndrome. Investigations revealed a normal WBC, hyperglobulinaemia ESR >100, CRP zero, ANA positive, DNA binding normal, positive antiRo antibodies and a lip gland biopsy showing widespread lymphoid infiltration.*

After a poor response to corticosteroids, he appeared to respond rapidly to i.v. cyclophosphamide and, apart from a relapse at 1 year, has remained well. The antiRo antibodies persist.

Myositis is well described, though whether this represents part of the accompanying connective tissue disease is uncertain. The infiltrate is predominantly mononuclear (Bloch *et al.* 1965). As in SLE, myasthenia gravis is occasionally associated with Sjøgren's syndrome (Downes, Greenwood & Wray 1966).

Case report. *A 63-year-old female developed ptosis, diplopia and generalized muscle weakness. Myasthenia gravis was confirmed and the patient responded well to neostigmine 60 mg daily. One year later the patient presented with a history of left parotid gland enlargement and dryness of the eyes. Xerostomia and keratoconjunctivitis sicca were confirmed and sialography revealed atrophy of the intraparotid duct system. At the age of 66 years the patient developed seropositive, erosive rheumatoid arthritis. Serological testing revealed rheumatoid factor antinuclear factor and thyroid microsomal and gastric parietal cell antibodies. DNA binding was normal.*

A series of reports from Johns Hopkins University have broadened the spectrum of neurological disease in Sjøgren's syndrome, to include hemiparosis, transverse myelopathy, seizures, movement disorders and multiple sclerosis. (Alexander, 1987). Their presence does not appear to relate to anti-Ro positivity (Heitaharju *et al.* 1992). While much discussion has centred on the frequency of these features, the possibility that a subset of 'M.S.' patients may have a different (and identifiable) pathogenesis raises intriguing possibilities.

Respiratory disease (Table 4.6)

Pulmonary function test abnormalities are common in Sjøgren's (Oxholm *et al.* 1982). The submucous glands of the larynx, trachea and bronchi may be infiltrated with lymphocytes and plasma cells with resultant atrophy leading to hoarseness, persistent cough and difficulty in expectorating thick, tenacious sputum. This leads in turn to recurrent pneumonitis and atelectasis. Chest infection has been found to be more frequent in patients with rheumatoid arthritis (Walker 1967). It may be that the sicca syndrome contributes to this tendency (Shearn 1971). It would appear likely, for example, that postoperative chest infections would be more prevalent in patients with dry respiratory tracts — another reason for clinical awareness of Sjøgren's syndrome.

Case report. *A 65-year-old patient with a long history of seropositive rheumatoid arthritis had complained of dryness of the eyes and mouth for approximately 5 years associated with winter bronchitis for the first time in her life. She was a non-smoker. More recently, she had undergone a series of minor orthopaedic operations, following each of which she developed chest infection with areas of atelectasis.*

An interrelationship between the sicca syndrome and fibrosing alveolitis occurs (Tomasi, Fudenberg & Finby 1966; Turner-Warwick 1968, 1974).

Table 4.6 Respiratory tract complications in Sjøgren's syndrome

Tracheitis
Bronchitis
Pneumonitis
Atelectasis
Pleurisy
Diffuse interstitial pulmonary fibrosis
Fibrosing alveolitis

Shearn (1971) observed 11 cases of fibrosing alveolitis in his series of 80 patients with Sjøgren's syndrome. Three of these patients had sicca syndrome without another connective tissue disease. Mason *et al.* (1970) reported 9 patients with the sicca syndrome, fibrosing alveolitis and renal tubular acidosis, none of whom had coexisting connective tissue disease. Pulmonary hypertension is also described. The subject has been reviewed by Fairfax *et al.* (1981) and by Moutsopoulos & Talal (1989).

Vascular changes

During our studies of the vasculopathy associated with anticardiolipin (see Chapter 3), we observed patients with widespread 'idiopathic' arterial and venous thromboses who also had Sjøgren's syndrome but no evidence of SLE.

Raynaud's phenomenon is seen in up to one-third of patients with sicca syndrome, being found equally frequently in those with an accompanying connective tissue disease in our series (Whaley *et al.* 1972b). In these patients Raynaud's was not associated with cryoglobulinaemia.

Of more significance is the occurrence of purpura and hyperglob-ulinaemia and these features have, if anything, been underemphasized in the literature.

Case report. *A 31-year-old mother gave birth to an infant with congenital heart block. On investigation, the mother had antiRo and antiLa antibodies and moderately raised IgM antibodies. She had a dry Schirmer's test.*

Her only symptoms were of frequent calf pains, and regular lower limb purpura, especially after playing tennis.

Although only a minority of patients develop this complication it has, on the other hand, been suggested that 20−30% of patients with purpura hyperglobulinaemia have, or will develop, Sjøgren's syndrome (Talal 1966). Significantly, it has been noted that Sjøgren's patients who develop malignant lymphoreticular neoplasms have an unduly high incidence of purpura hyperglobulinaemia (Talal, Sokoloff & Barth 1967).

Blood

A mild normochromic, normocytic anaemia is seen in about half the cases. Leukopenia is occasionally seen, but this is rarely marked (Bloch *et al.* 1965; Shearn 1971). The rare rheumatoid arthritis complication of Felty's syndrome is, however, almost invariably accompanied by Sjøgren's syndrome (Barnes, Turnbull & Vernon-Roberts 1971). Eosinophilia is also described; in the series reported by Bloch *et al.* (1965) 50% were noted to have this feature though our own figure is nearer 5–10% (Whaley *et al.* 1972b). The presence of eosinophilia should alert the physician to the possibility of drug sensitivity, a feature of this condition (see later).

DRUG ALLERGY

As in the case of SLE, a predisposition to drug allergy has been noted in Sjøgren's syndrome. Bloch *et al.* (1965) found that 71 out of 83 patients with Sjøgren's syndrome treated with gold salts developed an allergic skin rash. Williams *et al.* (1969) in a survey of penicillin allergy in patients with rheumatoid arthritis found that when these patients had accompanying sicca syndrome, the incidence of penicillin allergy trebled to over 40%. These findings, if substantiated, again argue for the routine testing of all rheumatoid patients for Sjøgren's syndrome.

Gharavi & Hughes (1980), in a simple but clinically useful study, found that gold hypersensitivity reactions were twice as common in rheumatoid arthritis patients with dry Schirmer's tests.

In our department, we have a clinical nugget called the 'Septrin provocation test'. It has never been published — until now. Almost 100% of our patients with primary Sjøgren's syndrome who have ever received the antibiotic Septrin (trimethoprim/sulphamethoxazole) have been allergic — sometimes with severe flares of rashes and polyarthritis.

Other associated features

Autoimmune thyroid disorders are commoner in Sjøgren's syndrome — up to 50%. Sjøgren's patients having antithyroid antibodies (Karsch 1980). Inflammatory synovitis is common and after intermittent. The interrelationships between Sjøgren's syndrome and rheumatoid arthritis are discussed elsewhere (p. 102).

LYMPHORETICULAR NEOPLASIA

In 1951, Rothman, Bloch & Hauser reported Sjøgren's syndrome in association with lymphoblastoma and hypersplenism. Workers in Bethesda subsequently reported the development of extrasalivary reticulum cell sarcoma in 3 out of 58 patients with Sjøgren's syndrome as well as a further patient with raised IgM levels and atypical lymphoid infiltrates in the lymph nodes and lung. The Bethesda group went on to report 8 other cases with extrasalivary lymphoid abnormalities; 2 had primary (Waldenström's) macroglobulinaemia and 5 had a significant increase of serum IgM (Bloch

Table 4.7 Summary of lymphoproliferative disorders associated with Sjøgren's syndrome (from Anderson & Talal 1972)

Diagnosis	Number of cases
Pseudolymphoma	8
Reticulum cell sarcoma	13
Waldenström's macroglobulinaemia	7
Malignant lymphocytic lymphoma	1
Giant follicular lymphoma	1
Lymphosarcoma	3
Hodgkin's disease	1
Lymphoma of vocal cords	1
Thymoma	3
Total	38

et al. 1965; Talal, Sokoloff & Barth 1967). The reported cases have been reviewed by Anderson and Talal (1972). These malignancies may be divided into intrasalivary (Azzopardi & Evans 1971) and extrasalivary (Talal, Sokoloff & Barth 1967; Anderson & Talal 1972; Whaley *et al.* 1972b), the spectrum of lymphoid proliferation varying from the highly malignant reticulum cell sarcoma and lymphosarcoma to the more benign giant follicular lymphoma and pseudolymphoma. A case of Sjøgren's terminating in acute myeloblastic leukaemia has been described (De Coteau *et al.* 1975).

Two clinical points should lead to a suspicion of malignant change: a progressive fall in levels of serum immunoglobulins, especially IgM, frequently accompanies and may precede the clinical appearance of malignancy. Secondly, the now abandoned practice of irradiation of the salivary glands may predispose to the development of such malignancy (Anderson & Talal 1972).

It certainly has been noticeable that in recent years reports of lymphoma development in Sjøgren's patients have become rare.

Sjøgren's and AIDS

Some patients with human immunodeficiency disease develop Sjøgren's-like features, including enlarged parotids, xerostomia, dry eyes, positive ANA and RF tests and even focal lymphocytic infiltrates on lip biopsy. However, these patients do not normally have antiRo or antiLa, and the CD4/CD8 ratio in tissues is 0·66 (compared to >3 in Sjøgren's syndrome) (Moutsopoulos & Talal 1989).

IMMUNOLOGICAL FINDINGS

Sjøgren's syndrome, like SLE, is characterized by the presence of multiple autoantibodies. It differs from SLE in that organ-specific antibodies are more prominent. The changes are summarized in Table 4.8.

Immunoglobulins. Sjøgren's syndrome is characterized by hyperglobulinaemia, sometimes marked. Significant increases in IgM, IgA and secretory IgA levels are usually observed (Gumpel & Hobbs 1970). Macroglobulinaemia and cryoglobulinaemia are also described though the latter is uncommon.

Serum hyperviscosity is, surprisingly, an unusual finding. In four patients, hyperviscosity has been associated with the presence of serum IgG—IgG rheumatoid factor complexes (Alarcon—Segovia *et al.* 1974).

Rheumatoid factors. In RA with sicca syndrome, the incidence of positive latex tests for IgM rheumatoid factor approaches 100%. In patients with the sicca syndrome alone, the figure varies between 50 and 80%.

IgA rheumatoid factors were found in 7 of 10 patients with systemic sicca syndrome and only 5 of 59 patients with other connective tissue diseases, raising the possibility that abnormalities of the mucosal immune system may be important in this condition (Elkon *et al.* 1981).

Antinuclear antibody. Positive ANA tests are found in the majority of patients with Sjøgren's syndrome, indeed the finding of a positive ANA

Table 4.8 Immunological findings of Sjøgren's syndrome

Finding	Percentage
Non-organ-specific antibodies	
Rheumatoid factor (IgM)	75—100
ANA	40—70
LE cells	10
DNA antibody (low titre)	10
ENA (antiRo)	75
Mitochondrial and smooth muscle antibodies	5—10
Organ-specific antibodies	
Thyroid microsomal antibodies	20—50
Thyroglobulin	25—33
Gastric parietal cell	3—30
Salivary duct cell	10—65
(Coombs' test)	10

test in a patient with rheumatoid arthritis should lead to a search for Sjøgren's syndrome. While the commonest nuclear immunofluorescence pattern is homogeneous, speckled and nucleolar patterns may also be seen (Whaley *et al*. 1972b). LE cells are found in about 10% of cases.

Extractable nuclear antigens

The development of tests for the recognition of antibodies against 'extractable nuclear antigens' — ENAs — (see Appendix) has helped to define Sjøgren's syndrome a little more precisely. Of the 20 or so antiENAs now recognized, two — antiRo and antiLa — are regularly found in Sjøgren's syndrome. Some 75% of patients with primary Sjøgren's syndrome possess antiRo compared with 3% of RA patients (Hughes 1984).

AntiDNA antibodies. DNA binding values are normal in the majority of cases of Sjøgren's syndrome including those with strongly positive ANF and LE cell tests (Hughes 1973).

Mitochondrial and smooth muscle antibodies. Mitochondrial antibodies are found in 5–10% of patients (see above). Smooth muscle antibodies are occasionally found, though they have little clinical significance (Whaley *et al*. 1972b).

Organ-specific antibodies

Thyroid antibodies. Antibodies against thyroglobulin and thyroid microsomes may be seen in up to 50% of patients, although the larger series of Sjøgren's patients include approximately 10% with thyroid disease (Bloch *et al*. 1965; Shearn 1971; Karsh 1980). It has been shown that patients with thyroid disease do not have an increased prevalence of Sjøgren's syndrome (Williamson *et al*. 1967).

Gastric parietal cell antibody. The prevalence of gastric parietal cell antibody may be increased in Sjøgren's syndrome (see above) though the relationship of Sjøgren's syndrome to pernicious anaemia is still unclear.

Salivary duct antibody. This can be demonstrated in roughly half the patients, though its pathogenic significance is unknown (Bertram & Halberg 1964; MacSween *et al*. 1967). Strangely, it appears to be confined to those cases with rheumatoid arthritis, and is absent in patients with sicca syndrome alone.

Antiphospholipid antibodies

In a study of 65 patients with primary Sjøgren's, increased levels of antiphospholipid antibodies were found in 13 (20%). They were mainly of the IgA isotype and were not significantly associated with arterial or venous thrombosis (Asherson *et al.* 1992).

C-reactive protein

Like SLE, and unlike RA, patients with primary Sjøgren's syndrome appear unable to mount a high CRP response, and the high ESR/low CRP ratio is a useful clinical pointer (Moutsopoulos *et al.* 1983).

ASSOCIATION WITH OTHER CONNECTIVE TISSUE DISEASE

The main reason for describing Sjøgren's syndrome before rheumatoid arthritis is to emphasize the interrelationships of these diseases (Fig. 4.3). Many of the systemic features of rheumatoid arthritis, such as vasculitis, pulmonary disease, Felty's syndrome, and the presence of hyperglo-bulinaemia and circulating autoantibodies are related as much to the presence of Sjøgren's syndrome as to rheumatoid arthritis itself. Rheumatoid arthritis is the most frequent disease accompanying the sicca syndrome; the overall incidence of the association is not known. In the series of 57 patients with Sjøgren's syndrome studied at the NIH, Bethesda, 30 had rheumatoid arthritis, 2 had possible rheumatoid arthritis, 3 had scleroderma and 4 had polymyositis. Conversely, reports of the incidence of keratoconjunctivitis sicca in rheumatoid arthritis have ranged from 10 to 58.4%, the high figure being obtained from a survey of 250 patients using careful slit-lamp examination.

The association with other connective tissue diseases is discussed in the relevant chapters. A proportion of patients with the sicca syndrome alone suffer arthralgia or a non-erosive arthritis, thus making a true assessment of the frequency of the association even more difficult.

DIAGNOSIS

Schirmer's test (Fig. 4.4)

This test should be standard procedure in all rheumatic disease patients, being the simplest screening test for keratoconjunctivitis sicca. A strip of filter paper 35-mm long and 5-mm wide (standardized commercially

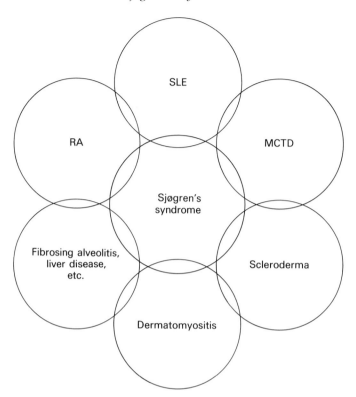

Fig. 4.3 Interrelationships of Sjøgren's syndrome.

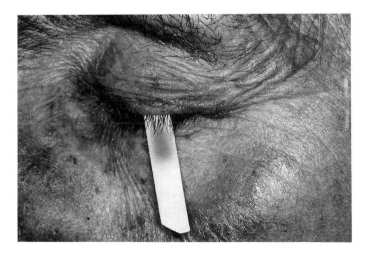

Fig. 4.4 Schirmer's test. Wetting of less than 15 mm of the test paper in 5 min is regarded as abnormal.

produced papers are available) is bent 5 mm from one end and hooked over the lower eyelid at the junction and the middle and outer thirds. The length of wetting is measured at 5 min. Less than 15 mm is regarded as abnormal. Subnormal results may occasionally be obtained in healthy elderly persons (Whaley *et al.* 1972a). If the Schirmer test gives equivocal results, it can be repeated after the stimulation of lacrimation by sniffing ammonia.

This routine bedside test may have even more clinical value in rheumatology than presently appreciated. For example:

Case report. *A 64-year-old man developed acute polymyalgia rheumatica. The only unexpected finding was of a bone-dry Schirmer's test. Despite the absence of synovitis at presentation, the patient went on to develop rheumatoid arthritis.*

Slit-lamp examination

A drop of 1% Rose Bengal dye instilled into the conjunctival sac facilitates the detection of superficial corneal scarring. Slit-lamp examination provides the most sensitive test for filamentous keratitis.

Tests of salivary function

In view of the difficulty in the clinical detection of xerostomia, it is perhaps not surprising that a battery of tests of salivary gland function have been advocated (Cummings *et al.* 1971) including salivary flow measurements, sialography (Fig. 4.5) and salivary scintigraphy. The latter method records the uptake concentration and excretion of ^{99m}Tc pertechnetate by the major salivary glands. The method is claimed to be sensitive, especially where asymmetry of parotid function is observed (Arrago *et al.* 1984).

Lip gland biopsy

This has become an important procedure in the diagnosis of Sjøgren's syndrome, following the observation that pathological changes occurring in the major salivary gland are mirrored in the minor salivary glands of the lip (Chisholm & Mason 1968). These glands can often be felt as small pin-head-sized lumps inside the lower lip. Under local anaesthesia, a gland can be removed through a small incision. More recent studies still show labial gland biopsy to be more practicable than parotid biopsy (Wise *et al.* 1988).

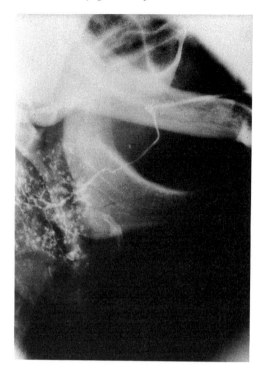

Fig. 4.5 Lateral oblique sialogram showing globular sialectasis of parotid gland in a patient with Sjøgren's syndrome. (Dr D.M. Chisholm, Glasgow Dental Hospital.)

TREATMENT

Keratoconjunctivitis sicca

Most patients obtain symptomatic relief from the regular use of methyl cellulose eye drops. Superinfection is a major problem which requires prompt local antibiotic therapy. Surgical procedures such as occlusion of the lower lacrimal punctum are rarely indicated.

Xerostomia

This may prove extremely difficult to alleviate, and regular sips of water or unsweetened lemon juice may be needed. Regular expert dental care is required to offset the marked tendency to caries. Superinfection in sialectatic parotids requires systemic antibiotic therapy.

Other sicca manifestations

Vaginitis sicca may be troublesome, and superinfection with *Candida* may occur. The tendency to bronchitis sicca and atelectasis requires extra vigilance in patients undergoing general anaesthesia.

Systemic therapy

Small doses of prednisone undoubtedly lessen many of the troublesome symptoms of Sjøgren's syndrome, and higher doses (over 10 mg prednisone daily) may benefit the complications of pulmonary fibrosis or peripheral neuropathy. Antimalarial (e.g. hydroxychloroquine 200 mg daily) are often helpful in the arthralgia or synovitis of Sjøgren's syndrome. In other patients, azathioprine is an effective steroid-sparing agent in Sjøgren's syndrome. In some cases, particularly in severe sicca syndrome not associated with rheumatoid arthritis, cyclophosphamide has proved beneficial though, fortunately, such cases are extremely rare.

REFERENCES

Alarcon-Segovia D., Fishbein E., Abruzzo J.L. & Heimer R. (1974) Serum hyperviscosity in Sjøgren's syndrome. *Annals of Internal Medicine*, **80**, 35.

Alexander E. (1987) Neurologic aspects of Sjøgren's. In: *Sjøgren's Syndrome: Clinical and Immunological Aspects*. pp. 102–125. Springer-Verlag, Berlin.

Anderson L.G. & Talal N. (1972) The spectrum of benign to malignant lympho-proliferation in Sjøgren's syndrome. *Clinical and Experimental Immunology*, **10**, 199.

Arrago J.P., Rocher F., Vigneron N., Pecking A. & Najean Y. (1984) Sjøgren's syndrome: a functional study of salivary glands. *Presse Medicale*, **13**, 209–213.

Asherson R.A., Fei H.-M., Staub H.L., Khamashta M.A., Hughes G.R.V. & Fox R.I. (1992) Antiphospholipid antibodies and HLA associations in primary Sjøgren's syndrome. *Annals of the Rheumatic Diseases*, **51**, 495–498.

Azzopardi J.G. & Evans D.J. (1971) Malignant lymphoma of parotid associated with Mikulicz disease (benign lymphoepithelial lesion). *Journal of Clinical Pathology*, **24**, 744.

Barnes C.G., Turnbull A.L. & Vernon-Roberts B. (1971) Felty's syndrome. *Annals of the Rheumatic Diseases*, **30**, 359.

Bertram U. & Halberg P. (1964) A specific antibody against the epithelium of the salivary ducts in sera from patients with Sjøgren's syndrome. *Acta Allergologica*, **19**, 458.

Bloch K.L., Buchanan W.W., Wohl M.J. & Bunim J. (1965) Sjøgren's syndrome: a clinical pathological and serological study of 62 cases. *Medicine*, **44**, 187.

Buchanan W.W. (1966) Gastric studies in Sjøgren's syndrome. *Gut*, **7**, 351.

Chisholm D.M. & Mason D.K. (1968) Labial salivary gland biopsy in Sjøgren's disease. *Journal of Clinical Pathology*, **21**, 656.

Chused T.M., Hardin J.A., Frank M.M. & Green I. (1974) Identification of cells infiltrating the minor salivary glands in patients with Sjøgren's syndrome. *Journal of Immunology*, **112**, 641.

Cummings N.A., Schall G.L., Asofsky R., Anderson L.G. & Talal N. (1971) Sjøgren's syndrome – newer aspects of research, diagnosis and therapy (NIH conference). *Annals of Internal Medicine*, **75**, 937.

Daniels T.E., Sylvester R.A., Silvermann S., Polando V. & Talal N. (1974) Tubulorecticular structures within labial salivary glands in Sjøgren's syndrome. *Arthritis and Rheumatism*, **17**, 593.

De Coteau W.E., Katakkar S.B., Skinnider L., Hayton R.C. & Somerville E.A. (1975) Sjøgren's syndrome terminating in acute myeloblastic leukaemia. *Journal of Rheumatology*, **2**, 331.

Doig J.A., Whaley K., Dick W.C., Nuki G., Williamson J. & Buchanan W.W. (1971) Otolaryngeal aspects of Sjøgren's syndrome. *British Medical Journal*, **4**, 460.

Downes J.M., Greenwood B.M. & Wray S.H. (1966) Autoimmune aspects of myasthenia gravis. *Quarterly Journal of Medicine*, **35**, 85.

Elkon K.B., Caeiro F., Gharavi A.E. & Hughes G.R.V. (1981) Radioimmunoassay profile of antiglobulins in connective tissue diseases: Elevated level of IgA antiglobulin in systemic sicca syndrome. *Clinical and Experimental Immunology*, **46**, 547−556.

Fairfax A., Haslam P., Pavia D. *et al.* (1981) Pulmonary disorders associated with Sjøgren's syndrome. *Quarterly Journal of Medicine*, **50**, 279−295.

Fielder A.H.L., Walport M.J., Batchelor J.R. *et al.* (1983) Family study of the major histocompatibility complex in patients with SLE: importance of null alleles of C_4A and C_4B in determining disease susceptibility. *British Medical Journal*, **286**, 425−429.

Fox R.I., Howell F.V., Bone R.C. *et al.* (1984) Primary Sjøgren's syndrome: clinical and immunopathologic features. *Seminars in Arthritis and Rheumatism*, **14**, 77−105.

Gharavi A.E. & Hughes G.R.V. (1980) The Schirmer's test and drug allergy in rheumatoid arthritis. *Journal of Rheumatology*, **7**, 428.

Golding P.L., Bown R., Mason A.M.S. & Taylor N. (1970) Sicca complex in liver disease. *British Medical Journal*, **4**, 430.

Greenspan J.S., Gutman G.A., Weismann I.L. & Talal N. (1974) *Clinical Immunology and Immunopathology*, **3**, 16.

Gumpel J.M. & Hobbs J.R. (1970) Serum immunoglobulins in Sjøgren's syndrome. *Annals of Rheumatic Diseases*, **29**, 681.

Heitaharju A., Korpele M., Ilonen J. & Frey H. (1992) Nervous system disease, immunological features and HLA phenotype in Sjøgren's syndrome. *Annals of the Rheumatic Diseases*, **51**, 506−509.

Henderson J.W. (1950) Keratoconjunctivitis sicca. A review with a survey of 21 additional cases. *American Journal of Ophthalmology*, **33**, 197.

Hradsky M., Bartos V. & Keller O. (1967) Pancreatic function in Sjøgren's syndrome. *Gastroenterologia (Basel)*, **108**, 252.

Hughes G.R.V. (1973) The diagnosis of systemic lupus erythematosus. *British Journal of Haematology*, **25**, 409.

Hughes G.R.V. (1984) Autoantibodies in lupus and its variants: experience in 1000 patients. *British Medical Journal*, **289**, 339−342.

Kaltreider H.B. & Talal N. (1969) The neuropathy of Sjøgren's syndrome. *Annals of Internal Medicine*, **70**, 751.

Karsh G. (1980) Autoimmune thyroid diseases in Sjøgren's patients. *Arthritis and Rheumatism*, **23**, 1326−1329.

Kassan S.S. & Gardy M. (1978) Sjøgren's syndrome: An update and overview. *American Journal of Medicine*, **64**, 1037.

Kilpi A., Bergroth V., Konttinen Y.T. *et al.* (1983) Lymphocyte infiltrations in the gastric mucosa in Sjøgren's syndrome: an immunoperoxidase study using monoclonal antibodies in the avidin–biotin–peroxidase method. *Arthritis and Rheumatism*, **26**, 1196–1200.

MacSween R.N.M., Goudie R.B., Anderson J.R. *et al.* (1967) Occurrence of antibody to salivary duct epithelium in Sjøgren's syndrome, rheumatoid arthritis and other arthritides. A clinical and laboratory study. *Annals of the Rheumatic Diseases*, **26**, 402.

McFarlane I.G., Wojcicko B.M., Tsantoulas D.C. *et al.* (1976) Cellular immune responses to salivary antigens in autoimmune liver disease with sicca syndrome. *Clinical and Experimental Immunology*, **25**, 389.

Mason A.M.S., McIllmurray M.B., Golding P.L. *et al.* (1970) Fibrosing alveolitis associated with renal tubular acidosis. *British Medical Journal*, **4**, 596.

Mason D.K. & Chisholm D.M. (1975) *Salivary Glands in Health and Disease*. Saunders, Philadelphia.

Meltzer M. & Franklin E.C. (1968) Cryoglobulins, rheumatoid factors and connective tissue disorders. *Arthritis and Rheumatism*, **10**, 489.

Miyasaka N., Seaman W., Bakshi A., Sauvezie B., Strand V., Pope R. & Talal N. (1983) Natural killing activity in Sjøgren's syndrome. *Arthritis and Rheumatology*, **26**, 954.

Morris C., Johnson L. & Fudenberg H.H. (1964) Studies on renal acidification in hyperglobulinaemic nonmyelomatous states. *Journal of Clinical Investigation*, **43**, 1293.

Moutsopoulos H.M. & Talal N. (1989) New developments in Sjøgren's syndrome. *Current Opinion in Rheumatology*, **1**, 332–338.

Moutsopoulos H.M., Balow J.E., Lawley T.J., Stahl N.I., Antonovych T.T. & Chused T.M. (1978) Immune complex glomerulonephritis in sicca syndrome. *American Journal of Medicine*, **64**, 955.

Moutsopoulos H.H., Elkon K.B., Hughes G.R.V. & Pepys M.B. (1983) C-Reactive protein levels in Sjøgren's syndrome. *Clinical and Experimental Rheumatology*, **1**, 57–59.

Oxholm P., Bundgaard A., Madsen E.B., Manthorpe R. & Rasmussen F.V. (1982) Pulmonary function in patients with primary Sjøgren's syndrome. *Rheumatology International*, **2**, 179–181.

Pedersen B.K., Oxholm P., Manthorpe R. & Anderson V. (1986) Interleukin II augmentation of the defective natural killer cell activity in patients with primary Sjøgren's syndrome. *Clinical and Experimental Immunology*, **63**, 1–7.

Rothman S., Bloch M. & Hauser F.V. (1951) *Archiv für Dermatologie und Syphilis*, **63**, 642.

Seifert G. & Geiler G. (1957) Speichel, Drusen und rheumatismus. *Deutsche medizinische Wochenschrift*, **82**, 1415.

Shearn M.A. (1971) *Sjøgren's Syndrome*. Saunders, Philadelphia.

Shearn M.A. & Tú W.H. (1965) Nephrogenic diabetes insipidus and other defects of renal tubular function in Sjøgren's syndrome. *American Journal of Medicine*, **39**, 312.

Shearn M.A. & Tú W.H. (1968) Latent renal tubular acidosis in Sjøgren's syndrome. *Annals of the Rheumatic Diseases*, **27**, 27.

Shioji R., Furuyama T., Onodera S. *et al.* (1970) Sjøgren's syndrome and renal tubular acidosis. *American Journal of Medicine*, **48**, 456.

Sjøgren H. (1933) Zur Kenntnis der Keratoconjunctivitis Sicca (Keratitis Filiformis bei Hypofunktion der Tranendrusen). *Acta Ophthalmologica (Kbh)*, **II**, Suppl. 2, 1.

Talal N. (1966) Sjøgren's syndrome. *Bulletin of Rheumatic Diseases*, **16**, 404.

Talal N., Sokoloff L. & Barth W.F. (1967) Extrasalivary lymphoid abnormalities in Sjøgren's syndrome (reticulum cell sarcoma, pseudolymphoma, macroglobulinaemia). *American Journal of Medicine*, **43**, 50.

Talal N., Sylvester R.A., Daniels T.E., Greenspan J.S. & Williams R.C. (1974) T & B lymphocytes in peripheral blood and tissue lesions in Sjøgren's syndrome. *Journal of Clinical Investigation*, **53**, 180.

Talal N., Zisman E. & Schur P.H. (1968) Renal tubular acidosis glomerulonephritis and immunologic factors in Sjøgren's syndrome. *Arthritis and Rheumatism*, **11**, 774.

Tomasi T.B., Fudenberg H.H. & Finby N. (1966) Possible relationship of rheumatoid factors and pulmonary disease. *American Journal of Medicine*, **33**, 243.

Turner-Warwick M. (1968) Fibrosing alveolitis and chronic liver disease. *Quarterly Journal of Medicine*, **37**, 133.

Walker W.C. (1967) Pulmonary infections and rheumatoid arthritis. *Quarterly Journal of Medicine*, **36**, 239.

Waterhouse J.P. & Doniach I. (1966) Postmortem prevalence of focal lymphocytic adenitis of the submandibular salivary gland. *Journal of Pathology and Bacteriology*, **91**, 53.

Whaley K., Webb J., McAvoy B.A., Hughes G.R.V., Lee P., MacSween R.N.M. & Buchanan W.W. (1972a) Sjøgren's syndrome. *Quarterly Journal of Medicine*, **42**, 513.

Whaley K., Williamson J., Wilson T., McGavin M.M., Hughes G.R.V., Hughes H., Schmulian L.R., MacSween R.N.M. & Buchanan W.W. (1972b) Sjøgren's syndrome and autoimmunity in a geriatric population. *Age and Ageing*, **1**, 197.

Williams B.O., St Onge R.A., Prentice A. *et al.* (1969) Penicillin allergy in rheumatoid arthritis with special reference to Sjøgren's syndrome. *Annals of Rheumatic Diseases*, **48**, 607.

Williamson J., Cant J.S., Mason D.K. *et al.* (1967) Sjøgren's syndrome and thyroid disease. *British Journal of Ophthalmology*, **51**, 721.

Williamson J., Paterson R.W.W. & McGavin D.D.M. *et al.* (1970) Sjøgren's syndrome in relation to pernicious anaemia and idiopathic Addison's disease. *British Journal of Ophthalmology*, **54**, 31.

Wise C.M., Agudelo C.A., Semble E.L., Stump T.E. & Woodruff R.D. (1988) Comparison of parotid and minor salivary gland biopsy specimens in the diagnosis of Sjøgren's syndrome. *Arthritis and Rheumatism*, **31**, 662–666.

5: *Rheumatoid Arthritis*

Rheumatoid arthritis (RA) holds a unique position among the connective tissue diseases. As well as being the commonest, and by far the most important in socioeconomic terms, it differs fundamentally from the others in its predominant localization to the musculoskeletal system. The reasons for this pattern of disease are unknown. In particular, one important question remains unanswered. Why is it that patients with RA, in which immune complexes play a pathogenetic role both in the synovitis and the arteritis, largely succeed in localizing the disease to their joints, sparing for the most part other organs such as the kidney?

EPIDEMIOLOGY

Prevalence (the number of cases in a community at a certain time) has proved easier to assess than incidence (the number of new cases occurring during a given period). Nonetheless, the epidemiology of RA has proved a muddier field than most, largely because of the difficulty in obtaining satisfactory classification criteria. Interviews, and even many clinical surveys have been bedevilled by the inclusion of other forms of 'rheumatism'. The commonly accepted prevalence is 1–2%, though in a survey carried out in the USA in 1951 the prevalence was approximately 6·9% (reviewed by Wolfe & Masi 1968). A major health examination in the USA in 1959–62 showed that an estimated 3·6 million adults (3·2%) had RA. In a UK study comparing a 'rural' (Wensleydale) and 'urban' (Leigh) population, 2·1% of men and 5·1% of women were found to be afflicted. There was little difference in radiological or serological evidence of RA between the two communities.

Neither, surprisingly, does climate affect the prevalence. In a Jamaican study (Lawrence *et al.* 1966), the prevalence of 'definite' (ARA criteria) RA was 1·7% while that of 'probable' RA was 9·0%. A clinical study of rheumatic disease patients in Jamaica confirmed the prevalence of the disease on the island (Wilson & Hughes 1979). The disease also appears to be equally prevalent among whites and negroes. Females are affected three times more frequently than males.

There is little concrete evidence of increased familiar aggregation of RA, although rheumatoid factor is positive in four times the number of first degree relatives of probands with RA compared with controls (O'Brien 1967).

One of the more baffling aspects of the disease is that it appears to be a disease of modern times. While ankylosing spondylitis, ochronosis, osteoarthrosis and gout have been identified in human remains dating back several thousand years, no such evidence of RA has been found. Also, as Boyle and Buchanan lucidly point out (1971). 'Perspicacious lay observers have also failed to comment on rheumatoid deformities: there is no reference to the disease either in the Bible or in the works of Shakespeare, nor do the paintings of the classical masters of the Dutch, French, Italian or Spanish schools depict it, although the changes of many other chronic afflictions, including osteoarthrosis, are seen.'

It is possible that the disease as now recognized was first described by a French medical student, Augustin-Jacob Landre-Beauvais, in 1800 (see Parish 1963).

It has been suggested that, recently, at least in certain countries, RA is becoming less common. Only time will tell.

PATHOLOGY (see Firestein 1992)

Synovium

The normal synovium consists of a layer of synoviocytes lining the joint cavity and resting on connective tissue and fat. At high magnification, two main types of synovial lining cells may be distinguished: Type A (phagocytic cells) and less numerous Type B cells (non-phagocytic and with prominent endoplasmic reticulum) (Norton & Ziff 1966). The lining, as well as acting as an active phagocyte barrier, also acts as a barrier to the transfer of high molecular weight proteins such as α- and β-macroglobulins and fibrin into the synovial cavity. The main pathological changes in RA are listed in Table 5.1.

The earliest change appears to be capillary damage (Schumacher & Kitridou 1972) with leakage of plasma constituents and fibrin. Early in the course of the disease the synovium becomes oedematous. Vascular congestion occurs and an infiltrate of cells — a few polymorphs initially, small lymphocytes and plasma cells later — is seen throughout the synovium (Fig. 5.1). Immunochemical staining has shown that a number of distinct HLA DR +ve cell types exist, one of which has the characteristics of the interdigitating cells of the lymph node paracortex (Poulter *et al.* 1982). The synovial cell layer reduplicates and becomes hypertrophied and the lymphocytes and plasma cells aggregate into follicle-like collections, surrounded by

Table 5.1 Pathological changes in RA (from Zvaifler 1973)

Histology
Oedema of synovium
Villous hypertrophy
Hyperplasia and hypertrophy of synovial lining cells
Giant cells
Vascular congestion and dilatation
Cellular infiltrates (lymphocytes and plasma cells)
Pannus (granulation) formation

Immunofluorescence
Increased fibrinogen deposition
Abundant IgG in lymphocytes and plasma cells
Extracellular complement and immunoglobulin
Perivascular complement and immunoglobulin
IgM in adult seropositive RA

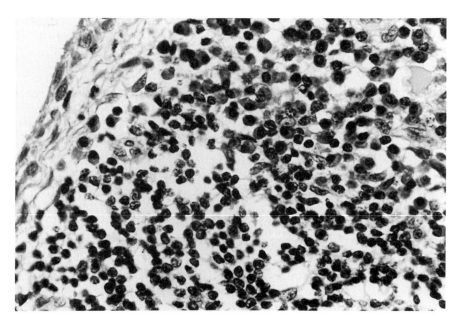

Fig. 5.1 Synovium in active RA, showing predominantly plasma cell (top) and lymphocyte infiltration. (H & E × 520). (Dr Shirley Amin, University Hospital of the West Indies.)

fibrous connective tissues (Fig. 5.2). A profuse granulation tissue consisting of proliferating fibroblasts (containing fibronectin (Matsuhara *et al.* 1983)), blood vessels and chronic inflammatory cells, so-called 'pannus', spreads over the surface of articular cartilage (Fig. 5.3), leading, through the mediation of proteases, collagenases and mechanical factors, to cartilage and bone erosion.

In active RA synovial fluid, the viscosity is decreased and the protein content increased. The cellular exudate consists largely of polymorphs, the numbers of which may be enough to render the synovial fluid frankly purulent. Some of these cells contain intracytoplasmic 'inclusions' consisting of immunoglobulins, complement and antigammaglobulins (rheumatoid factors). The synovial fluid contains cryoprecipitates with DNA and IgG–antiIgG complexes (Zvaifler 1973). The haemolytic complement activity of active RA synovial fluid is lowered in proportion to the amount of these complexes (see later).

For a comprehensive monograph on the anatomy and pathology of joints and synovial fluid see Sokoloff (1978).

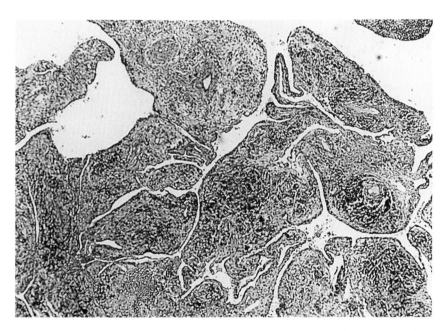

Fig. 5.2 Hypertrophied villi of synovial membrane due to chronic inflammation with lymphoid follicle formation. (H & E × 54.) (Dr Shirley Amin, University Hospital of the West Indies.)

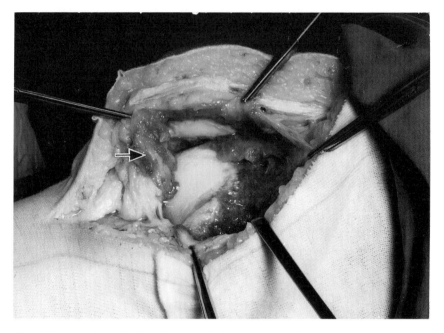

Fig. 5.3 Synovectomy for RA. The dark fleshy pannus can be seen spreading over the articular surface. (Professor E.G.L. Bywaters, Hammersmith Hospital.)

Nodules

Rheumatoid nodules, found mainly on the extensor surfaces such as the elbows, and along tendons, have a characteristic histological picture, with three distinct zones (Fig. 5.4): an inner necrotic area surrounded by palisades of radially arranged mononuclear inflammatory cells including histiocytes and monocytes. Many of these cells contain rheumatoid factor. The outer layer consists of chronic inflammatory cells (plasma cells and lymphocytes) and fibroblasts. (In some nodules, arteritis is seen, though this is by no means the rule.)

Vasculitis

Vasculitis, when it occurs, affects smaller arteries, and is most commonly seen clinically on the fingers as small periungal or finger pad infarcts. The vasculitis may be widespread, resulting in skin ulceration and neuropathy. More rarely, in a larger vessel, florid necrotizing vasculitis resembling polyarteritis nodosa may occur, with bowel or myocardial infarction or even peripheral gangrene. This form of 'malignant' RA carries a poor prognosis, though its activity may fluctuate markedly.

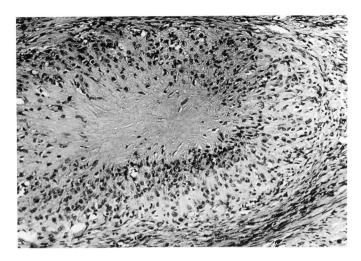

Fig. 5.4 Subcutaneous nodule in RA, showing inner necrotic zone, surrounding palisades of mononuclear inflammatory cells and an outer layer of chronic inflammatory cells and fibroblasts. (H & E × 160.) (Dr Shirley Amin, University Hospital of the West Indies.)

AETIOLOGY

The aetiology of RA is unknown, and although much of what has been said in the previous chapters has also been suggested in RA, the identification of aetiological factors seems remote at present. Nevertheless, advances have been made, both in the finding of HLA associations and in relationship to a possible infectious aetiology (reviewed by Bennett 1978 and Hicks 1992).

Immunological factors

Comprehensive reviews of this subject have been published (Clot & Sany 1975; Sheinberg 1983). The lymphocytes in RA synovium are predominantly B cells (Mellbye *et al.* 1972) though T cells are also present (Frøland, Natvig & Husby 1973). In the peripheral blood, it has been shown that a depression in the relative proportions of T cells during flares of disease activity may occur, though the many studies of lymphocyte populations have not yielded consistent results, and earlier reports of increased percentages of B cells, based on the demonstration of surface immunoglobulins were probably artefactual, resulting from the presence of cold-reactive antilymphocyte antibodies (Winchester *et al.* 1975). Other studies have demonstrated an as yet unexplained increase in RA synovial fluid of a population of 'null' cells — lymphocytes which lack surface markers of either T or B lymphocytes (Winchester *et al.* 1975; Williams *et al.* 1973; Firestein 1992).

Genetic factors (reviewed by Salmon 1992)

Although there is no strong evidence for familial aggregation of RA (Masi & Shulman 1965; O'Brien 1968), HLA work has provided strong clues to the influence of genetic factors in the disease (Stastny 1978). While no HLA A, B, or C locus associations were found, a strong association with the HLA-D locus DR4 has been demonstrated. A number of studies have confirmed Stastny's original observation. In one such study of 129 patients, HLA DR4 was increased in RA, whilst HLA DR2 was decreased. HLA DR3 patients had a higher prevalence of antinuclear antibodies (Gram, Husby & Thorsby 1983).

The relative risk of DR4 individuals for developing RA in most studies is about fourfold. There are however notable exceptions, e.g. in groups of Israeli Jews, Kuwaiti Arabs and in one group of Asian Indians in the UK. These exceptions could indicate that DR4 is merely a genetic marker in close linkage disequilibrium with the true susceptibility locus.

Infective agents (Hicks 1992)

Despite enormous effort, no agent has been unequivocally implicated in the infectious aetiology of RA, though the history of RA research has closely paralleled the history of microbiology, ranging from tubercule, streptococci and pneumococci, *Proteus* through diphtheroids and myocoplasma to viruses, including rubella. Parallels drawn from the findings in SLE, however (see Chapter 2), still suggest that the initial stimulus which results in the chronic inflammatory process in RA is exogenous, and may be a latent virus. One contender, following the observations of Alspaugh *et al.* (1978), is the Epstein–Barr (E–B) virus. This group demonstrated that certain lymphocytes, when transformed by E–B virus, possessed a nuclear antigen ('RANA') which was found to be reactive with antibody in rheumatoid arthritis (RA protein; 'RAP'). Other data, however, have suggested that RANA more likely represents another result of impaired T-cell function in RA (Dipper, Bluestein & Zvaifler 1981) leading to a secondary disturbance of E–B virus–host balance (Yao *et al.* 1986).

Bacterial cell-wall antigens

Following the observation that arthritis may follow bypass surgery for obesity, attention has once again focused on the possible links between the possible absorption of bacterial antigens through the gut wall and the development of arthritis (Bernstein *et al.* 1984).

Evidence is accumulating that the arthritogenic properties of bacterial adjuvants reside within the peptidoglycan dimers. In most bacteria, peptidoglycans are found within the capsule and outer membrane.

It is a theoretical possibility that under certain circumstances peptidoglycans cross the gut wall and either elicit an antibody response, forming either 7S immune complexes or, alternatively, become associated with the Fc regions of normal IgG and initiate a rheumatoid factor response (Bennett 1978; Levy *et al.* 1986).

Heat shock proteins

Heat shock proteins (HSP) are a group of polypeptides produced by cells of all species in response to stressful stimuli (including heat). The HSP response is remarkably uniform. The proteins themselves are remarkably preserved, often sharing more than 50% identity in bacteria and humans.

In animal models remarkably specific recognition of HSP can occur. For example, in adjuvant arthritis the T lymphocytes recognized an epitope of mycobacterial HSP 65 formed by amino acids 180–188. Prior administration of soluble HSP 65 caused resistance to subsequently induced adjuvant arthritis. It is conceivable that humans, following microbial infection, develop cross-reactive immunity to similar HSPs.

The reader is referred to a review by Kauffmann (1990).

The role of rheumatoid factor and immune complex formation

Rheumatoid factors (RF) do not appear to play a primary aetiological role in RA, but may affect the course of the disease, and are associated with vasculitis (Conn, McDuffie & Dyck 1972; Stage & Mannik 1971), nodules and pulmonary lesions (De Horatius, Abruzzo & Williams 1972). The pathogenetic role of RFs in the vasculitic and inflammatory synovitis of RA is unclear, though they may play a part in localising disease within the synovial cavity (Zvaifler 1973).

CLINICAL FEATURES

The disease may start at any age, and with any permutation of joint involvement. The commonest age of onset is in the forties, and the most frequent mode of presentation is of an insidious, symmetrical polyarthritis. Large joints are affected as frequently as small, though the patient frequently complains more initially about the small joints of the hands, the feet or the wrist. Systemic manifestations such as myalgia, weight loss, oedema, lymphadenopathy or anaemia (see later) may be prominent, but usually parallel the degree and rapidity of joint involvement. Detailed descriptions of patterns of joint involvement are dealt with in the larger rheumatology texts, but particular features and complications applicable to selected joints are mentioned here as each may contribute to the clinical picture of RA.

Joints

Hand. Synovitis of the metacarpophalangeal (MCP) joints is best detected by filling in of the 'hollows' normally visible between the metacarpal heads when the fingers are flexed at 90° (Fig. 5.5). There may be distension of the veins of the dorsum of the hand or in the immediate vicinity of the inflamed joints. Synovial swelling of the extensor tendon sheaths is an important finding in early RA. It may result in weakening and finally in rupture of the extensor tendon with finger drop. This may be disastrous in a patient with already severely compromised hand function and requires urgent repair. Distal interphalangeal involvement in RA is extremely rare and, if present, should lead to inspection of the nails and consideration of the possibility of psoriasis (Fig. 5.6).

The commonest late deformities are ulnar drift (often causing less disability than might be expected), 'swan neck' and 'boutonnière' deformity, and subluxation.

Wrists. The wrists are the joints most frequently clinically affected in RA. The earliest sign may be carpal tunnel syndrome, due to synovial hypertrophy. Indeed EMG studies have revealed delayed median nerve conduc-

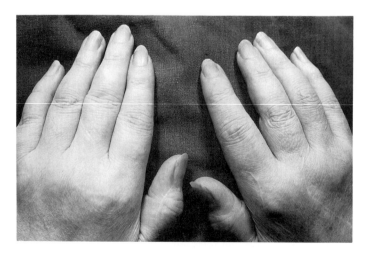

Fig. 5.5 Hands in active RA.

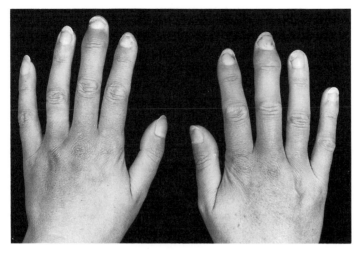

Fig. 5.6 Distal interphalangeal joint involvement (seronegative) arthritis.

tion in up to 50% of patients with early RA (Barnes & Currey 1967). The wrist is one of the earliest sites of radiological involvement, particularly erosion of the ulnar styloid. In patients who continue to perform heavy manual work despite active RA, cyst formation, especially in the distal ends of the ulna and radius, may be prominent (Fig. 5.7). Bony fusion is a feature of Still's disease both in children and in the adult (Fig. 5.8), but rarely of RA.

Cervical spine. Generalized RA almost invariably involves the cervical spine. The odontoid peg is surrounded by synovium and inflammation at this region and may result in two pathological lesions:
1   Erosion of the odontoid peg leading to a total dissolution of the prominence, with resultant instability at the base of the skull.
2   Weakness and slackening of the transverse ligament of the atlas, leading to atlanto-axial subluxation, detectable in up to 25% of RA patients (Conlon, Isdale & Rose 1966) (Fig. 5.9, A, B).
Either of these may result in direct pressure on the spinal cord. While some examples, such as those following surgery, present acutely, in others the neurological features may develop insidiously, and in a patient already handicapped with RA the additional weakness of an upper motor neurone lesion may be missed. A surprising degree of improvement may be obtained with treatment.

Case report. A 60-year-old Martinique woman was transferred to the University Hospital in Jamaica for possible orthopaedic surgery. She had long-standing RA,

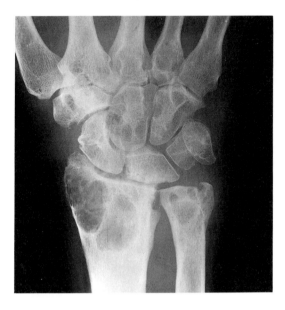

Fig. 5.7 Wrist in RA with erosion and prominent cyst formation.

but for almost 1 year had been confined to bed because of generalized weakness, attributed to active RA. On examination, the degree of synovitis was mild but the patient was quadriplegic with moderate spasticity and marked weakness in all four limbs. Lateral radiographs of the neck in flexion revealed a space of 8 mm between the ondontoid peg and anterior arch of the atlas.

Initial treatment consisted of immobilization of the neck in a collar. Within 2 to 3 days there was lessening of the amount of clonus and during the ensuing 3 weeks, the patient gained a surprising degree of strength and reversal of the quadriplegia. Though some degree of spasticity remained, the patient was able to walk and, following surgery, return to part-time employment as a housekeeper.

Not all cases of radiographically proved atlanto-axial subluxation progress to neurological complications though all patients with RA undergoing surgery should receive lateral X-rays of the neck in flexion prior to anaesthesia (Smith, Benn & Sharp 1972; Bland 1974). It has now become apparent that many of these cases, while alarming clinically, may not have the uniformly poor prognosis which might be expected (Matthews 1974).

The remainder of the spine is not clinically affected in RA, though Bywaters (1982) has shown that all the synovial joints of the spine may be involved histologically and in some patients the interspinous bursae. Sacroilitis is extremely rare in seropositive RA.

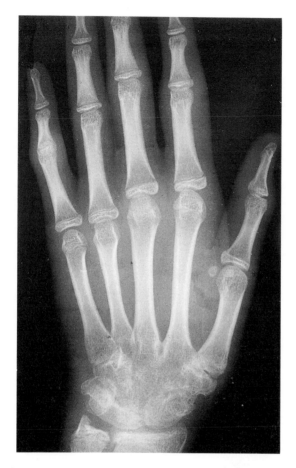

Fig. 5.8 Bony fusion of the wrist in long-standing Still's disease.

Hips. Aseptic (avascular) necrosis of the hip, while often less dramatic than that occurring in patients with SLE, is nonetheless, a significant complication of RA though it rarely occurs without the use of corticosteroid therapy. Approximately one in four RA patients develop significant hip involvement, ranging in radiological severity from no abnormality to prostrusio acetabuli.

Knees. Knee involvement poses major problems in management, dealt with in more detail in larger rheumatology texts. Three specific complications are mentioned here:
1 Aseptic necrosis of one or both of the condyles or tibial plateaus may occur.

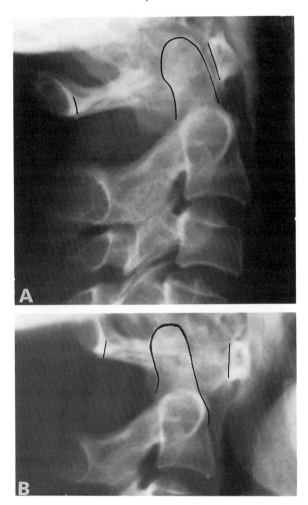

Fig. 5.9 RA cervical spine. A, Normal position of the odontoid peg in extension. B, Wide separation of the odontoid on full flexion of the neck.

2   A complication sometimes posing diagnostic problems is that of super-infection. Joint infection is more frequent in RA than in normal joints (probably due to a number of factors including lowered synovial fluid complement levels).

3   Effusions of the knee joint may result in popliteal distension and enlargement (Baker's cyst). A well-known complication of knee effusions (and less commonly in effusions of other joints) is rupture of the synovial sac into adjacent tissues (Fig. 5.10). Jayson & Dixon (1969) showed that,

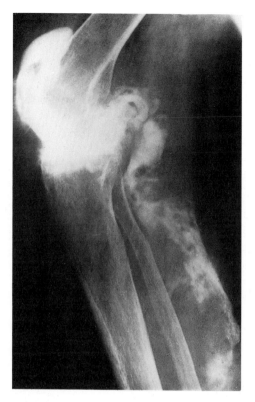

Fig. 5.10 Arthrogram showing rupture of the synovial sac posteriorly and tracking of contrast medium into the calf.

particularly in the presence of effusions, the pressures reached within the knee joint may exceed arterial pressures, with muscular effort. The acute presentation of synovial rupture may exactly mimic deep vein thrombosis, with calf tenderness, a positive Homan's sign, and swelling of the lower leg (Hughes & Pridie 1970).

Case report. *A 44-year-old man with a 5-year history of RA controlled by salicylates had an exacerbation of symptoms, with swelling and increase of pain in the knees and shoulders for 2 months prior to admission to hospital with deep vein thrombosis of the left calf.*

Whilst walking, he had experienced a sudden sharp pain in his left calf, which on examination was tender and 2·5 cm greater in circumference than the right. Both knees were swollen as was the left ankle. Homan's sign was positive on the left. Arthrography showed that contrast medium extravasated from the popliteal cyst into the calf, indicating the presence of synovial membrane rupture.

Feet. Involvement of the metatarsophalangeal (MTP) joints may be one of the earliest manifestations of RA (Fig. 5.11). Erosion of MTPs, leading to pain under the ball of the foot, and ultimately to subluxation, 'clawing' and callus formation is one of the most potent causes of disability in RA, and one of the most amenable to surgery (Fig. 5.12).

An occasional accompaniment of RA involving the ankle or foot joints is oedema which may, on occasion, be marked, and rarely is the presenting manifestation (Gandy, Ansell & Bywaters 1965).

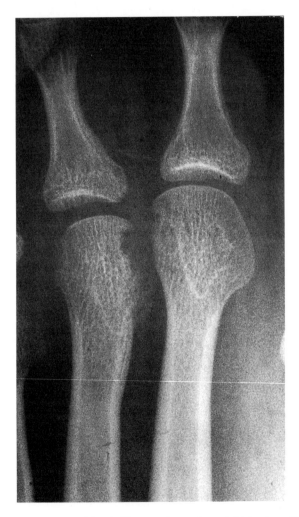

Fig. 5.11 Erosion of metatarsal head. There is also periosteal thickening of both phalanges.

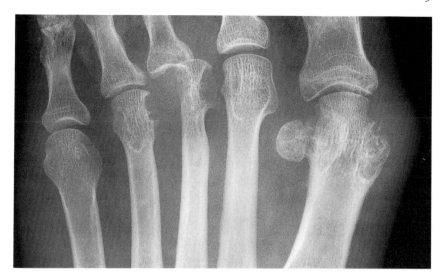

Fig. 5.12 Advanced RA with metatarsophalangeal erosions and subluxation. The patient successfully underwent resection of the metatarsophalangeal joints (Fowler's operation).

Cricoarytenoid joint. Involvement of this joint may, at its most severe, result in acute dysphagia.

SYSTEMIC MANIFESTATIONS (Table 5.2)

Nodules. Rheumatoid nodules are most commonly subcutaneous though they may be intradermal, subperiosteal or in a variety of organs including the heart, spleen and lung.

The commonest sites are at pressure points, in particular the elbow (Fig. 5.13), the fingers (especially in writers) over the ischial tuberosities in patients confined to a chair, on the bridge of the nose in those wearing spectacles, or around the scapular regions.

They may also occur in a variety of other sites, especially along the course of tendons, where they may occasionally interfere with normal tendon functions, or on the scalp.

Case report. *A 25-year-old housewife developed acute polyarthritis over the course of 3 days. At the time, she complained of small multiple painless nodules in the scalp, discovered whilst combing her hair. There were no peripheral nodules. The scalp nodules were firm, immobile and 1–2 mm in diameter. Over the course of the next 2 years, the disease persisted with the development of high-titre rheumatoid factor and joint erosions.*

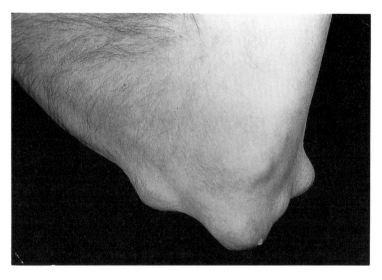

Fig. 5.13 Multiple subcutaneous RA nodules on the elbow.

Table 5.2 Extra-articular features of RA

Systemic Malaise, fever, myalgia, tiredness, anaemia, weight loss	*Lung* Pleurisy ± effusion Interstitial fibrosis Pneumoconiosis (Caplan's syndrome) Pulmonary nodules
Nodules	
RES Lymphadenopathy Splenomegaly Felty's syndrome	*Eye* Keratoconjunctivitis sicca Scleritis or episcleritis Scleromalacia perforans Iritis (rare in adults)
Vasculitis ['Systemic' features (above)] Nail fold lesions and finger pulp infarcts Raynaud's phenomenon and gangrene Chronic leg ulcers Neuropathy Large vessel arteritis (coronary, mesenteric, cerebral)	*Blood* Anaemia Thrombocytosis *Amyloid*
Heart Pericarditis Cardiomyopathy and conduction defects Valvular granulomata	

Visceral nodules result in some of the more serious sequelae in RA. In the heart they may lead to mitral or aortic valve disease (though aortic valve disease is extremely rare in RA; its association is with the seronegative arthritides). Involvement of the sclera of the eye by a nodule leads to weakening and rupture of the sclera (scleromalacia perforans). In the vocal cords they lead to hoarseness, whilst in the lungs (see below) they pose a difficult differential diagnosis from carcinoma. They may erode underlying bone. They are usually associated with seropositivity.

Vasculitis. Some of the difficulties in the classification of vasculitis are referred to in Chapter 10. In RA a variety of patterns of vasculitis are seen, and at least two histological varieties (inflammatory and non-inflammatory or obliterative) are known to occur (Fig. 5.14).

The most common clinical manifestation of vasculitis in RA is periungal infarcts (Fig. 5.15), seen as black or reddish-brown spot-like areas 0·5—1 mm in diameter, usually at the side of the finger-nail. They are a most important physical sign, for while they may represent localized vascular involvement only, they may also be a symptom of more widespread vasculitis — the development of 'malignant' RA. Capillary changes, detectable by nail fold microscopy, include tortuosity and elongation of loops (Redisch, Messina & Hughes 1970).

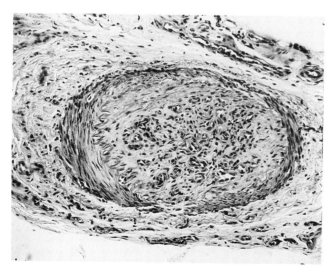

Fig. 5.14 Active vasculitis in RA with obliteration of the lumen. (H & E × 150.) (Professor E.G.L. Bywaters, Hammersmith Hospital.)

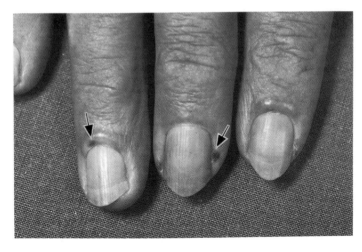

Fig. 5.15 Typical periungal infarcts.

Such vasculitis occurs almost exclusively in patients with seropositive and often very active RA, and is frequently associated with other systemic manifestations such as pleurisy, pericarditis or neuropathy.

One study has also suggested an association with HLA DR3 (Cunningham *et al.* 1982). The vasculitis may take the form of acute, major vessel disease, with neuropathy, bowel or coronary ischaemia or limb ischaemia. Sometimes, however, it may present in a less dramatic way, and elude appropriate treatment.

Case report. *A 68-year-old spinster with mild, long-standing RA developed anorexia, low-grade fever, myalgia and weight loss. She became cachexic, and developed large ulcers on the lateral sides of both legs. She was receiving salicylates only.*

On admission to hospital she was emaciated, with lymphadenopathy, bilateral 4-in diameter lacteral leg ulcers, and vasculitic lesion on the elbows.

Laboratory tests revealed an ESR of 150 mm/hour, a C1q binding of over 250 µg/ml (an important finding — see later) and RF titre of over 1 in 10 000.

She was treated with prednisolone and intermittent pulse cyclophosphamide. Six months later she was completely mobile and the leg ulcers (with the help of grafts) were healed.

An interesting group of patients (most commonly middle-aged men) appear to develop increasingly severe vasculitis at the same time as a diminution of the arthritis to minimal proportions and the clinical distinction of such cases from the polyarteritis nodosa presenting with arthritis is fine.

Case report. *A 61-year-old man had been known to suffer from mild, erosive, seropositive RA for 15 years. For 3 years he had suffered periodic attacks of widespread vasculitis, developing over the course of 2−3 days, with periungal, elbow, palmar and lower limb lesions, some 2 mm in diameter. Each crop of vasculitic lesions was associated with general malaise, and on three occasions evidence of systemic vasculitis was present. The episodes responded rapidly to 10−20 mg prednisone, but during a widespread attack the patient developed severe chest pain with ECG changes and died 2 hours later. Autopsy was not performed.*

Raynaud's phenomenon, when present, is almost invariably mild in RA. Small vessel involvement, resulting in livedo reticularis, also occurs.

Neuropathy. Neurological involvement in RA is frequent and principally involves the peripheral nervous system. A number of patterns may be distinguished (Table 5.3).

Entrapment neuropathy, especially carpal tunnel syndrome, is almost certainly the commonest. Mononeuritis multiplex is rare and related to arteritis of the vasa nervorum (Chamberlain & Bruckner 1970). In some of these patients immunoglobulin and complement are demonstrable in the vascular lesions (Conn *et al.* 1972).

More common than mononeuritis multiplex caused by infarction of individual nerves is a symmetrical peripheral neuropathy. Two main types are distinguished — a distal sensory neuropathy, with good prognosis, by far the commonest, and a fulminating sensorimotor neuropathy with a very bad prognosis. Both groups, especially the latter, are associated with seropositivity, nodules and vasculitis (Pallis & Scott 1965; Chamberlain & Bruckner 1970).

Table 5.3 Neurological involvement in RA

Entrapment neuropathy
Peripheral neuropathy
Autonomic neuropathy
Mononeuritis multiplex
Cranial nerve neuropathy (?related to Sjøgren's syndrome)
Drug-induced (e.g. chloroquine)
Cervical cord compression
(Cerebral vasculitis)

Despite the clinical association with vasculitis, the histology of the nerves in some cases is more suggestive of a 'metabolic', i.e. non-vascular origin (Weller, Bruckner & Chamberlain 1970). There is nothing to suggest that corticosteroids predispose either to vasculitis or neuropathy. Cranial nerve lesions are rare in RA, but have been described in Sjøgren's syndrome (see Chapter 4). Occasional RA patients with widespread vasculitis develop evidence of cerebral ischaemic episodes.

Heart. Cardiac involvement in RA is usually subclinical, consisting either of granulomatous inflammation, arteritis or pericarditis, most commonly detected at autopsy (Sokoloff 1953).

The commonest clinical abnormality is pericarditis, manifest by a symptomless friction rub. In one review which included data from 400 patients and eight postmortem series, an overall incidence of pericarditis of 30% was observed. In this series, of 33 patients with RA and pericarditis, only 8 complained of pericardial pain. Six developed effusions and 2 constrictive pericarditis (Kirk & Cosh 1969). Surgery may be required for chronic constrictive pericarditis (Liss & Bachman 1970).

As in SLE, complement levels in rheumatoid pericardial effusions may be low (Franco, Levine & Hall 1972). Aortic or other value disease is extremely rare in seropositive RA (Bonfiglio & Atwater 1969; Van Valkenburgh, Georges & Irby 1972). It is probable that most earlier series included ankylosing spondylitis, though an interesting subgroup of RA patients with widespread RA granulomata, scleromalacia perforans and, in some cases, aortic root disease, has been described (Zvaifler & Weintraub 1962).

Lungs. Table 5.14 lists some of the pulmonary manifestations of RA. Pleurisy and pleural effusions are increasingly recognised as a feature of RA, and, as in the case of SLE, may be the presenting manifestation of the disease. This clinical picture in older patients may result in diagnostic difficulties.

Table 5.4 Pulmonary manifestations of RA

Pleurisy ± effusion
Pulmonary nodules
Caplan's syndrome
Pulmonary fibrosis
Pulmonary arteritis
Sjøgren's syndrome

Case report. *A 67-year-old man was admitted to hospital with a suspected diagnosis of carcinoma of the lung. For 3 weeks he had complained of fatigue, dyspnoea, cough, chest pain. He had lost over 12 lb in weight and complained of 'aching all over', with both muscle and joint pain. He had smoked 10—15 cigarettes a day for years. On examination, he was wasted, with slight generalized muscle tenderness and small effusions in both knees and wrists. All joints were painful on extremes of movement, including the cervical spine and TM joints. There were moderate bilateral pleural effusions, and rubbery enlargement of the inguinal axillary and cervical lymph nodes.*

Investigations included an ESR of over 100, polyclonal increase of γ-globulins, latex test weakly positive, and normal muscle enzymes. There was no radiological evidence of joint erosion. Bronchoscopy was normal and pleural fluid aspirate revealed a clear yellow fluid, with no malignant cells, protein of 3 g% and glucose 16 mg%. The initial diagnosis of carcinoma of the lung with an associated arthralgia or polymyalgia rheumatica was changed to one of RA with a 'systemic' onset. The patient developed progressive, strongly seropositive, erosive polyarthritis requiring steroid therapy.

The reason for the very low glucose level frequently seen in RA pleural effusions is obscure, though it may be secondary to impaired entry of glucose through a thickened pleura (Pettersson, Klockars & Hellstrom 1982). The test is not infallible, and possibly of more diagnostic use is the determination of pleural fluid complement, which is reduced, due possibly to consumption by local immune complexes (Hunder, McDuffie & Hepper 1972). Cytology of the fluid shows a predominance of lymphocytes, polymorphs and large mononuclear cells containing immunoglobulin and complement (Boddington, Spriggs & Morton 1971) and pleural biopsy may show rheumatoid granulation tissue. However, even these diagnostic aids may not help distinguish rheumatoid from other pleural effusions as in the following case:

Case report. *A 34-year-old barman was admitted to hospital with a 2-week history of polyarthritis, cough and dyspnoea. He had complained of a dry cough for 4 weeks and tired more easily than before. He smoked 40 cigarettes daily. His son and daughter had both been receiving treatment for tuberculosis. There was a strong family history of psoriasis, but none of arthritis. On examination, he had a large right pleural effusion and a small left effusion. There was widespread arthralgia but no joint effusion. Investigations included a weakly positive latex test (1 in 40), normal white cell count and differential count and an ESR of 67. The chest X-ray showed pleural effusions but the lung fields were otherwise normal. The pleural fluid showed both a low glucose (40 mg%) and C3 (48 mg%). No acid-fast bacilli were seen. Mantoux testing was*

positive at 1 in 1000. A differential diagnosis of acute onset RA or of pulmonary
tuberculosis was made. A second pleural aspirate revealed acid-fast bacilii. He
was started on antituberculous therapy together wiin view of the size of the
effusion. His improvement was dramatic, the joint pains, needless to say,
improving with corticosteroid therapy. At 3 years follow-up and off all drugs,
the patient has shown no signs of recurrence of the polyarthritis or of the
tuberculosis.

Isolated pulmonary RA nodules provide a difficult diagnostic problem.
They occur almost invariably in association with subcutaneous nodules
and are most commonly peripheral.

A specific condition first described in coal miners by Caplan (1953) and
referred to as Caplan's syndrome, is the existence of multiple pulmonary
nodules, often confluent, varying in size from 0·5 to 5 cm and occasionally
cavitating or calcifying (Fig. 5.16). There may be accompanying moderate
or severe pulmonary fibrosis. Rheumatoid factor is present in high titre
and may be found in patients with little or no peripheral joint disease
(Shroeder, Franklin & McEwen 1962). The syndrome may be related to

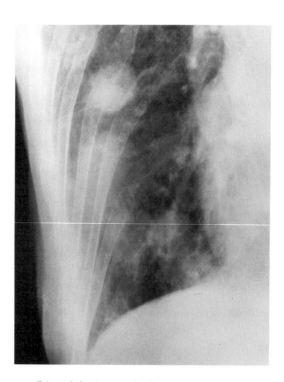

Fig. 5.16 Pulmonary RA nodules in a coal miner.

exposure to silica dusts and to asbestos in addition to coal dust and it is suggested that the silica acts as a local focus for rheumatoid nodule formation in those developing RA. The possibility that RF may augment this process is suggested by animal studies, where adjuvant-induced pulmonary granulomas are exaggerated by i.v. administration of IgM RF (De Horatius & Williams 1972).

Chronic fibrosing alveolitis is a rare complication of RA and has a poor prognosis (Stack & Grant 1965). It usually occurs in established RA, late in the course of the disease, and is difficult to distinguish from primary fibrosing alveolitis, in which positive RF tests may be found (Fig. 5.17).

Milder forms of pulmonary fibrosis are being recognized using full pulmonary function tests (Oxholm *et al.* 1982). In one such study, 10 of 30 RA patients were found to have evidence of interstitial rheumatoid lung disease with impaired diffusing capacity (Popper, Bogdonoff & Hughes 1972). Immunofluorescent studies of lung tissue in 5 patients with rheumatoid pulmonary fibrosis showed deposits of IgM and RF (but not complement) in pulmonary arterioles, alveolar walls and adjacent to cavitary nodules (De Horatius, Abruzzo & Williams 1972).

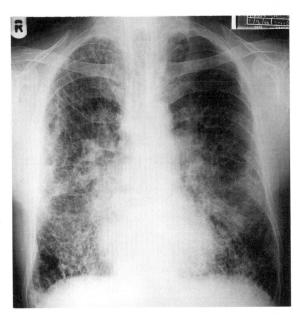

Fig. 5.17 Chest X-ray in RA. There are bilateral changes affecting particularly the middle and lower zones which consist of extensive linear opacities and characteristic loss of definition of normal pleural outlines. (Professor D. Allison, Hammersmith Hospital.)

Finally, Sjøgren's syndrome itself may result in dryness of the respiratory tract mucosa, with a tendency to bronchitis, atelectasis and chest infections (see Chapter 4).

Gastrointestinal tract. Apart from the manifestation of Sjøgren's syndrome (see Chapter 4) of rare cases of arteritis of the abdominal vessels and of amyloid disease, the main causes of GI tract involvement in rheumatoid disease are iatrogenic, from steroids, aspirin, gold (diarrhoea) or the non-steroidal anti-inflammatory drugs. Mild degrees of malabsorption may be detected (Dyer, Kendall & Hawkins 1972) and minor changes in liver function, especially a rise in liver alkaline phosphatase are seen early in the course of the disease, but these are of little clinical significance (Petterson, Wegelius & Skifvars 1970; Webb *et al.* 1975). The hepatotoxic effects of salicylates reported in juvenile RA and in SLE are rarely seen in adult RA.

Kidney. The kidney is not affected in uncomplicated RA, though rare cases of renal vasculitis have been reported. A group of patients with hypocomplementaemia and renal disease in RA have been reported by Franco & Schur (1972). An interstitial nephritis, related to Sjøgren's syndrome, is rare. Phenacetin is a well-known cause of renal papillary necrosis, and aspirin has more recently been implicated in the production of renal damage, although the evidence is weak.

Eyes. Ask any group of students the commonest ocular manifestation of RA and the answer is almost invariably iritis. While iritis certainly is a feature of the seronegative arthritides, particularly ankylosing spondylitis and juvenile chronic polyarthritis, it is rare in RA, probably occurring with the same frequency as in the general population. Table 5.5 lists the ocular complications of RA.

Keratoconjunctivitis sicca, part of Sjøgren's syndrome, is by far the commonest, and is described in Chapter 4.

Mild degrees of episcleritis are occasionally seen in seropositive RA patients and require specialist ophthalmological care (Lyne & Pitkeathly 1968). The rare and potentially blinding complication of scleritis also

Table 5.5 Ocular manifestations of RA

Keratoconjunctivitis sicca
Episcleritis and scleritis
Scleromalacia perforans
Drug effects (steroids and chloroquine)

requires urgent attention. The clinical features are tenderness of the eye, pericorneal vascular injection (as opposed to mainly peripheral vascular injection in conjunctivitis) and a cellular exudate in the anterior chamber usually requiring slit-lamp diagnosis (Jayson & Jones 1971). The condition may also be associated with uveitis and the development of glaucoma. The sclera develops a bluish discoloration possibly due to alteration of its proteoglycan structure (rather than due to thinning) allowing the blackish uveal tract to show through.

The rare complication of scleromalacia perforans (Fig. 5.18) is due to the development of a rheumatoid nodule in the sclera, resulting in a point of weakness at which perforation may occur.

Haematological changes

Anaemia. Although anaemia is one of the best indices of disease activity in RA, its nature has yet to be fully elucidated. The reader is referred to a review by Mowat (1972) of some of the contributing factors.

The commonest picture is that of a normochromic normocytic anaemia. The serum iron is low, and responses to oral iron poor. Unlike iron-deficiency anaemia, the total iron-binding capacity (or transferrin) level, is also low. Despite this, total body iron is normal or high in most patients and considerable amounts are sequestered in synovium and reticuloendo-thelial cells elsewhere (Muirden 1970; Bennett *et al.* 1972). Stores of iron in the marrow are adequate. The factors leading to failure of incorporation of

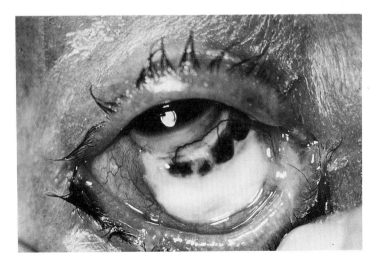

Fig. 5.18 Scleromalacia perforans. (Mr Peter Wright, Moorfield's Hospital.)

iron into the red cells are poorly understood, though the presence of inflammation is clinically associated with a direct inhibitory effect on this process. Corticosteroid treatment can result in a rise of mean haemoglobin levels of up to 2g in 2 weeks (Mowat, Hothersall & Aitchison 1969). There is no clear association between RA and pernicious anaemia (see Chapter 4).

White cells. Polymorph counts are usually normal in RA (the rare complication of Felty's syndrome is discussed below). Occasional cases of RA, in particular those with vasculitis and circulating complexes, demonstrate eosinophilia (Panush, Franco & Schur 1971).

Platelets. Platelet counts (with rare exceptions in Felty's syndrome) are normal or high in RA — indeed it is not uncommon during active RA to see counts approaching 750 000 per mm^3. The cause of these high counts is unknown.

FELTY'S SYNDROME

The white cell count and differential count are usually normal in RA, unlike SLE, where lymphopenia is common. However, a very small number of patients develop a clinical syndrome first described by Felty in 1924, consisting of rheumatoid arthritis, splenomegaly and neutropenia. Other less regular features of the syndrome are lymphadenopathy, thrombocytopenia, chronic leg ulceration and skin pigmentation. There is a strong association between Felty's syndrome and the presence of ANF, strongly positive RF tests and Sjøgren's syndrome. DNA binding values are often slightly raised and tests for immune complexes usually positive.

Patients with early RA in whom the spleen may often be tipped should *not* be described as having Felty's syndrome. The syndrome generally occurs after many years of disease and has a poor prognosis. The neutrophil count may fall to less than 500 per mm^3 and death from infection is common.

Leucocytes may, in addition to a decrease in numbers, show impaired chemotactic or granulopoietic function (Louise & Pearson 1971; Gupta, Robinson & Albrecht 1975). A few patients demonstrate polymorph specific ANFs, though their aetiological role is not fully known (Wiik 1975).

The vast majority of cases are HLA DR 4. A recent interesting observation claimed that 20 of 24 patients with Felty's syndrome had anti-histone antibodies (Cohen & Webb 1989).

Splenectomy is helpful in only half of the patients and steroid therapy is only partially helpful and usually at high doses (Barnes, Turnbull &

Vernon-Roberts 1971). The disease has a poor prognosis (Thorne & Urowitz 1982) though recent more aggressive approaches to treatment may offer improvement in outlook. We recently reported a patient with active RA and Felty's syndrome who responded to treatment with methotrexate (Hughes 1989).

INFECTION IN RA

It is almost certain that RA patients have not only an increased susceptibility to intra-articular infection, but to infection in general (Baum 1971; Huskisson & Hart 1972). As in the case of SLE, a variety of factors probably contribute, including therapy, and reduced chemotactic properties of the polymorphs.

HYPERVISCOSITY SYNDROME

One of the most satisfying diagnoses in RA is hyperviscosity syndrome, because of its dramatic response to plasmapheresis. Increased serum viscosity is caused by high concentration and polymerization of macromolecules such as IgM, fibrinogen and rheumatoid factors and related to the formation of intermediate complexes, formed, for example, by the self-association of IgG rheumatoid factors (Pope *et al*. 1975).

However, marked increases in serum viscosity, in which the serum appears more like synovial fluid to the naked eye, are rare in RA. The clinical features consist of dyspnoea, epistaxis, heart failure and the characteristic appearance of 'trucking' of the engorged retinal veins (Jason, LoSpalluto & Ziff 1970).

AMYLOIDOSIS

The incidence of amyloidosis in RA varies between series, ranging from 5 to 60% in long-standing RA.

The pattern of amyloidosis in RA is that of 'secondary' amyloid, with deposition in kidney, liver, spleen, GI tract, and occasionally other organs. It is now being increasingly realised that the condition does not have a uniformly poor prognosis, and that spontaneous clinical regression may occur. The measurement of serum amyloid-A protein may prove to have some predictive value in the determination of risk of amyloidosis (De Beer *et al*. 1982). The reader is referred to reviews by Franklin (1975), and Kyle and Bayrd (1975) for accounts of the structure, classification, pathogenesis and treatment of amyloidosis. Amyloidosis seems to be becoming distinctly rare in RA.

PALINDROMIC RHEUMATISM

Palindromic means recurrent, and this form of synovitis is intermittent, leaving the patient symptom-free between attacks. The attack is usually sudden, and often severe in intensity. One or many joints may be involved and there may be associated oedema, periarticular swelling and, rarely, low grade fever. Attacks last between several hours and 1–2 weeks and occur at irregular intervals, sometimes up to a year or more.

In some, though not all, patients the syndrome appears to be a form of RA, albeit unusual in its presentation. In a 7·4-year follow-up study of 35 patients diagnosed initially as having palindromic rheumatism, 19 had developed persistent arthritis (mostly seropositive) and 3 had developed rheumatoid nodules (Williams *et al.* 1971).

JUVENILE RHEUMATOID ARTHRITIS
(reviewed by Ansell 1992)

Still's disease is a useful eponym for juvenile chronic polyarthritis, for it clearly covers a group of arthritic diseases of which juvenile rheumatoid arthritis is one (Ansell 1976). By definition it occurs before the age of 17. Girls are affected more frequently than boys.

Still, in 1897, described 22 children with chronic polyarthritis and drew attention to a number of features distinguishing it from adult RA. In particular, he noted the systemic features such as lymphadenopathy, splenomegaly, rash and fever, and commented on the pattern of large joint involvement and the early occurrence of muscle wasting.

Clinical features

There are at least three distinct modes of onset: acute febrile: polyarticular and monoarticular. These patterns of onset tend to be associated with distinct courses, and some of the major features are listed in Table 5.6.

The disease will not be dealt with in detail in this volume.

Five points are worthy of emphasis however:

1 Salicylate hepatotoxicity has been described in juvenile rheumatoid arthritis (Rich & Johnson 1973) as in SLE.

2 IgM rheumatoid factor determination is of prognostic value in children with arthritis. In those children ultimately developing a clinical disease pattern similar to adult RA, the majority are persistently IgM RF positive early in the disease (Ansell 1976).

3 Iritis occurs in between 5 and 20% of patients and is not necessarily associated with more widespread arthritis — indeed the children appar-

Table 5.6 Clinical features of juvenile RA.

Acute febrile	Polyarticular	Monoarticular
Rash, leucocytosis, pericarditis and fever	Prognosis worst	Seen in one-third of patients
One-quarter develop progressive arthritis	Usually continuing polyarthritis	Insidious onset
Younger children	IgM RF when present is associated with worst	Knee commonest
Fever may antedate arthritis	prognosis (older children)	Pain mild
	May develop amyloid	Systemic features mild
		Usually remains confined to four joints or less
		Good prognosis but danger of iritis

ently most at risk are those with one or only a few joints affected (Calabro, Parrino & Marchesano 1970). Thus slit-lamp examination of the eye is mandatory in all children diagnosed as having juvenile RA. An important contribution was made by Schaller *et al.* (1974) who noted a strong association between positive ANA tests and chronic iridocyclitis in juvenile RA (Table 5.7).

4 Circulating immune complexes and free antinuclear antibody are seen more frequently in severe disease.

5 For all concerned the most worrying complications of juvenile RA is amyloidosis, which occurs in approximately 2–6% of patients (Smith, Ansell & Bywaters 1968; Antilla & Laaksonen 1969). Although amyloid characteristically complicates chronic progressive polyarticular disease, it is being recognized that amyloid may develop after many years in milder cases, as in the following case:

Case report. A 31-year-old man was admitted for management of hypertension associated with renal failure. Renal biopsy showed extensive amyloid deposition. Prior to the development of headaches and visual symptoms several months previously, he had felt perfectly well. Eighteen years previously he had been under the care of Professor Bywaters at Taplow with polyarticular, seronegative

Table 5.7 Positive tests for ANA in Still's disease (from Schaller *et al.* 1974)

Group	Positive (%)
JRA with iridocyclitis	75
JRA without iridocyclitis	30
Ankylosing spondylitis	9
Controls	0

Still's disease which had lasted for 4 years before going into spontaneous remission, leaving minimal residua.

Determination of serum amyloid-A levels may prove of prognostic value for amyloidosis (De Beer *et al*. 1982; Gwyther *et al*. 1982).

LABORATORY TESTS

Rheumatoid factor

What is the value of RF testing in rheumatoid arthritis? In general, patients with positive RF tests (IgM RF) have more severe RA as a group than those without (Franco & Schur 1972). Secondly, patients with high titres of RF have more severe joint disease. Thirdly, the complications of nodules, vasculitis, neuropathy, ulcers, Felty's syndrome and Sjøgren's syndrome are almost totally confined to the seropositive group of patients. Finally in a study of children with rheumatoid arthritis, those with increased IgG, IgA and IgM RFs had more chronic, active disease and lower serum and synovial fluid complement depression and a worse prognosis than those patients with only IgG and IgA RFs (Bianco *et al*. 1971).

Having said all this, most rheumatologists would agree that amongst their most disabled patients, a small group of seronegative patients feature prominently.

There is still reason for considering RF production as a possible defence mechanism — for example in facilitating the clearance of immune complexes.

Antinuclear antibodies

Positive ANA tests are found in up to 40% of RA patients, though generally at low titres; they give a 'homogeneous' pattern. High titre ANA in RA should lead to a search for Sjøgren's syndrome (see Chapter 4). Positive ANA tests are also more frequent in Felty's syndrome (see p. 136) and in patients with more severe RA, both articular and systemic. AntiDNA antibodies are absent or present at low titres only (Hughes 1971).

Complement

Serum complement levels are usually normal or high in RA, the high level having little diagnostic significance other than as an 'acute phase' reactant. Rare patients with aggressive RA, vasculitis, and usually with Sjøgren's syndrome have been described with lowered serum complement levels. In a study by Franco & Schur (1972), 11 of 250 consecutive RA patients had depressed total complement levels.

In RA synovial fluid, on the other hand, total complement activity is reduced (see later) — an important differentiation from seronegative arthritis effusions, where normal or high levels are found (Zvaifler 1973). Measurement of complement components suggests activation both of the classical and alternative pathways.

Cryoprecipitates and immune complexes

The majority of RA synovial fluids contain proteins which precipitate on standing at 4°C. These cryoprecipitates contain immunoglobulins, ANA and RF activity. They have anticomplementary activity suggesting that they contain immune complexes. Winchester, Agnello & Kunkel (1970) showed that the gammaglobulin complexes exist as a continuum of high molecular weight components, ranging from 9S to 30S.

Measurement of circulating serum immune complexes, though waning in popularity, *does* have a place in the management of RA. High titres (usually measured by C1q binding) are found in systemic RA and Felty's syndrome. In the RA patient with weight loss, or with leg ulcers, very high C1q levels point somewhat towards rheumatoid disease, rather than to another diagnosis such as malignancy (where circulating immune complex levels are usually unremarkable).

Synovial fluid analysis

Normal synovial fluid has been characterized as 'a dialysate of plasma to which hyaluronate protein has been added' (Sandson & Hammerman 1962), though it is now known that synthesis of IgG by the cells of the rheumatoid synovial membrane also occurs (Sliwinski & Zvaifler 1970). There is also a decrease in the degree of polymerization of synovial fluid mucopolysaccharides, leading to a decrease in viscosity.

Apart from examination for bacteria and crystals, joint fluid examination has been a disappointing tool in the investigation of rheumatic diseases.

DIFFERENTIAL DIAGNOSIS

The diagnosis of typical RA presents little difficulty. Far more important than diagnosis in such cases is the appreciation of the full spectrum of complications of the disease, the detection of which may contribute significantly to the management of RA patients. Table 5.8 and Fig. 5.19 attempt a synopsis of features which the clinician might see in RA patients.

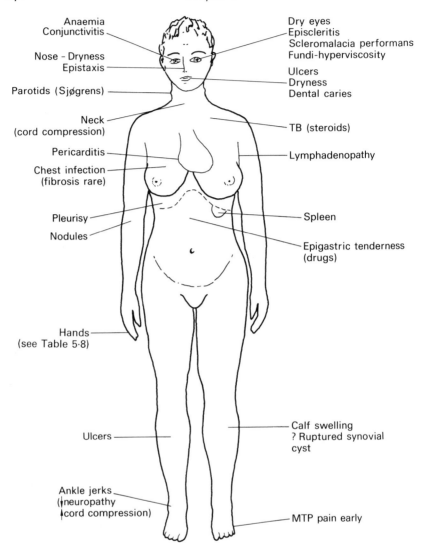

Anaemia
Conjunctivitis

Nose - Dryness
Epistaxis

Parotids (Sjøgrens)

Neck
(cord compression)

Pericarditis

Chest infection
(fibrosis rare)

Pleurisy

Nodules

Hands
(see Table 5·8)

Ulcers

Ankle jerks
(↑neuropathy
↓cord compression)

Dry eyes
Episcleritis
Scleromalacia performans
Fundi-hyperviscosity

Ulcers
Dryness
Dental caries

TB (steroids)

Lymphadenopathy

Spleen

Epigastric tenderness
(drugs)

Calf swelling
? Ruptured synovial
cyst

MTP pain early

Fig. 5.19 Examination of the RA patient.

MANAGEMENT

RA is a long and demoralizing disease. Management centres on a con-
tinuing positive attitude regarding therapy, even when such therapy
requires frequent and discouraging alteration. Psychosomatic factors are
of paramount importance — the successes and cures effected by everything
from yoga to copper bracelets testify to this. Claims for the efficacy of new

Table 5.8 An approach to the examination of the RA hand

Colour	Palmar erythema. Anaemia (skin creases)
Skin	Oedema, texture, prominent veins
Nails	Exclude psoriasis. Nailfold vasculitis
Muscles	Wasting 2° to synovitis. Thenar wasting, carpal tunnel syndrome
Sensation	Neuropathy rare. Carpal tunnel syndrome common
Tendons	Synovitis, rupture, nodules
Nodules	Especially on tendons and between fingers
Carpal tunnel syndrome	In 50% of early RA
Joints	Synovitis: acute or chronic
	Deformity:
	subluxation, ulnar deviation
	swan neck deformity
	boutonnière deformity
Hand function	Movements (and abnormal mobility), grip, pinch
Others	Psoriasis, gold dermatitis, clubbing (pulmonary fibrosis in RA rare)

antirheumatic drugs must be tempered by the knowledge that in patients motivated to get better, placebos will result in up to 60% of improvement by some of the yardsticks used to measure disease activity.

Times are changing for the better. The advent of low-dose methotrexate used earlier in the disease is already radically changing the prognosis for many RA patients.

Rest or exercises?

Activity is important and the patient should exercise within the bounds of pain. Physiotherapy services are vital to the management of RA and even in the patient with severe disease, gentle active exercises should be carried out. As in so many other situations 'taking to one's bed' can have dire consequences in RA, especially regarding stiffness.

Case report. A 74-year-old widow with long-standing, moderately active RA receiving salicylates and 5 mg daily of prednisone had been attending the physiotherapy department. Following one session, she was knocked down near her home and sustained a fractured femur. When next seen in the rheumatology department 6 months had elapsed and she was wheelchair-bound with 45° flexion contractures in both knees, and marked immobility in almost all joints. During the previous 6 months she had been confined to bed, with no active exercise treatment. Despite the efforts of the physiotherapists, the patient was

*unable to return to her independent existence in her flat and had to be admitted
to a home for the chronically ill.*

For the patient with acute RA, or with a severe generalized flare, however,
the situation is different.

While occupational therapists, social workers, and rehabilitation
specialists all play important roles in the management of RA patients, it is
important to remember that some independent people prefer to fight their
battle on their own. Most milder RA is managed by general practitioners,
and for those fortunate enough not to progress to more serious disease,
the avoidance of hospital outpatient departments is a goal in itself. The
social and rehabilitative aspects of rheumatoid arthritis are dealt with in
standard rheumatology texts.

Diet (see Walport, Parke & Hughes 1982)

Despite the observations of many RA patients, the role of diet in RA
has received little scientific attention. Nevertheless, there are theoretical
reasons why antigens entering via the GI tract might well exacerbate pre-
existing disease. In Sjøgren's syndrome, for example, mucosal abnormalities (Parke & Hughes 1981; Gendre *et al.* 1982), including IgA rheumatoid
factor production (Elkon *et al.* 1982) are prominent. Occult bowel disease
may be commoner in arthritic disease than hitherto recognized and techniques such as indium scanning or absorption of macromolecules (Sun-
dqvist *et al.* 1982) may throw further light on the subject. We recently
reported three patients with RA or coeliac disease, in whom the bowel
pathology might be implicated (Parke *et al.* 1983).

As always, the most dramatic evidence comes from the study of individual patients, such as the patient reported in the *British Medical Journal*
(Parke & Hughes 1981).

Salicylates

Aspirin has anti-inflammatory activity, though it is not known whether
this influences the long-term course of RA. Salicylates were once the first
line of drug treatment in RA. The dose varies between 3–6 g daily (10–20
300 mg tablets). In most adults, toxicity is heralded by the development of
tinnitus, and in some patients the desired blood level of 20–25 mg% may
be attainable. In children, toxicity may be more serious, and the early
subtle signs of hyperventilation or abnormal behaviour may be missed.

The side effects of salicylates are well known and will not be dealt with
here in detail. Perhaps the major drawback of aspirin therapy is its famili-

arity — the patient who goes through the various stages leading to an appointment with a specialist in rheumatic diseases is often disappointed with the bottle of aspirin which he or she collects from the pharmacy. The second drawback is the number of tablets required (up to 7300 per year!) and more realistic surveys suggest that few patients take the full prescribed dose (Geersten, Gray & Ward 1975). For this reason, there is an important place for variations in aspirin formulation, such as Benorylate (a para-cetamol ester of acetylsalicylic acid).

Non-steroidal antiinflammatory drugs

These traditionally provide the 'second line' of drug therapy, and include the fenamates, the propionic acid derivatives (ibuprofen, fenoprofen, naproxen, ketoprofen), indomethacin, phenylbutazone, diclofenac, azapropazone piroxicam, tenoxicam, etodolac, etc. The reader is referred to reviews by Huskisson (1977) & Simon (1990).

Indomethacin. This is one of the best tried of the antiinflammatory drugs and has powerful antiinflammatory properties. The commoner side effects are dyspepsia, headaches, giddiness and nightmares. Gastrointestinal haemorrhage occasionally occurs. The drug has been a major contribution to the management of inflammatory arthritis, and has been especially useful given at night orally (or as a suppository) for morning stiffness, though it must be remembered that up to 80% of the suppository is absorbed.

Case report. *A 77-year-old man with many years' RA had been noticed by his wife to be behaving strangely for 4−5 days. On the morning of admission he was confused and overactive. He deteriorated, and on admission to casualty was shouting, disoriented, and hyperactive, and had to be restrained. He was sedated and over the following 48 hours improved. In retrospect the only likely cause of his toxic confusional state was indomethacin. He had found marked relief of his morning stiffness by taking indomethacin suppositories and for the week prior to his illness had been taking four suppositories each night — an approximate absorbed dose of 320 mg daily.*

The lack of major haematological side effects and its potency make indomethacin an early choice in an increasing number of RA patients, especially for the relief of night pain.

Slow-release indomethacin, 75 mg nocte (or occasionally b.d.) has proved a major advance, being tolerated better than the 25 mg preparation.

A drug chemically related to indomethacin, sulindac (Clinoril), has already proved useful in the management of RA, possibly having fewer side effects than its parent drug, though it seems less effective.

Propionic acid derivatives. (ibuprofen, ketoprofen, fenoprofen and naproxen). Minor differences in potency and side effects are noted between the different members of the group. Ibuprofen has been in use in the UK for a long time and achieved considerable popularity because of its low incidence of gastrointestinal side effects. Naproxen, one of the most useful of these drugs, is also available in suppository form.

A useful trend has been in the development of sustained release preparations such as Oruvail, with fewer GI side effects and better patient compliance.

Despite attacks by the media and others, the development of the NSAIDs has proved a major advance for the patient with arthritis.

Gold

Although gold salts were discovered to have therapeutic effects in RA in 1927, the first controlled trial of gold salts was in 1961 when gold therapy was shown to suppress inflammation in some 75% of cases of RA. Conventional therapy consists of weekly i.m. injections of 50 mg of sodium aurothiomalate (Myocrisin) for 8 weeks (400 mg) thereafter 50 mg monthly. It is usual to continue for as long as therapeutic benefit is apparent. Serum levels have not proved useful in the monitoring of gold regimes, though Lorber *et al.* (1973) suggested that personalized regimes aimed at maintaining serum gold levels greater than 300 μg% may be more effective. It is also possible that free circulating gold, as opposed to albumin-bound gold, is the therapeutically active form. Injected gold is, as expected, largely taken up by the reticuloendothelial system (RES) or excreted in urine and faeces, and of that remaining in the circulation 95% is albumin bound.

Side effects occur in 30% of patients and usually consist of skin rashes or mouth ulcers. Far the commonest early warning of gold toxicity is skin itching, often between the fingers. Rarer, more serious complications include proteinuria and renal damage, marrow suppression (especially thrombocytopenia) and diarrhoea. With careful monitoring these side effects are largely avoidable. Eosinophilia is a common accompaniment or antecedent of other side effects and serum IgE levels often reach very high levels in patients with mucocutaneous side effects, suggesting a type I hypersensitivity mechanism (Fig. 5.20) (Davis *et al.* 1973). In a small number of patients who developed nephrotic syndrome an immune-complex mechanism has been postulated (Skrifvars *et al.* 1974). The mechanism by

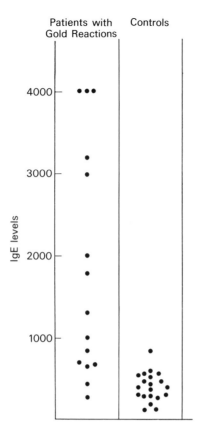

Fig. 5.20 Raised IgE levels in patients with mucocutaneous reactions to gold. (From Davis & Hughes 1973.)

which gold acts is unknown though the possibility that it might have an adjuvant effect is suggested by the common complaint of patients receiving gold of a transient worsening of the arthritis following each injection. This side effect may be sufficiently severe to result in withdrawal of the drug.

Case report. *A 41-year-old woman social worker with active RA was started on weekly gold injections. She complained of a marked increase in pain and stiffness following each injection. A series of careful observations made in hospital revealed a definite disease pattern. Within 24 hours of each injection not only was an increase in stiffness and synovitis documented but fresh vasculitic lesions were seen at the elbows and nail folds. Placebo injections failed to cause the changes. After perseverance for several further injections gold was stopped.*

D-Penicillamine

This drug, first used in RA by Griffin in 1960, on the assumption that it would dissociate the macromolecular rheumatoid factor, was shown by Jaffe in the USA to be therapeutically effective in RA. The dose recommended is 125–250 mg daily initially usually reaching a ceiling of 500 mg daily. Side effects of nausea and metallic taste are less if the drug is introduced slowly. More serious are thrombocytopenia and nephrotic syndrome, the latter again associated with IgG and complement deposits in the glomerulus. Rarer side effects include fever, myasthenia gravis (Delamere *et al.* 1983), a lupus-like illness, and Goodpasture's syndrome. Food reduces bioavailability of penicillamine markedly (Schuna *et al.* 1983).

The mechanism whereby the drug exerts its effect in RA is unknown.

As experience with penicillamine has increased, it has become accepted that doses higher than 750 mg (some would say 500 mg) are rarely needed. The subject has been reviewed by Jaffe (1978).

Antimalarials. These drugs stabilize lysosomal membranes and reduce the titre of rheumatoid factor in the serum. Although among the few anti-rheumatic drugs free from GI side effects, they almost fell into disuse in RA because of the ocular side effects. However, well on the heels of success in the treatment of SLE, antimalarials are now once again in increasing use (reviewed in the *American Journal of Medicine* 1983 and *Lupus* 1993).

Sulphasalazine

Two double-blind controlled studies have suggested that sulphasalazine (Salazopyrine) compared favourably with gold in RA (Neumann *et al.* 1983; Pullar, Hunter & Capell 1983). Widely used in the UK, but less popular in the USA, sulphasalazine lack the efficacy of methotrexate & has higher toxicity ratio. It might be more appropriately used in gut-associated and seronegative arthritis.

Corticosteroids

What are the current indications for prednisone in RA in view of the long list of side effects? Table 5.9 lists the major indications.

Items 2–5 in the list are relatively rare and clear cut in interpretation. Item 1, however, is open to variable interpretation. Situations regularly arise where 'rules' cannot apply, such as the young parent in whom

Table 5.9 Indications for systemic steroid therapy in RA

1 Progressing disease which has not responded to adequate trials of salicylates, other non-steroidal antiinflammatory agents, gold or penicillamine
2 Progressive rheumatoid vasculitis
3 Scleritis and iritis
4 Pericarditis and pleuritis
5 Felty's syndrome

morning stiffness unimproved by conventional therapy limits the ability to get the children to school, or the elderly patient with acute inflammatory disease in whom the known side effects of steroids may be thought worth the risk in order to produce an acceptable quality of life (Jasani 1975).

For those with serious, fulminant disease, pulses of i.v. methylprednisolone may have short-term benefit (Williams, Baylis & Shipley 1982), and is frequently used in the acute RA patient first admitted to hospital.

The pros and cons of corticosteroid therapy are reviewed by Kimberly (1992).

Intra-articular (IA) steroids. Despite the theoretical dangers of IA steroid, this form of therapy has been widely practised for years with little conclusive detriment. Infection has been rarely documented, and chondrolysis (seen following high-dose IA steroid injection in rabbits) has not been adequately demonstrated in man. This being said, the indications for IA steroids are still limited in RA. The two commonest indications are:
1 The acutely inflamed knee, where physiotherapy to a weak quadriceps muscle is hampered until aspiration and injection have been performed.
2 The painful shoulder — a non-weight-bearing joint where morale as well as joint mobility are improved by successful injection.

Cyclophosphamide (reviewed by McCune & Friedman 1992)

Like all alkylating agents, cyclophosphamide kills cells whether or not they are dividing. It thus differs from azathioprine which primarily affects dividing cells only. In dosage of 2·5 mg/kg/day, commonly used in RA and SLE, it reduces the absolute number of B cells in the blood (Santos, Owens & Sensenbrunner 1964; Horowitz 1974), immunoglobulin synthesis (Levy, Whitehouse & Barnett 1972) and T-cell function (Arinoviche & Levy 1970; Winkelstein, Mikulla & Nankin 1972; Clements *et al.* 1974). Clinically, it has been shown to result in improvement in standard criteria for disease activity, diminution in steroid requirement, and, somewhat surprisingly, a reduction in the development of erosions (Cooperating Clinics of the ARA 1970; Currey, Harris & Mason 1974).

Unfortunately, the drug is highly toxic even at therapeutic doses with alopecia in up to 90%, ovarian suppression in 30% of women, and azoospermia in males. Of even more importance is bladder toxicity, resulting in haemorrhagic cystitis and in persistent bladder fibrosis requiring cystectomy in some patients. Perhaps most important is the increased risk of long-term malignancy (Baltus *et al.* 1983). For these reasons this drug has little place in the longterm management of the vast majority of RA patients.

Having said this, the use of intermittent, short-term i.v. 'pulse' cyclophosphamide is now seen as having an important place in the management of fulminant disease, especially vasculitis and will be discussed in more detail in Chapter 10.

Azathioprine

This, also in dosage of 2·5 mg/kg/day, has been shown to have beneficial effects in RA (Urowitz, Gordon & Smythe 1971; Mason, Currey & Barnes 1972; Levy, Whitehouse & Barnett 1972; Currey, Harris & Mason 1974; Hunter, Urowitz & Gordon 1975). Whether its effect is entirely immunosuppressive is arguable as the drug probably has a slight additional anti-inflammatory effect. While it has many of the toxic properties of cyclophosphamide, bladder toxicity is not a feature and its therapeutic ratio is much more acceptable for use in non-lethal conditions such as RA.

It is probable that immunosuppression, by whatever means, is potentially carcinogenic, and the emergence of malignancy, particularly of the RES, may complicate treatment with these drugs.

Methotrexate

One of the true advances in rheumatology this decade has been the widespread use of 'low-dose' methotrexate in inflammatory arthritis (RA, Reiter's, psoriatic arthritis) (Wilkens & Watson 1982). This treatment, in countries throughout the world, has eclipsed other second line agents, quite simply because of its lower toxicity and greater efficacy.

The commonest starting dose is 7·5 mg orally weekly, often given in three divided doses 12 hours apart, e.g. Friday p.m., Saturday a.m. and Saturday p.m.

Side effects include nausea, cytopenia and liver function abnormalities, thus regular blood test monitoring is required. Rarely, a hypersensitivity pneumonitis may occur. The drug is contraindicated in pregnancy. Hawley & Wolfe (1991) reviewed over 120 trials of second-line agents and clearly demonstrated that patients remain on methotrexate for a longer period of time than patients on intramuscular gold, D-penicillamine, sulphasalazine or azathioprine.

For reviews, see Hughes (1990), Weinblatt *et al*. (1991) and Brooks (1992).

Other treatment

Other treatments, attempted in fulminant RA, include plasmapheresis (Dwosh *et al*. 1983), leukopheresis (Wahl *et al*. 1983) total lymphoid irradiation (Field *et al*. 1983), and, possibly most logically of all, the use of combination DMARDs.

Immunotherapy

Immunotherapy — the specific inhibition of an immune response involved in the pathogenesis of disease — is now under study in rheumatoid arthritis. Agents under investigation, and clearly still in the experimental stage, include antiHLA-DR monoclonal antibodies, anti-T-cell vaccines, blocking peptides and antibodies directed against T-cell accessory molecules such as CD4, CD7, CD5 and IL-2 receptors (Panayi, Kingsley & Lanchbury 1992).

Surgery

Orthopaedic and plastic surgery plays a considerable role in the management of RA and combined orthopaedic–rheumatology clinics are an important facet of care. However, the enthusiastic claims for surgical manoeuvres must be tempered by conservatism. Of the scores of operations performed in RA patients, three stand out in terms of success:

1 *Fowlers' operation*. Removal of the metatarsal heads with fibrous ankylosis, provides marked relief and an increase in functional capacity in patients with MTP erosions and deformities. As the synovium is removed, the relief provided is lifelong.

2 *Fusion of the wrist*. The wrist is frequently the worst affected joint in RA and active inflammation here severely limits grip strength and hand function. The patient is often left with 5–10° of painful movement. While wrist splinting or synovectomy in this situation may help, wrist fusion results in permanent pain relief.

3 *Total hip replacement*. This operation developed by Charnley and others has contributed more than any other advance in therapy to improvement of functional capacity in RA (Charnley 1971).

Other operations. Synovectomy of the knee is still widely performed, though the physician can give the patient no firm promise of success. As the years go by, increasing numbers of RA patients turn up in clinic with recurrent synovitis in the operated knee. Nevertheless, in other patients the operation clearly halts the active process of joint destruction. Synovectomy of other joints draws the same comments.

Joint replacements. The hip apart, silastic and plastic joint replacement is being performed at a variety of sites. Knee joint replacement is now a standard procedure and experience of other joint replacement, particularly the shoulder, is increasing greatly.

PROGNOSIS

Despite the high morbidity of RA, no representative mortality figures are available. Cobb, Anderson and Bauer in 1953 reviewed mortality data in 583 patients followed at the Massachusetts General Hospital and showed earlier mortality than in the overall population. This figure represents the precorticosteroid era, and whether the advent of corticosteroids has improved mortality figures by decreasing deaths from Felty's syndrome, pericarditis or vasculitis, or contributed to them by the increase in infection and peptic ulceration is unknown. Perhaps more figures will be obtained when RA is broken down into subsets for analytical purposes (Abruzzo 1982).

One of the major changes in our attitude to the prognosis — and thus to management — has come about following the studies of Ted Pincus and his colleagues (Pincus *et al.* 1990) who showed how serious the prognosis in RA can be. The impact of this disease on life span, earning capacity and functional capabilities may be just as severe as is the effect on joints.

This changing perspective of RA (Kushner & Dawson 1992) has signalled a sea change away from the old 'pyramid' treatment of RA towards the earlier use of more effective therapy. It may be that the widespread, earlier use of agents such as methotrexate will prove one of the genuine advances in the management of RA.

REFERENCES

Abruzzo J.L. (1982) Rheumatoid arthritis and mortality. *Arthritis and Rheumatism*, **25**, 1020–1030.

Alspaugh M.A., Jensen F.C., Robin H. & Tan E.M. (1978) Lymphocytes transformed by Epstein–Barr virus. Induction of nuclear antigen reactive with antibody in rheumatoid arthritis. *Journal of Experimental Medicine*, **147**, 1018.

Ansell B. (1992) Juvenile rheumatoid arthritis, juvenile chronic arthritis and juvenile spondylarthropathies. *Current Opinion in Rheumatology*, **4**, 706–712.

Antilla R. & Laaksonen A. (1969) Renal disease in juvenile rheumatoid arthritis. *Acta Rheumatologica Scandinavica*, **15**, 99.

Arinoviche R. & Levy J. (1970) Comparison of the effects of two cytotoxic drugs and of antilymphocyte serum on immune and non-immune inflammation in experimental animals. *Annals of the Rheumatic Diseases*, **29**, 32.

Baltus J.A.M., Boersma J.W., Hartman A.B. & Vanderbrouke J.P. (1983) The occurrence of malignancies in patients with RA treated with cyclophosphamide: a controlled retrospective follow-up. *Annals of the Rheumatic Diseases*, **42**, 368–373.

Barnes C.G. & Currey H.L.F. (1967) Carpal tunnel syndrome in rheumatoid arthritis. A clinical and electrodiagnostic survey. *Annals of the Rheumatic Diseases*, **26**, 226.

Barnes C.G., Turnbull A. & Vernon-Roberts B. (1971) Felty's syndrome: A clinical and pathological survey of 21 patients and their response to treatment. *Annals of the Rheumatic Diseases*, **30**, 359.

Baum J. (1971) Infection in rheumatoid arthritis. *Arthritis and Rheumatism*, **14**, 135.

Bennett J.C. (1978) The infectious aetiology of rheumatoid arthritis. *Arthritis and Rheumatism*, **21**, 531.

Bennett R.M., Hughes G.R.V., Bywaters E.G.L. & Holt P.J.L. (1972) Studies of a popliteal synovial fistula. *Annals of the Rheumatic Diseases*, **31**, 482.

Bernstein R.M., Mackworth-Young C.G., Saverymutu S.H., Gupta S. & Hughes G.R.V. (1984) *Yersinia* arthritis: demonstration of occult enteritis by [111]indium leucocyte scanning. *Annals of the Rheumatic Diseases*, **43**, 493–494.

Bianco N.E., Panush R.S., Stillman J.S. & Schur P.H. (1971) Immunologic studies of juvenile rheumatoid arthritis. *Arthritis and Rheumatism*, **14**, 685.

Bland J.H. (1974) Review: Rheumatoid arthritis of the cervical spine. *Journal of Rheumatology*, **1**, 319.

Boddington M.M., Spriggs A.U. & Morton J.A. (1971) Cytodiagnosis of rheumatoid pleural effusions. *Journal of Clinical Pathology*, **24**, 95.

Bonfiglio T. & Atwater E.D. (1969) Heart disease in patients with seropositive rheumatoid arthritis. *Archives of Internal Medicine*, **24**, 714.

Boyle J.A. & Buchanan W.W. (1971) *Clinical Rheumatology*, p. 74. Blackwell Scientific Publications, Oxford.

Brooks P. (1992) Current issues of methotrexate and cyclosporine. *Current Opinion in Rheumatology*, **4**, 309–313.

Bywaters E.G.L. (1982) Rheumatoid and other diseases of the cervical interspinous bursae, and changes in the spinous processes. *Annals of the Rheumatic Diseases*, **41**, 360–370.

Calabro J.J., Parrino G.R. & Marchesano J.M. (1970) Monoarticular onset juvenile rheumatoid arthritis. *Bulletin on the Rheumatic Diseases*, **21**, 613.

Caplan A. (1953) Certain unusual radiological appearances in the chest of coalminers suffering from rheumatoid arthritis. *Thorax*, **8**, 29.

Chamberlain M.A. & Bruckner F.E. (1970) Rheumatoid neuropathy, clinical and electrophysiological features. *Annals of the Rheumatic Diseases*, **29**, 609.

Charnley J. (1971) Present status of total hip surgery. *Annals of the Rheumatic Diseases*, **30**, 559.

Clements P.J., Yu D.T.Y., Levy J., Paulus H.E. & Barnett E.V. (1974) Effects of cyclophosphamide on B and T lymphocytes in rheumatoid arthritis. *Arthritis and Rheumatism*, **17**, 347.

Clot J. & Sany J. (Eds) (1975) *Rheumatology. An Annual Review, 6. Immunological Aspects of Rheumatoid Arthritis*. Karger, Basel.

Cobb S., Anderson F. & Bauer W. (1953) Length of life and cause of death in rheumatoid arthritis. *New England Journal of Medicine*, **249**, 553.

Cohen M.G. & Webb J. (1989) Antihistone antibodies in rheumatoid arthritis and Felty's syndrome. *Arthritis and Rheumatism*, **32**, 1319–1324.

Conlon P.W., Isdale I.C. & Rose B.S. (1966) Rheumatoid arthritis of the cervical spine. An analysis of 333 cases. *Annals of the Rheumatic Diseases*, **25**, 120.

Conn D.L., McDuffie F.C. & Dyck P.J. (1972) Immunopathologic study of sural nerves in rheumatoid arthritis. *Arthritis and Rheumatism*, **15**, 135.

Cooperating Clinics of the American Rheumatism Association (1970) A controlled trial of cyclophosphamide in rheumatoid arthritis. *New England Journal of Medicine*, **283**, 883.

Cunningham T.J., Tait B.D., Mathews J.D. & Muirden K.D. (1982) Clinical rheumatoid vasculitis associated with the B8 DR3 phenotype. *Rheumatology International*, **2**, 137–139.

Currey H.L.F., Harris J. & Mason R.M. (1974) Comparison of azathioprine, cyclophosphamide, and gold in the treatment of rheumatoid arthritis. *British Medical Journal*, **3**, 763.

Davis P. & Hughes G.R.V. (1973) Immunological studies on the mechanism of gold hypersensitivity reactions. *British Medical Journal*, **ii**, 767–769.

Davis P., Ezeoke A., Munro J., Hobbs J.R. & Hughes G.R.V. (1973) Immunological studies on the mechanism of gold hypersensitivity reactions. *British Medical Journal*, **2**, 676.

De Beer F.C., Mallya R.K., Fagan E.A., Lanham J.G., Hughes G.R.V. & Pepys M.B. (1982) Serum amyloid-A protein concentration in inflammatory diseases and its relationship to the incidence of reactive systemic amyloidosis. *Lancet*, **ii**, 231–234.

De Horatius R.J., Abruzzo J.L. & Williams R.C., Jr (1972) Immunofluorescent and immunologic studies of rheumatoid lung. *Archives of Internal Medicine*, **129**, 441.

De Horatius R.J. & Williams R.C., Jr (1972) Rheumatoid factor accentuation of pulmonary lesions associated with experimental diffuse proliferative lung disease. *Arthritis and Rheumatism*, **15**, 293.

Delamere J.P., Jobson S., Mackintosh L.P., Wells L. & Walton K.W. (1983) Penicillamin-induced myasthenia in rheumatoid arthritis: its clinical and genetic features. *Annals of the Rheumatic Diseases*, **42**, 500–504.

Dipper J.M., Bluestein H.G. & Zvaifler N. (1981) Impaired regulation of Epstein–Barr virus-induced lymphocyte proliferation in rheumatoid arthritis is due to AT cell defect. *Journal of Immunology*, **127**, 1899–1902.

Dyer N., Kendall M.J. & Hawkins C.F. (1972) Malabsorption in rheumatoid disease. *Annals of the Rheumatic Diseases*, **30**, 626.

Dwosh I.L., Giles I.R., Foro P.M., Pater J.L. & Anastassiades T.P. (1983) Plasmapheresis therapy in rheumatoid arthritis: a controlled, double blind crossover study. *New England Journal of Medicine*, **308**, 1124–1129.

Elkon K. *et al.* (1982) Immunoglobulin A and polymeric IgA rheumatoid factors in systemic sicca syndrome: partial characterisation. *Journal of Immunology*, **129**, 576–581.

Felty A.R. (1924) Chronic arthritis in the adult associated with splenomegaly and leucopenia. *Bulletin of the Johns Hopkins Hospital*, **35**, 16.

Field E.H., Strober S., Hoppe R.T. *et al.* (1983) Sustained improvement of intractable rheumatoid arthritis after total lymphoid irradiation. *Arthritis and Rheumatism*, **26**, 937–946.

Firestein G.S. (1992) Mechanisms of tissue destruction and cellular activation in rheumatoid arthritis. *Current Opinion in Rheumatology*, **4**, 348–354.

Franco A.E., Levine H.D. & Hall A.P. (1972) Rheumatoid pericarditis, report of 17 cases diagnosed clinically. *Annals of Internal Medicine*, **77**, 837.

Franco A.E. & Schur P.H. (1972) Hypocomplementaemia in rheumatoid arthritis. *Arthritis and Rheumatism*, **14**, 231.

Franklin E.C. (1975) Amyloidosis. *Bulletin on the Rheumatic Diseases*, **26**, 832.

Frøland S.S., Natvig J.B. & Husby G. (1973) Immunological characteristics of lymphocytes in synovial fluid from patients with rheumatoid arthritis. *Scandinavian Journal of Immunology*, **2**, 67.

Gandy R.H., Ansell B.M. & Bywaters E.G.L. (1965) Protein concentration of oedema fluid in rheumatoid arthritis. *Annals of the Rheumatic Diseases*, **24**, 234.

Geersten H.R., Gray R.M. & Ward J.R. (1975) Patient non-compliance within the context of seeking medical care for arthritis. *Journal of Chronic Diseases*, **26**, 689.

Gendre J.P., Luboinski J., Prier A., Camus J.P. & Le Quintrec Y. (1982) Jejunal mucosal abnormalities and rheumatoid arthritis: report of 30 cases. *Gastroenterology and Clinical Biology*, **6**, 772–775.

Gram J.T., Husby G. & Thorsby E. (1983) HLA DR antigens in rheumatoid arthritis. *Scandinavian Journal of Rheumatology*, **12**, 241–245.

Gupta R., Robinson W.A. & Albrecht D. (1975) Granulopoietic activity in Felty's syndrome. *Annals of the Rheumatic Diseases*, **34**, 156.

Gwyther M., Schwartz H., Howard A. & Ansell B.M. (1982) C-Reactive protein in juvenile chronic arthritis: an indicator of disease activity and possibly amyloidosis. *Annals of the Rheumatic Diseases*, **41**, 259–262.

Hawley D.J. & Wolfe F. (1991) Are the results of controlled clinical trials and observational studes of second-line therapy in RA valid? *Journal of Rheumatology*, **18**, 1008–1014.

Horowitz D.A. (1974) Selective depletion of Ig bearing lymphocytes by cyclophosphamide in rheumatoid arthritis and systemic lupus erythematosus. *Arthritis and Rheumatism*, **17**, 363.

Horowitz D.A. (1974) Selective depletion of Ig bearing lymphocytes by cyclophosphamide in rheumatoid arthritis and systemic lupus erythematosus. *Arthritis and Rheumatism*, **17**, 363.

Hughes G.R.V. (1989) Methotrexate in RA. *Annals of the Rheumatic Diseases*, **49**, 275–276.

Hughes G.R.V. & Pridie R.B. (1970) Acute synovial rupture of the knee – a differential diagnosis from deep vein thrombosis. *Proceedings of the Royal Society of Medicine*, **63**, 587.

Hunder G.G., McDuffie F.C. & Hepper N.G.G. (1972) Pleural fluid complement in systemic lupus erythematosus and rheumatoid arthritis. *Annals of Internal Medicine*, **76**, 357.

Hunter T., Urowitz M. & Gordon D. (1975) Azathioprine and rheumatoid arthritis. *Arthritis and Rheumatism*, **18**, 15.

Huskisson E.C. (1977) Antiinflammatory drugs. *Seminars in Arthritis and Rheumatism*, **vii**, 1.

Huskisson E.C. & Hart F.D. (1972) Severe unusual and recurrent infections in rheumatoid arthritis. *Annals of the Rheumatic Diseases*, **31**, 118.

Jaffe I.A. (1978) D-Penicillamine. *Bulletin of the Rheumatic Diseases*, **28**, 948.

Jasani M.K. (1975) The importance of ACTH and glucocorticoids in rheumatoid arthritis.

In: *Clinics in Rheumatic Diseases*, Vol. 1, p. 335, Eds: W.C. Dick & C.M. Pearson. Saunders, Philadelphia.

Jason H.E., LoSpalluto J. & Ziff M. (1970) Rheumatoid hyperviscosity syndrome. *American Journal of Medicine*, **49**, 484.

Jayson M.I.V. & Dixon A.S. (1969) Ruptured synovial cysts. *Annals of the Rheumatic Diseases*, **25**, 32.

Jayson M.I.V. & Jones D.E.P. (1971) Scleritis and rheumatoid arthritis. *Annals of the Rheumatic Diseases*, **30**, 343.

Kaufmann S.H. (1990) Heat shock proteins and the immune response. *Immunology Today*, **11**, 129–136.

Kimberly R.P. (1992) Glucocorticoid therapy for rheumatic diseases. *Current Opinion in Rheumatology*, **4**, 325–331.

Kirk J.A. & Cosh J. (1969) The pericarditis of rheumatoid arthritis. *Quarterly Journal of Medicine*, **38**, 397.

Kushner I. & Dawson N.V. (1992) Changing perspectives in the treatment of RA. *Journal of Rheumatology*, **19** (12), 1831–1834.

Kyle R.A. & Bayrd E.D. (1975) Amyloidosis: Review of 236 cases. *Medicine*, **54**, 271.

Lawrence J.S., Bremmer J.A., Ball J. & Burch T.A. (1966) Rheumatoid arthritis in a subtropical population. *Annals of the Rheumatic Diseases*, **25**, 59.

Levy J., Whitehouse M.W. & Barnett E.V. (1972) Comparative immunosuppressive effects of azathioprine and cyclophosphamide in the treatment of arthritis. *Arthritis and Rheumatism*, **15**, 44.

Levy R.J., Haidar M., Park H., Tar L. & Levinson A.I. (1986) Bacterial peptidoglycan induces *in vitro* rheumatoid factor production by lymphocytes of healthy subjects. *Clinical and Experimental Immunology*, **64**, 311–317.

Liss J.P. & Bachman W.T. (1970) Rheumatoid constrictive pericarditis, treated by pericardectomy. Report of a case and review of the literature. *Arthritis and Rheumatism*, **13**, 869.

Lorber A., Atkins C.J., Chang C.C., Fee Y.B., Starrs J. & Bovy R.A. (1973) Monitoring serum gold levels to improve chrysotherapy in rheumatoid arthritis. *Annals of the Rheumatic Diseases*, **32**, 133.

Louise J.S. & Pearson C.M. (1971) Felty's syndrome. *Seminars in Haematology*, **8**, 216.

Lyne A.J. & Pitkeathly D.A. (1968) Episcleritis and scleritis associated with connective tissue diseases. *Archives of Ophthalmology*, **80**, 171.

McCune W.J. & Freidman A.W. (1992) Immunosuppressive drug therapy for rheumatic disease. *Current Opinion in Rheumatology*, **4**, 314–321.

Masi A.J. & Shulman L.S. (1965) Familial aggregation and rheumatic disease. *Arthritis and Rheumatism*, **8**, 418.

Mason M., Currey H.L.F. & Barnes C.G. (1972) Azathioprine in rheumatoid arthritis. *British Medical Journal*, **i**, 420.

Matsuhara T., Spycher M.A., Ruttner J.R. & Fehr K. (1983) The localisation of fibronectin in rheumatoid arthritis synovium by light and electron microscopic immunohistochemistry. *Rheumatology International*, **3**, 153–159.

Matthews J.A. (1974) Atlanto-axial subluxation in rheumatoid arthritis. A five-year follow-up study. *Annals of the Rheumatic Diseases*, **33**, 526.

Mellbye O.J., Messner R.P., DeBord J.R. *et al.* (1972) Immunoglobulin and receptors for C3 on lymphocytes from patients with rheumatoid arthritis. *Arthritis and Rheumatism*, **15**, 371.

Mowat A.G. (1972) Haematologic abnormalities in rheumatoid arthritis. *Seminars in*

Arthritis and Rheumatism, **3**, 195.

Mowat A.G., Hothersall T.E. & Aitchison W.R. (1969) Nature of the anaemia in rheumatoid arthritis. XI. Change in iron metabolism induced by the administration of corticotrophin. *Annals of the Rheumatic Diseases,* **28**, 303.

Muirden K.D. (1970) The anaemia of rheumatoid arthritis: the significance of iron deposits in the synovial membrane. *Australian Annals of Medicine,* **19**, 97.

Neumann V.C., Grindulis K.A., Hubball S., McConkey B. & Wright V. (1983) Comparison between penicillamine and sulphasalazine in rheumatoid arthritis: Leeds–Birmingham trial. *British Medical Journal,* **287**, 1099–1102.

Norton W.L. & Ziff M. (1966) Electron microscopic observation on the rheumatoid synovial membrane. *Arthritis and Rheumatism,* **9**, 589.

O'Brien W.M. (1967) The genetics of rheumatoid arthritis. *Clinical and Experimental Immunology,* **2**, 785.

O'Brien W.M. (1968) Twin studies in rheumatic disease. Current comment. *Arthritis and Rheumatism,* **11**, 81.

Oxholm P., Madsen E.B., Manthorpe R. & Rasmussen F.V. (1982) Pulmonary function in patients with RA. *Scandinavian Journal of Rheumatology,* **11**, 109–122.

Pallis C.A. & Scott J.T. (1965) Peripheral neuropathy in rheumatoid arthritis. *British Medical Journal,* **i**, 1141.

Panayi G.S., Kingsley G.H. & Lanchbury J.S.S. (1992) Immunotherapy of immune-mediated diseases. *Quarterly Journal of Medicine,* **84**, 489–495.

Panush R.S., Franco A.E. & Schur P.H. (1971) Rheumatoid arthritis associated with eosinophilia. *Annals of Internal Medicine,* **75**, 199.

Parish L.E. (1963) An historical approach to the nomenclature of rheumatoid arthritis. *Arthritis and Rheumatism,* **6**, 138.

Parke A.L., Fagan E.A., Chadwick V.S. & Hughes G.R.V. (1983) Coeliac disease and rheumatoid arthritis. *Annals of the Rheumatic Diseases,* **42**, 216.

Parke A. & Hughes G.R.V. (1981) Rheumatoid arthritis and food: a case study. *British Medical Journal,* **282**, 2027.

Pettersson T., Klockars M. & Hellstrom P.E. (1982) Chemical and immunological features of pleural effusions: comparison between RA and other disease. *Thorax,* **37**, 354–361.

Pettersson T., Wegelius O. & Skifvars B. (1970) Gastrointestinal disturbances in patients with severe rheumatoid arthritis. *Acta Medica Scandinavica,* **188**, 139.

Pincus T. & Callahan L.F. (1990) Remodelling the pyramid or remodelling the paradigms concerning RA. *Journal of Rheumatology,* **17**, 1582–1585.

Pope R.M., Mannik M., Gilliland B.C. & Teller D.C. (1975) The hyperviscosity syndrome in rheumatoid arthritis due to intermediate complexes formed by self-association of IgG rheumatoid factors. *Arthritis and Rheumatism,* **18**, 97–106.

Popper M.S., Bogdonoff M.L. & Hughes R.L. (1972) Interstitial rheumatoid lung disease. *Chest,* **62**, 243.

Poulter L.W., Duke O., Hobbs S., Janossy G. & Panayi G. (1982) Histochemical discrimination of HLA-DR positive cell populations in the normal and arthritic synovial lining. *Clinical and Experimental Immunology,* **48**, 381–388.

Pullar T., Hunter J.A. & Capell H.A. (1983) Sulphasalazine in rheumatoid arthritis: a double-blind comparison with placebo and sodium aurothiomalate. *British Medical Journal,* **287**, 1102–1105.

Redisch W., Messina E.J. & Hughes G. (1970) Capillaroscopic observations in rheumatic diseases. *Annals of the Rheumatic Diseases,* **29**, 244.

Rich R.R. & Johnson J.S. (1973) Salicylate hepatotoxicity in patients with JRA. *Arthritis and Rheumatism*, **16**, 1.

Salmon M. (1992) The immunogenetic component of susceptibility to rheumatoid arthritis. *Current Opinion in Rheumatology*, **4**, 342–347.

Sandson J. & Hammerman D. (1962) Isolation of hyaluronate protein from human synovial fluid. *Journal of Clinical Investigation*, **41**, 1817.

Santos G.W., Owens A.H. & Sensenbrunner L.L. (1964) Effect of selected cytotoxic agents on antibody production in man. *Annals of the New Academy of Science*, **114**, 404.

Schaller J.G., Johnson G.D., Holborow E.J., Ansell B.M. & Smiley W.K. (1974) The association of antinuclear antibodies with the chronic iridocyclitis of juvenile rheumatoid arthritis (Still's disease). *Arthritis and Rheumatism*, **17**, 409.

Schumacher H.R. & Kitridou R.C. (1972) Synovitis of recent onset: a clinicopathologic study during the first month of disease. *Arthritis and Rheumatism*, **15**, 465.

Schuna A., Osman M.A., Patel R.B., Welling P.G. & Sundstrom W.R. (1983) Influence of food on the bioavailability of penicillamine. *Journal of Rheumatology*, **10**, 95–97.

Sheinberg M.A. (1983) The pathogenesis of rheumatoid arthritis and the immune response. *Seminars in Arthritis and Rheumatism*, **13**, 99–101.

Shroeder W., Franklin E.C. & McEwen C. (1962) Rheumatoid factors in patients with silicosis with round nodular fibrosis of the lung in the absence of rheumatoid arthritis with a note on the failure to induce such factors in animals. *Arthritis and Rheumatism*, **5**, 10.

Simon, L.S. (1990) Toxicity of nonsteroidal anti-inflammatory drugs. *Current Opinion in Rheumatology*, **2**(3), 481–488.

Skrifvars B., Torriroth T., Tallqvist G. & Ahlqvist J. (1974) Gold induced immune complex nephritis in seronegative arthritis. Abstracts of VIth Pan American Congress on Rheumatic Diseases, Toronto. Abstract 207, p. 111.

Sliwinski A.J. & Zvaifler N. (1970) *In vivo* synthesis of IgG by rheumatoid synovium. *Journal of Laboratory and Clinical Medicine*, **76**, 304.

Smith M.E., Ansell B.M. & Bywaters E.G.L. (1968) Mortality and prognosis related to the amyloidosis of Still's disease. *Annals of the Rheumatic Diseases*, **27**, 137.

Smith P.H., Benn R.T. & Sharp J. (1972) Natural history of rheumatoid cervical luxations. *Annals of the Rheumatic Diseases*, **31**, 431.

Sokoloff L. (1953) The heart in rheumatoid arthritis. *American Heart Journal*, **45**, 635.

Sokoloff L. (1978) (Ed.) *The Joints and Synovial Fluids*. Academic Press, London.

Stack B.H.R. & Grant I.W.B. (1965) Rheumatoid interstitial lung disease. *British Journal of Diseases of the Chest*, **59**, 202.

Stastny P. (1978) HLA-D and Ia antigens in rheumatoid arthritis and systemic lupus erythematosus. *Arthritis and Rheumatism*, **21**, No. 5 (Suppl.), 139.

Still G.F. (1897) On a form of chronic joint disease in children. *Medico-Chirurgical Transactions*, **80**, 47.

Sundquist T., Lindstrom F., Magnusson K-E. & Skoldstam L. (1982) Influence of fasting on intestinal permeability and liver disease in patients with RA. *Scandinavian Journal of Rheumatology*, **11**, 33–38.

Thorne C. & Urowitz M.B. (1982) Long-term outcome in Felty's syndrome. *Annals of the Rheumatic Diseases*, **41**, 486–489.

Urowitz M.B., Gordon D.A. & Smythe H.A. (1971) Azathioprine treatment of rheumatoid arthritis, a double blind, cross over study. *Arthritis and Rheumatism*, **14**, 411.

Van Valkenburgh W.G., Georges L.P. & Irby R. (1972) Aortic insufficiency and pelvo-spondylitis in a seropositive female with rheumatoid nodules. *Arthritis and Rheumatism*, **15**, 544.

Wahl S.M., Wilder R.L., Katona I.M. *et al.* (1983) Leukapheresis in rheumatoid arthritis: association of clinical improvement with reversal of energy. *Arthritis and Rheumatism*, **26**, 1076–1084.

Walport M.J., Parke A.L. & Hughes G.R.V. (1982) Food and the connective tissue diseases. *Clinical Immunology and Allergy*, **2**, 113–120.

Waxman J., Lockshin M.D., Schnapp J.J. & Donesan I. (1973) Cellular immunity in rheumatic diseases. I. Rheumatoid arthritis. *Arthritis and Rheumatism*, **16**, 449.

Webb J., Whaley K., MacSween R.N.M. Nuki G., Dick W.C. & Buchanan W.W. (1975) Liver disease in rheumatoid arthritis and Sjøgren's syndrome. *Annals of the Rheumatic Diseases*, **34**, 70.

Weinblatt M.E. (1991) Methotrexate in RA: effects on disease activity in a multicentre prospective study. *Journal of Rheumatology*, **18**, 334–338.

Weller R., Bruckner F. & Chamberlain M. (1970) Rheumatoid neuropathy: a histological and electrophysiological study. *Journal of Neurology, Neurosurgery and Psychiatry*, **33**, 593.

Wiik A. (1975) Circulating immune complexes involving granulocyte specific ANFs in Felty's syndrome and rheumatoid arthritis. *Acta Petrologica et Microbiologica Scandinavica*, **83**, 354.

Williams I.A., Baylis E.M. & Shipley M.E. (1982) A double-blind placebo controlled trial of methylprednisolone pulse therapy in active rheumatoid disease. *Lancet*, **ii**, 237–240.

Williams M.H., Sheldon P.J.H.S., Torrigiani G., Eisen V. & Mattingley S. (1971) Palindromic rheumatism. *Annals of the Rheumatic Diseases*, **30**, 375.

Williams R.C., Jr., DeBord J.R., Mellbye O.J., Messner R.P. & Lindstrom F.D. (1973) Studies of T and B lymphocytes in patients with connective tissue diseases. *Journal of Clinical Investigation*, **52**, 283.

Willkens R.F. & Watson M.A. (1982) Methotrexate: a perspective of its use in the treatment of rheumatic diseases. *Journal of Laboratory and Clinical Medicine*, **100**, 314–321.

Wilson W.A. & Hughes G.R.V. (1979) Rheumatic diseases in Jamaica. A 3 year study. *Annals of the Rheumatic Diseases*, **38**, 320.

Winchester R.J., Agnello V. & Kunkel H.G. (1970) Gamma globulin complexes in synovial fluids of patients with rheumatoid arthritis. Partial characterization and relationship to lowered complement levels. *Clinical and Experimental Immunology*, **6**, 689.

Winchester R.J., Winfield J.B., Siegal F., Wernet P., Bentwich Z. & Kunkel H.G. (1975) Analysis of lymphocytes from patients with rheumatoid arthritis and systemic lupus erythematosus. Occurrence of interfering cold reactive antilymphocyte antibodies. *Journal of Clinical Investigation*, **54**, 1082.

Winkelstein A., Mikulla J.M. & Nankin H.R. (1972) Effects of cyclophosphamide on lymphocytes. *Journal of Laboratory and Clinical Medicine*, **80**, 506.

Wolfe A.M. & Masi A.T. (1968) The epidemiology of rheumatoid arthritis (Parts I & II). *Bulletin of the Rheumatic Diseases*, **19**, 518.

Yao Q.Y., Rickinson A.B., Gaston J.S.H. & Epstein M.A. (1986) Disturbance of the Epstein–Barr virus–host balance in RA patients: a quantitative study. *Clinical and Experimental Immunology*, **64**, 302–310.

Zvaifler N.J. (1973) The immunopathology of joint inflammation in rheumatoid arthritis. In: *Advances in Immunology*, Vol. 16, p. 265, Eds: F.J. Dixon & H.C. Kunkel. Academic Press, New York.

Zvaifler N.J. & Weintraub A.M. (1962) Aortitis and aortic insufficiency in the chronic rheumatic disorders: a reappraisal. *Arthritis and Rheumatism*, **6**, 241.

6: *Scleroderma*

Scleroderma (progressive systemic sclerosis — PSS) is a disease of unknown aetiology, characterized by widespread and diffuse sclerosis, affecting skin, gastrointestinal tract, heart and muscle. Pulmonary and renal involvement are common, and Raynaud's phenomenon is a regular and frequent early accompaniment. While in some patients the disease appears to remain confined to the skin for many years, in others it progresses steadily to visceral involvement and to death from pulmonary, cardiac or renal failure. Women are affected between three and five times more commonly than men, and blacks are frequently affected. The disease may occur at any age.

A number of variants of scleroderma are recognized and these will be dealt with separately. As well as being a multisystem disease, scleroderma is, in many cases, a multistage disease. Skin involvement may be minimal, and in some patients, absent (Rodnan & Fennell 1962).

The annual incidence of the disease in one large study was 2·7 new patients per million population (Medsger & Masi 1971).

PATHOLOGY

There are no pathognomonic features. The earliest changes in the skin include oedema, perivascular lymphocytic infiltrates, swelling and degeneration of collagen fibres which become eosinophilic. Dermal collagen increases and elastic tissue becomes reduced (Fig. 6.1) the combination leading to the thickening and immobility seen clinically. Despite the increase in collagen, fibroblast proliferation is not seen. The small blood vessels of the skin show some increase in cellularity, a basophilic 'mucoid' change in the intima and the deposition of an adventitial cuff of collagen. Some maintain that the small artery lesion is central to the widespread pathology. A myopathy or inflammatory myositis may occur. Fibrosis may occur in cardiac muscle. In the pulmonary capillaries, basement membrane thickening may be seen by electron microscopy and later there is widespread fibrosis. Later, cystic or 'honeycomb' change occurs with marked and excessive interstitial fibrosis.

Replacement of smooth muscle by fibrous tissue may also be seen in the oesophagus and in the small gut.

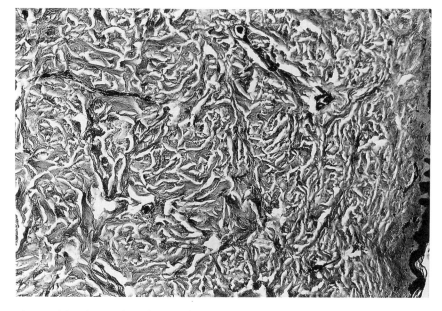

Fig. 6.1 Scleroderma skin, showing hypertrophied collagen and atrophy of dermal appendages (×54). (Dr Shirley Amin, University Hospital of the West Indies.)

The renal lesions resemble those seen in severe hypertension, with fibrinoid changes in the artery and arteriole walls (Fig. 6.2). Fibrinoid may also be seen in thickened glomerular capillary loops. Later changes, include thrombosis and cortical infarction or ultimately a small granular kidney.

AETIOLOGY

The aetiology is unknown, but three main lines of investigation into pathogenesis are currently being pursued: the factors leading to altered collagen synthesis, the role of capillary changes, and immunological aspects. These are discussed separately.

Changes in collagen (reviewed by Smith 1992)

Early studies of the connective tissue in scleroderma focused on the gross structural features of collagen. Scleroderma collagen was shown to be identical to normal collagen by amino acid composition (Neldner, Jones & Winkelmann 1966) and X-ray diffraction pattern (Fleischmajer 1964), and showed similar banded periodicity by electron microscopy (Fleischmajer, Damiano & Nedwich 1971). Studies of collagen solubility showed that

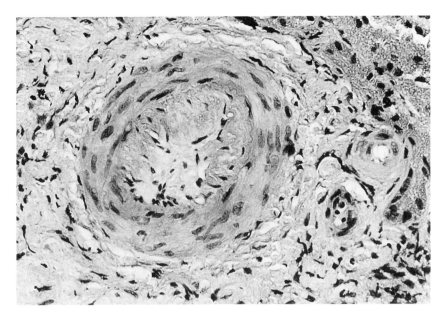

Fig. 6.2 Scleroderma renal biopsy (H & E ×54) showing onion-skin thickening of the media and basophilic intimal proliferation of an interlobular vessel. (Dr Shirley Amin, University Hospital of the West Indies.)

neutral salt-soluble collagen (i.e. newly synthesized) was increased in some scleroderma skin samples (Uitto, Ohlenschaeger & Lorenzen 1971).

The stability of the collagen fibre depends on the formation of inter-molecular crosslinks between the tropocollagen molecules making up the fibre. The crosslinks in newly synthesized collagen are labile, and not present in inactive disease. Herbert *et al.* (1974) found an increase in labile crosslinks in active scleroderma, suggesting an excess synthesis of collagen in this disease (Fig. 6.3). In an elegant series of experiments using cultures of dividing fibroblasts from normal and sclerodermatous human skin, LeRoy (1974) produced evidence for a basic increase in collagen synthesis by scleroderma fibroblasts.

In these studies, scleroderma fibroblasts even after 15 subcultures shared an increased capacity to synthesize collagen and fourfold more of their protein synthetic activity was directed to collagen production than in the normal skin fibroblast. At present the cellular nature of this abnormal synthesis is obscure.

Brady (1975) has demonstrated minimal or absent collagenase activity in involved skin in seven patients with scleroderma.

For a full review of the fibrosing processes, see Kallenberg (1992).

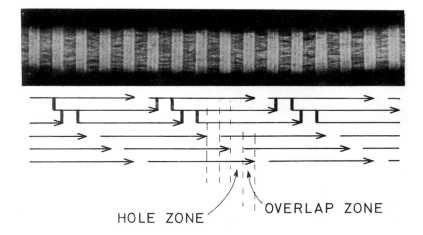

Fig. 6.3 Electron micrograph of the collagen fibre and the quarter-stagger arrangements of the fibre showing the intermolecular crosslinks. Collagen is a fibrous protein built up of essentially identical subunits. Under the light microscope, these fibres can be seen to consist of a large number of small fibrils, and with the electron microscope the fibrils appear as bundles of smaller identical and parallel molecules, aligned quarter-staggered with respect to each other. The newly formed fibres have little tensile strength and readily redissolve in neutral salt buffers. With time, however, the collagen fibres gradually become insoluble through the formation of stable covalent bonds between the tropocollagen molecules. Confirmation of the need for these intermolecular crosslinks is demonstrated in experimental lathyrism where the biosynthesis of the crosslinks is inhibited, resulting in an extremely fragile fibre due to the slippage of adjacent molecules under tension. (Dr Carol Black.)

Capillary changes (Lally 1992)

The simple technique of nailfold capillary microscopy has been used to identify patterns of capillary damage which can separate rheumatoid arthritis, SLE and scleroderma. The class of severity of the capillary pattern abnormality has been correlated with the presence of more widespread organ involvement (Maricq & LeRoy 1973; Thompson *et al.* 1984). A follow-up study has confirmed the predictive value of nailfold capillary microscopy in some patients. Five of ten Raynaud's patients initially showing sclero-derma patterns had developed scleroderma at follow-up (Maricq, Weinberger & LeRoy 1982). If these findings are upheld, the implications extend beyond diagnostic convenience and directly link the small artery lesion and the microvascular lesion. The suggestion that scleroderma may be a primary vascular disease also comes from some earlier histological findings. Norton, Hurd & Lewis (1969) noted the loss of up to 80%

of capillaries in skeletal muscle. Peripheral vascular changes have been detected by a variety of angiographic and plethysmographic studies and hyperreactivity to angiotensin, serotonin are well recognized.

Immunology (Kallenberg 1992)

In early scleroderma, a number of immunological abnormalities are frequently seen, including ANA (especially speckled or nucleolar), rheumatoid factors, positive tests for circulating immune complexes, and abnormal cell-mediated immunity to collagen. These have been reviewed in detail by Needleman (1992). One study showed a circulating factor influencing endothelial cell growth (Kahaleh & LeRoy 1983) but this was not confirmed in another study (Shanahan & Korn 1982). An interesting parallel to scleroderma is seen in some patients with graft-versus-host disease (Graham-Brown & Sarkany 1983).

A variety of antinuclear antibodies are seen in scleroderma. These include anticentromere (seen especially in the CREST syndrome), scl-70, and, occasionally, ENA (reviewed by Hughes 1984). DNA antibodies are usually absent.

The current value of antibody measurements in the differentiation of scleroderma from other overlapping and fibrosing conditions is reviewed by Kallenberg (1992).

Genetic factors (Fox & Kang 1992)

Major histocompatibility cell (MHC) studies have shown an association with class I alleles A9 and B8 and class II alleles DR5 and DR4, though the latter may be more attributable to their linkage with certain DQ alleles. Reveille *et al.* (1992) suggested that the MHC alleles are more closely associated with scleroderma autoantibodies than with clinical subgroups.

Environmental factors

Clusters of scleroderma cases, notably related to mining, have periodically been reported. In particular, silica, with its well-known adjuvant effects, has been strongly implicated. Other agents implicated include adulterated rape seed oil, vinyl chloride, certain drugs (including dapsone) and paraffin (reviewed by Fox & Kang 1992). Perhaps the most remarkable agent is the silicone breast implant, implicated not only in a systemic sclerosis-like disease, but also in myositis, Raynaud's and a variety of autoimmune phenomena including the production of autoantibodies including those against topoisomerase. The term 'human adjuvant disease' is widely used for the collection of features associated with silicone implants. So important has this 'disease model' become that at the annual scientific meeting of the American College of Rheumatology in September 1992, over 16 papers and abstracts on the topic were presented (*Arthritis and Rheumatism* **35**, no. 9, supplement).

CLINICAL FEATURES

Raynaud's phenomenon (reviewed by Lally 1992)

The disease most commonly starts in the thirties, forties or fifties. Raynaud's phenomenon occurs in over 90% of all cases and may precede other features by months and even years. The Raynaud's phenomenon is unequivocal and usually a prominent feature, a point of differentiation from the other connective tissue diseases, where severe Raynaud's is unusual. Another clinical aphorism is that Raynaud's developing in a patient over the age of 40 is due to scleroderma until proved otherwise. LeRoy in a recent review stated 'we have been increasingly impressed with the low incidence of intravascular (cryoglobulins, cold agglutinins, etc.) mechanical (jack hammer operation and other vibration-induced syndromes) or thoracic outlet causes for Raynaud's phenomenon .... A high proportion of patients with Raynaud's phenomenon, when followed carefully for several years eventually develop scleroderma or an overlapping variant of scleroderma. Because, Raynaud's syndrome may precede scleroderma by months or years, we consider patients with Raynaud's syndrome as the nearest thing to an identifiable population with a high incidence of scleroderma in whom observations can be made and therapies considered *before* the appearance of fibrosis' (LeRoy 1976).

One of the more dramatic sequelae of the Raynaud's phenomenon is tuft resorption, with loss both of tissue pulp and of the tip of the distal phalanx. Bone resorption may occur in patients with Raynaud's syndrome who have no other evidence of scleroderma. Conversely, resorption may appear to be out of all proportion to the severity of the Raynaud's phenomenon.

Skin

Some of the main dermatological features seen in scleroderma are listed in Table 6.1.

During the early stages of the disease there may be considerable oedema, distinguishable by its non-pitting character and sometimes by a clear line of demarcation. This may be difficult to distinguish from

Table 6.1 Dermatological features of scleroderma

Oedema (early)
Thickening and tightening
Dermal atrophy
Telangiectasis
Ulceration
Increased pigmentation
Areas of vitiligo
Calcification
Pulp atrophy
Loss of hair and skin appendages

scleroedema, a benign condition of localized cutaneous hardening which sometimes follows an upper respiratory infection and involves the upper part of the body. In some patients the scleroedema may last two years or more (Curtis & Shulak 1965) and its spread may be rapid. An early sign is hyperpigmentation.

The changes of skin tightness, tethering and shininess in the fingers result in decreased mobility of the whole hand. Tautness of the skin around the nose gives the face an almost characteristic bird-like appearance. The mouth becomes pinched and the patient or her dentist notices difficulty in opening the mouth wide. For those who perform Schirmer's tests routinely, an early sign of facial involvement is a tightness of the lower eyelid. The skin of the neck and of the chest may also become involved ('Roman breastplate'), while in occasional patients skin involvement is so widespread that all movements become compromised.

Alopecia occurs in scleroderma, though not as frequently as in SLE. It is usually associated with widespread skin involvement and may be severe.

Calcification in the skin and subcutaneous tissues is usually localized to the distal ends of the fingers (Fig. 6.4) though more widespread calcification may occur. Calcification, like distal bone erosion, may occur with or without Raynaud's phenomenon, and X-ray evidence of calcification may be seen early. Widespread calcification in scleroderma skin sometimes carries the eponym Thibierge–Weissenbach syndrome (Fig. 6.5).

Telangiectasia usually occurs on the cheeks and around the lips. It may occasionally be widespread and mimic that seen in hereditary telangiectasia. Pigmentation, including buccal pigmentation, may be prominent and resemble that seen in Addison's disease. Conversely, patches of depigmentation may occur, and especially in black patients, widespread vitiligo may be prominent.

Despite the widespread skin abnormality and circulatory problems, surgical wounds generally heal remarkably well.

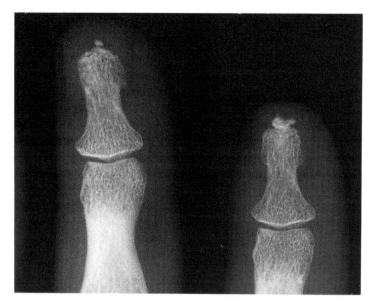

Fig. 6.4 Fingertip calcification in scleroderma.

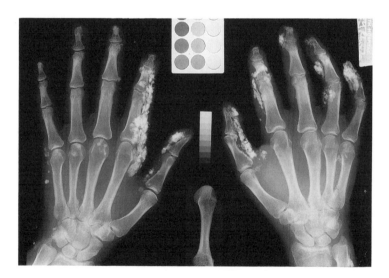

Fig. 6.5 Widespread calcification in skin and subcutaneous tissues in scleroderma. (Dr David Allison, Royal Postgraduate Medical School, Hammersmith Hospital.)

Gastrointestinal tract

Almost all the GI tract may be involved, from microstomia and sicca syndrome affecting the mouth to colonic diverticulosis.

Mouth. Sjøgren's syndrome occurs in scleroderma, and Alarcon-Segovia has drawn attention to the frequency with which Sjøgren's occurs in this disease (Alarcon-Segovia *et al.* 1974). The dryness of the mouth and oesophagus may provide an important contribution to the difficulties of swallowing in some patients. It is also seen in two-thirds of patients with CREST syndrome (Drosos *et al.* 1991).

An increase in collagen in the periodontal membrane may result in widening of this membrane, detectable on X-ray as an increase in trans-lucency around the roots of the teeth, particularly the molars (Fullmer & Witte 1962).

Oesophagus. Oesophageal involvement occurs in the majority of scleroderma patients and often proves to be the most distressing complaint. The most sensitive index of dysfunction is manometry which may detect motility abnormalities even in the absence of symptoms. In early scleroderma, oesophageal pressures are weak and there are incoordinated contractions in the smooth muscle portion (Creamer, Anderson & Code 1956). In advanced cases, a fibrotic change in the smooth muscle layers (predomi-nantly the distal two-thirds) occurs, though neural defects may play a role in pathogenesis. The main complaints are dysphagia and reflux oesoph-agitis. Barium swallow may show delayed or absent peristalsis (Fig. 6.6) and, more importantly, may reveal that swallowing is achieved only in the upright position. Shortening of the oesophagus, stricture and dilatation of the proximal two-thirds are later features. Hiatus hernia is a common finding and this may add to the reflux oesophagitis. Dilatation of the oesophagus is not as marked in achalasia, where sphincter spasm and oesophageal dilatation are far more prominent.

In a prospective study using oesophageal manometry, the course of oesophageal dysfunction was not related to the course or severity of skin or other visceral involvement. Progressive deterioration occurred in over one-half of the patients studied, and in none was improvement or reversal noted. It was pointed out that oesophageal dysfunction is not unique to scleroderma amongst the connective tissue diseases (Fig. 6.7) though the most frequent and gross abnormalities are seen in this condition particularly where Raynaud's phenomenon is marked (Tatelman & Keech 1966; Weiranch & Korting 1982; Takebyashi 1991).

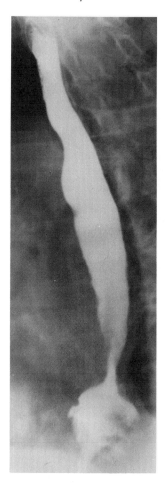

Fig. 6.6 Absent peristalsis and small hiatus hernia in scleroderma. These appearances in themselves are not pathonognomic, and screening or manometry are required to demonstrate the incoordinated contractions.

Stomach and duodenum. Fibrotic involvement of the stomach may lead to gastric dilatation. Duodenal atrophy may be striking (Fig. 6.8), leading to dilatation, and loss of folds (D'Angelo, Fries & Masi 1969; Peacher, Creamer & Pierce 1969).

Small bowel. Malabsorption syndrome and abdominal fullness and cramps are well-known features of scleroderma. As well as collagenous replacement of the muscularis, a number of other factors contribute to the small bowel involvement including deposition of collagen in the submucosal and serosal

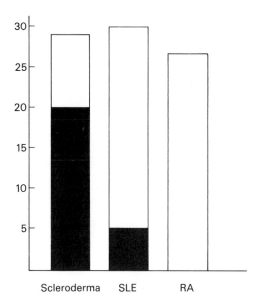

Fig. 6.7 Percentage of cases with abnormal oesophageal motility. (From Tatelman & Keech 1966.)

gut layers, lymphatic obstruction and diminished arterial blood supply leading in rare cases to gangrene. A considerable contribution to the steatorrhoea may be made by alterations in bowel flora due to a 'stagnant loop' syndrome, and broad spectrum antibiotics have proved helpful in some cases. In a series of barium follow-through examinations, Reinhardt and Barry (1962) reported 52 cases of scleroderma in which 44% had abnormalities of small bowel consisting of dilatation and prolongation of transit time. In particular, marked dilatation of the proximal jejunum may be seen radiologically. In one study jejunal sacculation was recognized in 8 of 10 patients with scleroderma (Queloz & Woloshin 1972). Almost all patients with small bowel involvement have oesophageal abnormalities but there is no correlation between small bowel involvement and overall severity, duration or frequency of other organ involvement in scleroderma.

Colon. Dilatation occurs, though in other cases the colon may be rigid in appearance. A very characteristic feature is the presence of wide-mouthed square-shaped pseudodiverticulae of the colon (Fig. 6.9) and some gastro-enterologists even advocate barium enema as a useful diagnostic procedure in scleroderma. The time incidence of these is unknown, however. Intestinal atony may be widespread (Greenberger *et al.* 1968). In one report (Strosberg, Peck & Harris 1977) two members of the same family developed fatal

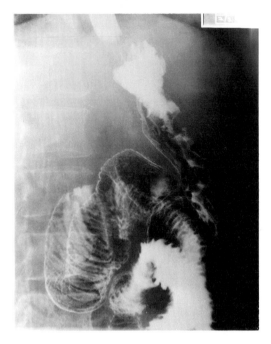

Fig. 6.8 Dilatation of the second part of the duodenum in scleroderma. (Dr David Allison, Royal Postgraduate Medical School.)

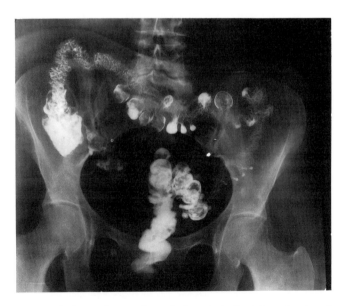

Fig. 6.9 Wide-mouthed sacculations ('pseudodiverticulae') of the colon in scleroderma.

complications of intestinal scleroderma. Faecal impaction can occur and it is common to see incomplete emptying of the barium after a barium enema. A rare, but well recognized, complication of scleroderma is pneumatosis cystoides intestinalis, recognized as radiolucent cysts or streaks of gas within the bowel wall and mesentery (White, Treece & Juniper 1970).

Liver disease

While earlier large series failed to demonstrate liver involvement in scleroderma, a number of subsequent reports have pointed to an association between portal hypertension and primary biliary cirrhosis and scleroderma or its variants (CREST syndrome and sclerodactyly). In 1971 Reynolds *et al.* described six female patients with pruritus, jaundice and hepatomegaly, associated with widespread telangiectasis, resembling those seen in the Rendu−Osler−Weber (hereditary telangiectasia) syndrome. Other features of the CREST syndrome (calcinosis, Raynaud's, and sclerodactyly) were present to a varying degree. Liver histology showed primary biliary cirrhosis.

The serological marker of those patients having primary biliary cirrhosis and scleroderma is the anticentromere antibody (Bernstein *et al.* 1982).

Pulmonary

Pulmonary involvement in scleroderma (Table 6.2) is an early and frequent finding. The fibrotic process which affects the lungs is concentrated predominantly in the lower lobes, often sparing the apices and hilar regions. Pulmonary function abnormalities may be detected well before the patient becomes symptomatic, and dyspnoea as a presenting complaint is uncommon (Godfrey, Bluestone & Higgs 1969). Arterial desaturation may develop during exercise. Pulmonary function tests do not necessarily correlate with

Table 6.2 Pulmonary manifestations of scleroderma

Pulmonary fibrosis
Honeycombing
Reflux pneumonitis
Chest infections
Pulmonary hypertension
Pleural thickening and calcification
Pneumoconiosis
Alveolar-cell carcinoma
Pulmonary vasculitis

the extent of clinical involvement with the disease. The commonest physical findings are of hyperventilation and of scattered medium crepitations in both lower lung fields. Later, heart failure and pulmonary hypertension may supervene (reviewed by Pronk & Swaak 1991). Clubbing is rare. Late changes include cystic changes, pleural thickening and bronchiectasis, the last possibly related to repeated chest infections. Aspiration pneumonia and opportunistic infection may occur.

Pulmonary function tests show restrictive ventilatory impairment, reduced transfer factor and compliance, and progressive hypoxaemia during exercise. Airway conductance and gas distribution are little affected (Laitinen, Salorinne & Poppius 1973). Chest X-rays in later stages show diffuse mottling and linear densities in the basal regions. Later a symmetrical pulmonary fibrosis occurs. In other patients small cystic changes occur in the periphery of the lung fields, which may become sufficiently numerous to lead to a honeycomb lung.

A rare complication of severe fibrotic lung disease is alveolar cell or bronchiolar carcinoma. These mainly peripheral tumours may remain small and undetected during life (Richards & Milne 1958; Tompkin 1969). Pulmonary hypertension is a frequent cause of death in scleroderma. In some cases it occurs in the absence of pulmonary fibrosis (Young & Mark 1978; Ungerer et al. 1983). It may develop insidiously and, rarely, is the presenting manifestation of the disease (Wade & Ball 1957). One interesting but unexplained finding is the high prevalence of scleroderma in coal miners, gold miners and stone masons (Rodnan et al. 1967).

Cardiovascular

The heart is involved in up to 50% of scleroderma patients. Primary myocardial fibrosis and conduction defects are described as well as fibrotic pericarditis (D'Angelo, Fries & Masi 1969). A variety of ECG abnormalities occur, including prolonged PR, QRS and QT intervals, ST and T wave abnormalities. Techniques such as thallium scans show abnormalities in over 80% of patients (Fallansbe et al. 1984). Prognostic cardiac features in scleroderma have been received by Clements et al. (1991).

Kidney

Clinical renal disease is usually a late manifestation of scleroderma. Its presence has severe prognostic implications (see below). The hallmark of renal involvement is hypertension, often sudden in onset. Malignant hypertension may develop rapidly, especially if the patient is treated with corticosteroids.

Case report. *A man in his fifties with active systemic sclerosis was admitted to hospital for investigation. He had active skin involvement with pulmonary abnormalities and clinical and EMG evidence of myopathy. His blood pressure was 160/100 and fundi showed nipping. He was started on 20 mg prednisone. Twenty-four hours later he complained of headache and visual impairment. He was found to have gross papilloedema. His blood pressure was 220/140. He responded to hypotensive therapy, but over the ensuing year showed marked deterioration in renal function.*

Less frequently there may be proteinuria for many years before the advent of other evidence of renal involvement.

The renal manifestations of scleroderma have been reviewed by Donohoe (1992).

Muscles and joints

Myopathy and inflammatory myositis are important features of scleroderma, and have, if anything, been underemphasized in their importance. Enzyme elevations are unusual and EMG abnormalities are predominantly seen in those with myositis. Muscle weakness may, however, be extreme, and an almost characteristic feature in some late cases is weakness and wasting of the neck muscles, particularly posteriorly, so that the unfortunate patient cannot hold her head up without the aid of a support collar. In a study of 53 patients with typical scleroderma, Medsger *et al.* (1968) found that the majority had clinical and biochemical features of a myopathy. Proximal weakness especially of the shoulder girdle was common. Microscopic involvement of muscle fibres or interstitium was present in 14 of 36 cases, the most consistent abnormality being interstitial fibrosis.

In another study, 23 out of 24 patients with systemic sclerosis were found to have muscular involvement and three had inflammatory muscle disease (Clements *et al.* 1978).

In one-quarter of scleroderma patients, a true polyarthritis occurs, usually early in the course of the disease, and involving predominantly small joints (Rodnan 1962). In later stages joint limitation and stiffness is mainly due to the rigidity of the surrounding tissues. A characteristic finding is leathery crepitus on movement, observed best in the patella and in the flexor and extensor tendons of the wrist.

Joint erosions do not usually occur. While bone changes are predominantly confined to the distal phalanges, osteolysis of the distal end of the radius and ulna, of the acromioclavicular joint, of the femoral head, and even of the cervical spine and ribs have been described (Haverbush *et al.* 1974), as well as resorption of the mandible (Siefert, Steigerwald & Cliff 1975).

Other

The anaemia of scleroderma is usually 'inflammatory' though autoimmune haemolytic anaemia and thrombocytopenia may also occur (Ivey, Hwang & Sheets 1971; Rosenthal & Sack 1971). In rare cases a systemic vasculitis is prominent and in such cases cardiac, cerebral and bowel infarctions may occur.

Trigeminal neuropathy was reported in five patients (Ashworth & Tait 1971). An association between progeria and scleroderma in infancy has been observed (Feingold & Kidd 1971) and between scleroderma and lichen sclerosis (Gordon, Kahn & Dove 1972).

Association with malignancy

Apart from the rare complication of alveolar cell carcinoma, no firm association of scleroderma with malignancy exists. A number of isolated cases of associated malignancy (especially breast) and scleroderma have been reported, and we were impressed some years ago in New York Hospital, by the simultaneous coincidence in two patients of breast cancer and rapidly developing scleroderma. In view of the similarities in some cases to dermatomyositis, an increased tendency to malignancy might be forecast in scleroderma, but at the present time aggressive investigation for occult neoplasms is unwarranted in these patients.

VARIANTS OF SCLERODERMA

Mixed connective tissue disease

This syndrome, in which features of SLE, dermatomyositis and scleroderma all occur is discussed in Chapter 8.

Scleroderma with positive LE cell tests. Dubois, in reviewing 81 cases of scleroderma and/or morphoea, noted 9 in whom features of SLE were also present (Dubois *et al*. 1971). It is possible that a number of these cases fitted the picture subsequently described as mixed connective tissue disease.

Localized scleroderma (reviewed by Clements 1992)

A number of forms of localized scleroderma are recognized in dermatological practice and these are dealt with briefly here.

Morphoea. Localized patches of scleroderma, sometimes violaceous or lilac and sometimes itchy, may appear on any part of the body. They are raised, clearly demarcated and often indurated. A 'guttate' form occurs, with 'raindrop' appearance. Morphoea may be widespread and chronic and may involve the fingers with acrosclerosis and contractures. Nonetheless, the condition does not involve internal organs, and therefore requires differentiation from systemic sclerosis proper. Only 1 of 44 patients with generalized morphoea reported by Christianson, Dorsey and O'Leary (1956) had systemic involvement.

Linear scleroderma. The most well-known area for this white, scar-like localized form of scleroderma is the forehead, stretching from the nose to the forehead ('coup de sabre') or sternum. A more widespread lesion on the face may be associated with hemiatrophy of the face.

CRST syndrome. A group of patients with prominent cutaneous manifestations of calcinosis, Raynaud's, sclerodactyly and telangiectasia is recognized, in whom visceral involvement (other than oesophageal) is absent or minimal. In the original group described by Winterbauer (1964), the telangiectasia was prominent and difficult to differentiate from Rendu–Osler–Weber syndrome, though bleeding from the telangiectasia was rare.

While a minority of patients with CRST syndrome have evidence of systemic sclerosis, widespread systemic involvement is rare. Oesophageal motility disturbances are common, leading to the alternative nickname CREST (or CROST in the UK, presumably).

This condition is not altogether benign — a late complication in some patients is pulmonary hypertension.

Eosinophilic fasciitis (Shulman's syndrome)

A further possible variant of scleroderma was described by Shulman (1974) who reported a group of patients with diffuse fasciitis, hyperglobulinaemia and eosinophilia. None of the patients had Raynaud's phenomenon, impaired oesophageal motility or visceral sclerosis. ANF or extractable nuclear antigen were not detected. Further cases are coming to light (Rodnan *et al.* 1975; Schumacher 1976) and the syndrome is yet to be fully defined. The prognosis appears to be more favourable than that in scleroderma, though rare cases have been reported in association with aplastic anaemia.

Acro-osteolysis

This rare condition, with Raynaud's and painful swelling of the distal phalanges and subcutaneous calcification, sometimes leading to a chalky discharge from the fingers, is sometimes associated with other congenital bony abnormalities.

An interesting association of this condition with industrial exposure to vinyl chloride has been described (Dinman, Cook & Whitehouse 1971). Twenty-five cases of acro-osteolysis were seen among 5011 employees in a plant employing a process of vinyl chloride cleaning of polymerizers. Clinical features included Raynaud's, joint pains, synovial and skin thickening, tendon thickening and oesophageal abnormalities. Radiological changes included marginal erosion and resorption in phalanges, transverse defects, and, interestingly, sacroiliac joint involvement (reviewed in the Symposium on the Fibrotic Processes 1977). One study has suggested a genetic predisposition, associated with HLA DR5 (Black *et al.* 1983).

Eosinophilia-myalgia syndrome; toxic oil syndrome

In 1989, an epidemic characterized by myalgia and eosinophilia, related to the ingestion of certain chemicals, notably L-tryptophan, was recognized. Some features of this syndrome were similar to the far more deadly toxic oil syndrome which occurred in Spain in 1981. The clinical features include muscle pain, fasciitis, eosinophilia, dyspnoea and cough, neuropathy and CNS involvement (reviewed by Silver 1992).

LABORATORY

Positive ANA tests are found in up to 60% of scleroderma patients (see Appendix). Anti-centromere antibodies are found both in scleroderma (Catoggio *et al.* 1983) and in a subset of patients with primary biliary cirrhosis and scleroderma (Bernstein *et al.* 1982, 1986).

An increasing number of antibodies are being detected in scleroderma. Their clinical significance is as yet uncertain.

DNA antibodies are not found in scleroderma, and there is little to suggest a major contribution of immune-complex formation to pathogenesis.

Raised gammaglobulin levels and positive tests for rheumatoid factor are found in one-third of patients. False-positive tests for syphilis are sometimes seen (Clark, Winkelmann & Ward 1971). The sedimentation rate is raised in one-third of scleroderma patients, raised values tending to be associated with the presence of myositis and with more rapidly progressive disease in general (Tuffanelli & Winkelmann 1961).

TREATMENT
(reviewed by Medsger 1991; Wiglem 1992)

'No drug has been proved totally ineffective until it has been tried in scleroderma'.

Sadly, this gloomy comment, introduced in the first edition, still holds true in the fourth.

This feeling is widespread amongst physicians. Few diseases in their advanced stages cause so much distress to patients and feelings of helplessness in their doctors. One review, for example, listed 35 drugs and 'therapeutic agents' which have been recommended for this disease. Table 6.3 lists some of the drugs in use in scleroderma, under the general headings 'vasoactive', 'antiinflammatory' and 'experimental'.

D-penicillamine has been used in scleroderma for a quarter of a century, but as yet there is no conclusive evidence that it is effective. Nevertheless, two studies in 1991 suggested benefits in skin scleroderma and possibly overall survival (Staen 1991; Jimenez & Sigal 1991). Other agents tried include photopheresis (Edelson 1991), methotrexate and cyclosporin A, though the last may have potentially hazardous additive effects as far as the vasculopathy is concerned (Bunchman & Brookshine 1991). One undoubted advance in the management of the ischaemic vascular problems of scleroderma has come with the use of infusions of the prostacyclin analogue Iloprost (Torley 1991). In our own practice at St Thomas', we repeatedly see a timely infusion of Ilioprost 'carrying the patient through' the cold months of January and February.

Corticosteroids are contraindicated in most cases. That being said, there are occasional patients in whom corticosteroid therapy is valuable, particularly where early inflammatory features predominate, or where myositis is active (Medsger 1991). Steroids are generally unhelpful in more advanced pulmonary fibrosis and in scleroderma renal disease. Broadspectrum antibiotics should be tried where malabsorption syndrome is prominent. Careful management of reflux oesophagitis is important, and the development of omeprazole has proved a major advance in this area.

PROGNOSIS

Survival in scleroderma varies from one month to 23 years (D'Angelo, Fries & Masi 1969). Bennett *et al.* (1971) reviewed the prognosis of 67 scleroderma patients using life-table methods. Five-year survival was 73%. The overall features found at initial diagnosis which suggested an adverse prognosis were age (especially over 40), trunk involvement, and, as expected, major visceral involvement. While renal involvement was of high prognostic significance, interestingly none of the patients for whom the cause of

Table 6.3 Drugs used in scleroderma (adapted from Winkelman *et al.* 1971)

Vasoactive drugs
Phenoxybenzamine
Tolazoline
Methyldopa
Guanethidine
Reserpine
Nicotinic acid
Procaine
Prostacyclin infusions

Antiinflammatory
Salicylates
p-Aminobenzoic acid
Indomethacin and phenylbutazone
Antimalarials
Corticosteroids
Azathioprine (? pure antiinflammatory effect)

Experimental
Calcium antagonists:
  Nifedipine
Oedema-reducing:
  p-Aminobenzoic acid
  ε-Aminocaproic acid
  Disodium etidronate
Hormones:
  Corticosteroids
  Relaxin
  Progesterone
Lathyrogens:
  Penicillamine
Immunosuppressives:
Alkylating agents
Azathioprine
Methotrexate
Cyclophosphamide
? Colchicine

death was known died of renal failure. It may be that renal involvement, like trunk involvement, is present only when there is extensive visceral involvement elsewhere. Somewhat different is the experience of LeRoy & Fleischmann (1978) who reported renal failure in 25 of 100 patients with scleroderma seen over a five-year period. Some encouragement was given by the survival of a patient in this series following renal transplantation.

A more recent prospective study of 264 patients showed a linear decline in survival. The cumulative survival rate was 80% at 2 years, 50% at 8.5 years and 30% at 12 years (Altman *et al.* 1991).

REFERENCES

Alarcon-Segovia D., Ibañez G., Kershenobich D. & Rojkind M. (1974) Treatment of scleroderma. *Lancet*, i, 1054.

Altman R.D., Medsger T.A. Jr, Bloch D.A. *et al.* (1991) Predictors of survival in systemic sclerosis. *Arthritis and Rheumatism*, **34**, 403–413.

Ashworth B. & Tait G.B.W. (1971) Trigeminal neuropathy in connective tissue disease. *Neurology*, **21**, 609.

Bennett R.M., Bluestone R.H., Holt P.J.L. & Bywaters E.G.L. (1971) Survival in scleroderma. *Annals of the Rheumatic Diseases*, **30**, 581.

Bernstein R.M., Callender M.E., Neuberger J.M. & Hughes G.R.V. (1982) Anticentromere antibody in primary biliary cirrhosis. *Annals of the Rheumatic Diseases*, **41**, 612–614.

Bernstein R.M., Morgan S.H., Bunn C.C., Gainey R.C., Hughes G.R.V. & Mathews M.B. (1986) The SL auto antibody–antigen system: clinical and biochemical studies: *Annals of the Rheumatic Diseases*, **45**, 353–358.

Black C.M., Welsh K.I., Walker A.C. *et al.* (1983) Genetic susceptibility to scleroderma-like syndrome induced by vinyl chloride. *Lancet*, i, 53–55.

Brady A.H. (1975) Collagenase in scleroderma. *Journal of Clinical Investigation*, **56**, 1175.

Catoggio L.J., Bernstein R.M., Black C.M., Hughes G.R.V. & Maddison P.J. (1983) Serological markers in progressive systemic sclerosis: clinical correlations. *Annals of the Rheumatic Diseases*, **42**, 23–27.

Christianson H.B., Dorsey C.S. & O'Leary R.A. (1956) Localized scleroderma: a clinical study of 235 cases. *Archives of Dermatology*, **74**, 629.

Clark J.A., Winkelmann R.K. & Ward L.E. (1971) Serologic alterations in scleroderma and sclerodermatomyositis. *Mayo Clinic Proceedings*, **46**, 104.

Clements P. (1992) Clinical aspects of localized and systemic sclerosis. *Current Opinion in Rheumatology*, **4**, 843–850.

Clements P.J., Furst D.E., Campion D.S., Bohan A., Harris R., Levy J. & Paulus H.E. (1978) Muscle disease in progressive systemic sclerosis. *Arthritis and Rheumatism*, **21**, 62.

Clements P.J., Lachenbruch P.A., Furst D.E. *et al.* (1991) Cardiac score: a semiquantitative measure of cardiac involvement that improves prediction of prognosis in systemic sclerosis. *Arthritis and Rheumatism*, **34**, 1371–1380.

Creamer B., Anderson H.A. & Code C.F. (1956) Esophageal motility in patients with scleroderma and related diseases. *Gastroenterologia*, **86**, 763.

Curtis A.C. & Shulak B.M. (1965) Scleroderma adultorum: not always a benign self-limiting disease. *Archives of Dermatology*, **92**, 526.

D'Angelo W.A., Fries J.F. & Masi A.T. (1969) Pathologic observations in systemic sclerosis (scleroderma). A study of 58 autopsy cases. *American Journal of Medicine*, **46**, 428.

Dinman B.D., Cook W.A. & Whitehouse W.M. (1971) Occupational acro-osteolysis. I. An epidemiological study. *Archives of Environmental Health*, **22**, 61.

Dononhoe J.F. (1992) Scleroderma and the kidney. *Kidney International*, **41**, 462–477.

Drosos A.A., Lagos G., Moutsopoulos H. *et al.* (1991) Sjogren's syndrome in patients with the CREST variant of progressive systemic scleroderma. *Journal of Rheumatology*, **18**, 1685–1688.

Dubois E.L., Chandor S., Friou G.J. & Bischel M. (1971) Progressive systemic sclerosis and localized scleroderma (morphoea) with positive LE cell test and unusual systemic manifestations compatible with SLE. *Medicine*, **50**, 199.

Edelson R.L. (1991) Photopheresis in the treatment of autoimmune disease. *Annals of the New York Academy of Science*, **636**, 209–216.

Fallansbe W.D., Curtis E.I., Medsger T.A. Jr *et al.* (1984) Physiologic abnormalities of cardiac function in progressive systemic sclerosis with diffuse scleroderma. *New England Journal of Medicine*, **310**, 142.

Feingold M. & Kidd R. (1971) Progeria and scleroderma in infancy. *American Journal of Diseases of Children*, **122**, 61.

Fleischmajer R. (1964) The collagen in scleroderma. *Archives of Dermatology*, **89**, 437.

Fleischmajer R., Damiano V. & Nedwich A. (1971) Scleroderma and the subcutaneous tissue. *Science*, **171**, 1019.

Fox R.J. & Kang H.I. (1992) Genetic and environmental factors in systemic sclerosis. *Current Opinion in Rheumatology*, **4**, 857–861.

Fullmer H.M. & Witte W.E. (1962) Periodontal membrane affected by scleroderma. A histochemical study. *Archives of Pathology*, **73**, 184.

Godfrey S., Bluestone R. & Higgs B.E. (1969) Lung function and the response to exercise in systemic sclerosis. *Thorax*, **24**, 427.

Gordon W., Kahn L.B. & Dove J. (1972) Lichen sclerosis et atrophicus and scleroderma. *South African Medical Journal*, **46**, 160.

Graham-Brown R.A.C. & Sarkany I. (1983) Scleroderma-like changes due to chronic graft-versus-host disease. *Clinical and Experimental Dermatology*, **8**, 531–538.

Greenberger N.J., Dobbins W.O., Ruppert R.D. *et al.* (1968) Intestinal systemic sclerosis. *American Journal of Medicine*, **45**, 301.

Haverbush T.J., Wilde A.H., Hawk W.A. & Sherbel A.L. (1974) Osteolysis of the ribs, and cervical spine in progressive systemic sclerosis (scleroderma). *Journal of Bone and Joint Surgery*, **56A**, 23.

Herbert C.M., Lindberg K.A., Jayson M.I.V. & Bailey A.J. (1974) Biosynthesis and maturation of skin collagen in scleroderma, and effect of D-penicillamine. *Lancet*, **i**, 187.

Hughes G.L. (1984) Autoantibodies in lupus and its variants: experience in 1000 patients. *British Medical Journal*, **289**, 339–342.

Ivey K.J., Hwang Y.F. & Sheets R.F. (1971) Scleroderma associated with thrombocytopenia and Coombs-positive haemolytic anaemia. *American Journal of Medicine*, **51**, 815.

Jimenez S. & Sigal S. (1991) A 15-year prospective study of treatment of rapidly progressive systemic sclerosis with D-penicillamine. *Journal of Rheumatology*, **18**, 1496–1503.

Kahaleh M.B. & LeRoy E.C. (1983) Endothelial injury in scleroderma: a protease mechanism. *Journal of Laboratory and Clinical Medicine*, **101**, 553–560.

Kallenberg C.G.M. (1992) Overlapping syndrome, undifferentiated connective tissue disease and other fibrosing conditions. *Current Opinion in Rheumatology*, **4**, 837–842.

Laitinen O., Salorinne Y. & Poppius H. (1973) Respiratory function in systemic lupus erythematosus, scleroderma and rheumatoid arthritis. *Annals of the Rheumatic Diseases*, **32**, 531.

Lally E.V. (1992) Raynaud's phenomenon. *Current Opinion in Rheumatology*, **4**, 825–836.

LeRoy E.C. (1974) Increased collagen synthesis by scleroderma skin fibroblasts *in vitro*. *Journal of Clinical Investigation*, **54**, 880.

LeRoy E.C. (1976) Scleroderma. In: *Topics in Rheumatology*. Ed: G.R.V. Hughes, Heinemann, London.

LeRoy E.C. & Fleischmann R.M. (1978) The management of renal scleroderma. *American Journal of Medicine*, **64**, 974.

Maricq H.R., Weinberger A.B. & LeRoy E.C. (1982) Early detection of scleroderma-spectrum disorders by *in-vivo* capillary microscopy: a prospective study of patients with Raynaud's phenomenon. *Journal of Rheumatology*, **9**, 289–291.

Maricq H.R. & LeRoy E.E. (1973) Patterns of finger capillary abnormalities in connective tissue diseases by 'wide field' microscopy. *Arthritis and Rheumatism*, **16**, 619.

Medsger T. (1991) Treatment of systemic sclerosis. *Annals of the Rheumatic Diseases*, **50**, 877–886.

Medsger T.A. & Masi A.T. (1971) Epidemiology of systemic sclerosis. *Annals of Internal Medicine*, **74**, 714.

Medsger T.A., Rodnan G.P., Moossy J. & Vester J.W. (1968) Skeletal muscle involvement in progressive systemic sclerosis (scleroderma). *Arthritis and Rheumatism*, **II**, 554.

Needleman B.W. (1992) Immunologic aspects of scleroderma. *Current Opinion in Rheumatology*, **4**, 862–868.

Neldner K.H., Jones J.D. & Winkelmann R.K. (1966) Scleroderma: dermal amino acid composition with particular reference to hydroxyproline. *Proceedings of the Society for Experimental Biology and Medicine*, **122**, 39.

Norton W.L., Hurd E.R. & Lewis D.C. (1969) Evidence of a microvascular injury in scleroderma and systemic lupus erythematosus: quantitative study of the microvascular bed. *Journal of Laboratory and Clinical Medicine*, **71**, 919.

Peacher R.D.G., Creamer B. & Pierce J.W. (1969) Sclerodermatous involvement of the stomach and the small and large bowel. *Gut*, **10**, 285.

Pronk L.C. & Swaak A. (1991) Pulmonary hypertension in connective tissue disease — report of three cases and review of the literature. *Rheumatology International*, **11**, 83–86.

Queloz J.M. & Woloshin H.J. (1972) Sacculation of the small intestine in scleroderma. *Radiology*, **105**, 513.

Reidhardt J.F. & Barry W.F. (1962) Scleroderma of the small bowel. *American Journal of Roentgenology*, **88**, 687.

Reveille J.D., Overbach D., Goldstein R. *et al.* (1992) Association of polar aminoacids at position 26 of the HLA-DQB1 first domain with the anticentromere autoantibody response in systemic sclerosis. *Journal of Clinical Investigation*, **89**, 1208–1213.

Reynolds T.B., Denison E.K., Frankel H.D., Lieberman F.L. & Peters R.L. (1971) Primary biliary cirrhosis with scleroderma, Raynaud's phenomenon and telangiectasia. *American Journal of Medicine*, **50**, 302.

Richards R.C. & Milne J.A. (1958) Cancer of the lung in progressive systemic sclerosis. *Thorax*, **13**, 238.

Rodnan G.P. (1962) The nature of joint involvement in progressive systemic sclerosis. *Annals of Internal Medicine*, **56**, 422.

Rodnan G.P., Benedek T.G., Medsger T.A. & Cammarata R.J. (1967) The association of progressive systemic sclerosis (scleroderma) with coal miners' pneumoconiosis and other forms of silicosis. *Annals of Internal Medicine*, **66**, 323.

Rodnan G.P., DiBartolomeo A., Medsger T.A. *et al.* (1975) Eosinophilic fasciitis — a report of six cases of a newly recognized scleroderma like syndrome (abstract). *Clinical Research*, **23**, 443.

Rodnan G.P. & Fennell R.H. Jr (1962) Progressive systemic sclerosis sine scleroderma. *Journal of the American Medical Association*, **180**, 665.

Rosenthal D.S. & Sack B. (1971) Autoimmune haemolytic anaemia in scleroderma. *Journal of the American Medical Association*, **216**, 2011.

Shanahan W.R. & Korn J.H. (1982) Cytotoxic activity of sera from scleroderma and other connective tissue diseases: lack of cellular and disease specificity. *Arthritis and*

Rheumatism, **25**, 1391–1395.

Schumacher H.R. (1976) A scleroderma like syndrome with fasciitis, myositis and oesinophilia. *Annals of Internal Medicine*, **84**, 49.

Shulman L.E. (1974) Diffuse fasciitis with hyperglobulinaemia and eosinophilia. A new syndrome? (abstract). *Journal of Rheumatology*, **1** (Suppl. 1), 46.

Siefert M.H., Steigerwald J.C. & Cliff M.M. (1975) Bone resorption of the mandible in progressive systemic sclerosis. *Arthritis and Rheumatism*, **18**, 507.

Silver R.M. (1992) Eosinophilia-myalgia syndrome, toxic-oil syndrome, and diffuse fasciitis with eosinophilia. *Current Opinion in Rheumatology*, **4**, 851–856.

Smith E.A. (1992) Connective tissue metabolism including cytokines in scleroderma. *Current Opinion in Rheumatology*, **4**, 869–877.

Steen V.D. (1991) D-Penicillamine treatment in systemic sclerosis. *Journal of Rheumatology*, **18**, 1435–1437.

Strosberg J.M., Peck B. & Harris E.D. (1977) Scleroderma with intestinal involvement: fatal in two of a kindred. *Journal of Rheumatology*, **4**, 46.

Symposium on the Fibrotic Processes (1977) *Annals of the Rheumatic Diseases* (Suppl. 2), **36**.

Takebayashi S. (1991) Cervical oesophageal motility: evaluation with US in progressive systemic sclerosis. *Radiology*, **179**, 389–393.

Tatelman M. & Keech M.K. (1966) Esophageal motility in SLE, RA and scleroderma. *Radiology*, **86**, 1041.

Thompson R.P., Harper F.E., Maize J.C. *et al.* (1984) Nailfold biopsy in scleroderma and related disorders: correlation of histologic, capillaroscopic and clinical data. *Arthritis and Rheumatism*, **27**, 97–104.

Tompkin G.H. (1969) Systemic sclerosis associated with carcinoma of the lung. *British Journal of Dermatology*, **81**, 213.

Torley H.I. (1991) A double blind, randomized, multicentre comparison of 2 doses of intravenous iloprost in the treatment of Raynaud's phenomenon secondary to connective tissue disease. *Annals of the Rheumatic Diseases*, **50**, 800–804.

Tuffanelli D.L. & Winkelmann R.K. (1961) Systemic scleroderma: a clinical study of 727 cases. *Archives of Dermatology*, **84**, 359.

Uitto J., Ohlenschaege K. & Lorenzen I. (1971) Solubility of skin collagen in normal human subjects and in patients with generalized scleroderma. *Clinica Chimica Acta*, **31**, 13.

Ungerer R.G., Tashkin D.P., Furst D. *et al.* (1983) Prevalence and clinical correlates of pulmonary arterial hypertension in progressive systemic sclerosis. *American Journal of Medicine*, **75**, 65–74.

Wade G. & Ball J. (1957) Unexplained pulmonary hypertension. *Quarterly Journal of Medicine*, **26**, 83.

Weiranch T.R. & Korting G.W. (1982) Manometric assessment of oesophageal involvement in progressive systemic sclerosis, morphea and Raynaud's disease. *British Journal of Dermatology*, **107**, 325–332.

White W.O., Treece T.R. & Juniper J. (1970) Pneumatosis scleroderma of the small bowel. *Journal of the American Medical Association*, **212**, 1068.

Wigley F.M. (1992) Treatment of systemic sclerosis. *Current Opinion in Rheumatology*, **4**, 878–886.

Winkelmann R.K., Kierland R.R., Perry H.O., Muller S.A. & Sams W.M. (1971) Management of scleroderma. *Mayo Clinic Proceedings*, **46**, 128.

Winterbauer R.H. (1964) Multiple telangiectasia, Raynaud's phenomenon, sclerodactyly and subcutaneous calcinosis: a syndrome mimicking hereditary haemorrhagic telangiectasia. *Bulletin of the Johns Hopkins Hospital*, **114**, 361.

Young R.H. & Mark G.J. (1978) Pulmonary vascular changes in scleroderma. *American Journal of Medicine*, **64**, 998.

7: *Polymyositis and Dermatomyositis*

Dermatomyositis, once thought to be a rare disease, is now considered to be one of the more common myopathies. Childhood myositis, because of frequent and prominent vasculitic complications, is usually considered as a distinct entity. Adult polymyositis may be acute or chronic in onset, with or without the characteristic rash, and associated in a proportion of cases with an underlying malignancy. In the large series reported by Pearson (1966), 70% presented primarily with muscle involvement, 25% cutaneous and 5% with 'systemic' features such as weight loss and fever. The disease is commonest in the fifties and sixties with a slight female predominance.

PATHOLOGY

In the skin there is collagenous thickening of the dermis, with epidermal atrophy. The dermis is infiltrated by lymphocytes, plasma cells and histiocytes, often in perivascular accumulations (Fig. 7.1, A, B). Chronic progression of skin changes may lead to a thin atrophic epidermis, with an increase in fibrosis resembling scleroderma. Calcium deposition may occur, sometimes in sheets.

In skeletal muscle there is widespread degeneration of muscle fibres, with hyalinization, swelling, vacuolation and disruption of muscle cells. At the same time, regeneration of other muscle cells may be seen. Between the muscle fibres there is a chronic inflammatory cell infiltrate, especially of lymphocytes. At a later stage there may be fibrosis and extensive muscle atrophy, often difficult to distinguish on muscle biopsy from muscular dystrophy. The myocardium may be similarly affected though florid involvement is unusual (Adams 1975).

AETIOLOGY

During the past few years a number of contributions to the understanding of the pathogenesis of this disease have been made.

Genetic

A number of reports of multiple cases within the same family have

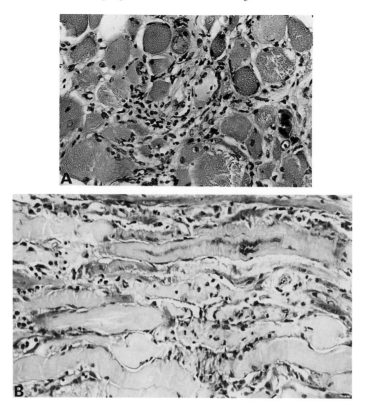

Fig. 7.1 A, Cross-section (× 340) and B, longitudinal section (× 210) of muscle in acute polymyositis, showing inflammatory cells and necrotic muscle fibres.

appeared. A patient with polymyositis associated with a deficiency of C_2 has been seen (Leddy *et al.* 1975) suggesting aetiology factors similar to some cases of SLE with genetic complement deficiencies. An association with the haplotype HLA B8, DR3, DRw52 has been suggested (reviewed by Miller 1991).

Cellular immunity (reviewed by Kalovidouris 1992)

Immunohistology of muscle biopsies in active disease shows T cells bearing activating matters such as major histocompatibility complex class II antigens in close proximity to muscle cells, and under certain experimental circumstances, direct cytotoxicity of these cells on autologous muscle can be demonstrated.

Studies using monoclonal antibodies have suggested that cytokines and adhesion molecules may play an important role in the accumulation of T cells in affected muscles.

Humoral immunity

Several autoantibodies have been demonstrated in the sera of patients with myositis. They fall into two main groups — tissue specific (directed against muscle antigens) and a second group that react with nuclear or cytoplasmic antigens of a variety of tissues (Table 7.1). The role of these autoantibodies is uncertain, but some, including some cases of anti-Jo1 antibody have been detectable months before the onset of disease. For an excellent review of the topic, the reader is referred to Miller (1991).

Malignancy

Some controversy exists over the exact strength of the association with malignancy, recognized for over 100 years. One study in 1960 noted that 12 out of 35 patients with dermatomyositis had malignancies and Barnes (1976) also reported that dermatomyositis presented a stronger association than myositis alone, the incidence of malignancy being five- to sevenfold that of the general population.

However, these figures have been questioned. Large prospective studies (Bohan *et al.* 1977) have found possibly associated malignancies in less

Table 7.1 Autoantibodies in myositis (adapted from Kalovidoursis 1992, with permission)

Specificity	Prevalence (%)
Anti-muscle (myosin, myoglobin)	80−90
ANA	25−70
AntiLa	5−20
AntiRo	10−15
Antithyroglobulin	6−10
Rheumatoid factor	4−8
Myositis-associated ANA	
AntiPM-Sd	8
AntiMi-2	5
Myositis-associated anticytoplasmic antibodies	
AntiJo-1 (histidyl t-RNA synthetase)	4
AntiPL7 (threonylt-RNAsynthetase)	3
AntiPL12 (alanyl t-RNA synthetase)	2

than 9%, the patients all being over 40 years of age. No clear pattern of disease or response to treatment of the tumour was seen.

In another study, 57 patients who had dermatomyositis with malignancies were analyzed. It was concluded that a 'blind' malignancy search was not of value, the diagnosis almost always being apparent clinically or on routine laboratory and X-ray screening (Callen 1982).

Inclusion particles

A variety of these particles has now been described, including nuclear micro-tubular inclusions in some cases of chronic progressive myositis (Schochet & McCormick 1973), endothelial tubuloreticular inclusions in a number of patients with dermatomyositis (Norton, Kelayos & Robinson 1970; Hashimoto *et al.* 1971), and crystalline picornavirus-like structures in cases of severe fulminant dermatomyositis (Chou & Gutmann 1970). Their significance, if any, is unknown.

We have observed raised Coxsackie B virus neutralization titres in patients with early polymyositis (Travers *et al.* 1977) and Coxsackie B virus has been implaced in polymyositis in certain neonatal mouse strains (reviewed by Miller 1991).

CLINICAL FEATURES
(see Table 7.2) (reviewed by Bohan & Peter 1975;
Bohan *et al.* 1977)

Myositis

In the most common presentation, there is progressive symmetrical muscle weakness. Despite the inflammatory nature, muscle pain is not prominent and may be absent. Proximal muscles are affected more severely, especially those of the thigh. Thus the presenting complaint may be of weakness on climbing stairs or on standing after a sitting position. In acute polymyositis, oedema overlying the affected muscles may be marked (Fig. 7.2).

As the weakness progresses, muscle wasting and atrophy occur and the tendon reflexes become difficult and ultimately impossible to elicit. The neck muscles are frequently involved. In more widespread disease, pharyngeal muscle involvement leads to dysphagia and a nasal voice. In adults, respiratory muscle involvement is a late stage, though in children it may occur early and insidiously. There is no sensory loss or muscle fasiculation and involvement of the ocular muscles is rare. In late chronic stages muscle contractures become a major problem.

Table 7.2 Percentage of clinical signs and symptoms in 133 cases of polymyositis (from Barwick & Walton 1963).

Sign/Symptom	Percentage
Musculature	
Weakness	
Proximal	99
arms	80
legs	35
Distal	65
Neck flexors	62
Dysphagia	5
Facial muscles	2
Extraocular muscles	48
Pain or tenderness	35
Contractures	35
Atrophy	
Skin	
Typical 'heliotrope' rash	40
'Atypical' rash	20
Other	
Raynaud's	30
Rheumatic features	35
Intestinal disorders	8
Pulmonary disorders	2

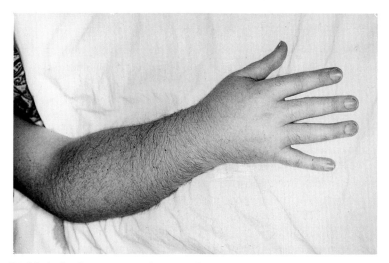

Fig. 7.2 Marked subcutaneous oedema overlying involved muscles in acute polymyositis.

Skin. The characteristic rash is unmistakable, with a purplish, dusky appearance, predominantly on the eyelids, cheeks and light-exposed areas. The rash may be patchy or confluent. In some cases, there is evidence of photosensitivity.

A rash may also be seen on the extensor surfaces of the knees, elbows and knuckles (MCP and PIP joints). These lesions are often violaceous, and may later become scaly. A late characteristic appearance is of atrophic cutaneous lesions on the knuckles and PIP joints. A rarer presentation is of acute scleroderma-like thickening and atrophy, making diagnosis more difficult. Periorbital oedema is an important physical finding in the diagnosis of dermatomyositis and may be seen in the absence of other skin lesions.

Ulceration of lesions may occur, and telangiectases are prominent in some cases.

Subungal splinter haemorrhages are sometimes seen in adult dermatomyositis, but in children are prominent and an important physical sign. Calcinosis of subcutaneous tissues and in the connective tissue of muscles, is a rare but dramatic complication (Figs 7.3, 7.4). Widespread sheets of

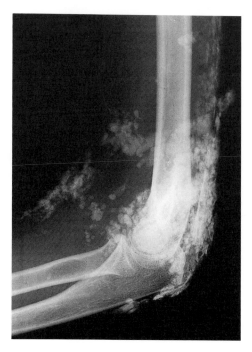

Fig. 7.3 Widespread subcutaneous and muscle calcification in long-standing polymyositis.

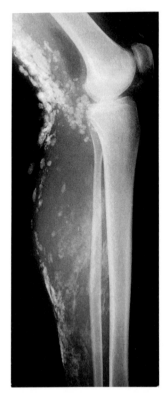

Fig. 7.4 Calcification in the lower limbs in polymyositis.

calcification, seen many years after the onset of childhood dermatomyositis, provide popular X-rays in examinations, but, perhaps surprisingly, often cause little in the way of major disability. Some cases develop troublesome ulceration.

Gastrointestinal tract. As in scleroderma, dysphagia and oesophageal dysfunction may be prominent. Oesophageal diverticulae also occur and are of some diagnostic importance if found in a patient with obscure muscle disease (Walton & Adams 1958).

Heart and blood vessels

Myocardial involvement, with ECG abnormalities, although to be expected, is somewhat uncommon (Diessner *et al.* 1966; Askari & Huettner

1982). Vascular disease and Raynaud's phenomenon are rare in adults. Renal disease is also rare.

Vasculitis, once thought to be confined to childhood dermatomyositis, is now recognized as a feature of some adult patients (Feldman *et al.* 1983).

Case report. A 37-year-old female presented with ischaemia of the fingertips of both hands, leading to loss of the tufts. Over the ensuing 2 months she developed marked muscle weakness. The disease progressed rapidly with marked inflammatory muscle disease and cardiac involvement.

Lung

Although dyspnoea is an important feature of dermatomyositis (Dubowitz & Dubowitz 1964), the incidence of primary lung involvement is unknown. A few cases of pneumonitis and fibrosis may relate to conditions where scleroderma or mixed connective tissue disease was the primary diagnosis. A subset of patients with antibodies against Jo-1 has now been distinguished, where the clinical features are myositis and pulmonary fibrosis (see below). In children, respiratory muscle weakness may develop insidiously and constitute a medical emergency. Death from aspiration pneumonia may occur in severe cases (Schwartz *et al.* 1976).

Joints

In up to one-third of patients, a mild and transient synovitis precedes the remainder of the disease, and in rare patients this synovitis becomes chronic and even erosive (Pearson 1966; Bohan *et al.* 1977).

The Jo-1 syndrome (Table 7.3)

A variety of precipitating antibody systems have been seen in the serum of patients with connective tissue diseases — notably in those with overlap syndromes.

Table 7.3 Features of the Jo-1 syndrome

Major	*Others*
Myositis	Raynaud's
Pulmonary fibrosis	Tenosynovitis
	Pericarditis and pleurisy
	Protracted course

In 1979, Nishikai and Reichlin reported a precipitating antibody system, which they called Jo-1, in a group of patients with polymyositis and dermatomyositis.

This particular system has proved both extremely interesting serologically, and remarkably specific clinically.

As distinct from many of the other 'ENA' systems, antiJo-1 antibodies appear to be confined largely to one group of patients. Those patients have myositis and pulmonary fibrosis (see Table 7.3).

In a study of 1200 sera, we demonstrated antiJo-1 antibodies in 19 cases. AntiJo-1 was demonstrated in 76% of patients with both myositis and lung disease but in only 3·5% of patients with either of these abnormalities alone (Bernstein *et al.* 1984; Hughes 1984).

The syndrome is quite distinctive and readily diagnosed clinically. 'Overlap' clinical features include Raynaud's, arthritis and tenosynovitis (sometimes a prominent early feature) and, occasionally, pleurisy and pericarditis. To date, none of our patients has had malignancy. Underscoring the place of the Jo-1 syndrome amongst the connective tissue diseases has been the finding of Sjøgren's syndrome in some of the patients.

Diagnostically, the recognition of the Jo-1 syndrome is very important —some patients in the author's experience had previously been labelled 'late onset lupus', while in others, the importance of the fibrosing alveolitis component was underestimated.

Serologically, the antibody is interesting. It is notably specific for this syndrome rarely being found, for example, in SLE (Hughes 1984), and was the first of the precipitating antibodies to be demonstrated against an intracellular enzyme, in this case histidyl-tRNA synthetase (Mathews & Bernstein 1983).

The reader is recommended to read the retailed review by Miller (1991).

DIAGNOSIS

Non-specific changes

The ESR is usually, though not invariably, elevated. Hypergammaglobulinaemia, rheumatoid factor, ANF and false-positive tests for syphilis may, as in almost all diseases discussed in this book, occasionally be found in dermatomyositis.

The interesting association between Jo-1 and the combination of polymyositis and pulmonary fibrosis (Bernstein *et al.* 1968) is described above.

Muscle enzymes

Of the three most widely used muscle enzyme determinations — SGOT, CPK and aldolase — any one may be normal even in acute disease. For this reason it is recommended that all three estimations be performed at each assessment. Muscle enzyme estimations (especially the CPK) provide the corner stone of outpatient management, and may forewarn of a clinical relapse by up to 6 weeks. In one comparative study of diagnostic methods (Vignos & Goldwyn 1972) serum aldolase and creatinine kinase were elevated in 24 of 44 and 16 of 20 patients, respectively. Creatinuria of greater than 6% of creatinine excretion in a 24-hour specimen was found in all 39 patients tested and was thereby the most sensitive laboratory measure of muscle injury. In subsequent management, creatinuria remained the most sensitive measure of improvement and recrudescence.

In childhood dermatomyositis, by contrast, muscle enzyme elevations may be unhelpful, both diagnostically and in monitoring disease progress (Dubowitz 1976).

Myoglobin

Myoglobinaemia was detected by radioimmunodiffusion in 23 cases of adult dermatomyositis (Kagen 1971). An extension of Kagen's original observation has come with the use of a radioimmunoassay for serum myoglobin (Nishikai & Reichlin 1977). In a study of 53 patients with polymyositis, 50% of patients had serum myoglobin values greater than 80 ng/ml. It was concluded that serum myoglobin values fluctuated more sensitively than CPK or SGOT values.

Muscle biopsy

As muscle involvement is patchy, 'false-negative' biopsies occur. While the procedure is desirable in adults, it is arguable in children whether the rewards justify the trauma involved — in the majority of children the diagnosis can be made on clinical grounds and the other diagnostic aids. In one study (Vignos & Goldwyn 1972) of 41 patients muscle biopsies, 33 specimens were compatible with polymyositis, 5 were suggestive, and 3 were negative. The need for the selection of a clinically involved but not severely weakened muscle is clear.

Needle muscle biopsy has now largely superseded open 'surgical' biopsy.

Electromyography

One of the situations where EMG comes into its own is in the differentiation of myositis from non-inflammatory myopathy. In the former, the combination of fibrillation, polyphasic action potentials and pseudomyotonic discharges is said to be almost pathognomonic (Pearson 1966).

Pulmonary function tests

These (or at very least vital capacity measurements) should be performed at the outset, serving as a baseline for further observations. The early recognition of intercostal muscle involvement may be life-saving in children.

Myometry

A variety of reproducible methods for measuring muscle strength are now available and are readily performed by physiotherapists or clinicians. These are extremely valuable for the serial monitoring of patients.

TREATMENT

Except in those in whom the resection of malignant tumours results in improvement, corticosteroids and immunosuppressives are the drugs of choice (Pearson 1963, 1966; Winkelmann *et al.* 1968). An initial dose of 60 mg prednisone daily (or higher in the more florid cases) results in improvement in the majority. However, in a 'hard core' minority of patients all known remedies are ineffective.

In children particularly, prednisone should be given as early as possible, following pulmonary function tests. Dubowitz (1976) and Miller, Heckmatt & Dubowitz (1983), suggest that moderate dosage, short-term treatment is preferable, and that clinical response is a more reliable guide to progress than serum enzyme levels.

Most physicians are agreed that, at least in adults, a combination of steroids and immunosuppressives has proved more effective than steroids alone (indeed in the author's recent practice, 'pulse' cyclophosphamide alone has proved dramatically effective in some cases of acute polymyositis).

The choice between methotrexate (the most widely used) and azathioprine or cylophosphamide is not clear cut, though methotrexate is rapidly gaining ground as the maintenance treatment of choice.

For fulminating or intractable polymyositis, plasma exchange and cyclo-

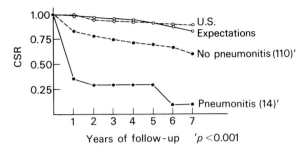

Fig. 7.5 Survival in polymyositis. (From Medsger, Robinson & Masi 1971.) CSR = cumulative survival rate.

sporin have been tried. An interesting, and promising approach in such cases is total body irradiation (Morgan, Bernstein & Hughes 1985). In four patients treated in this way, a marked and immediate improvement was seen; however the treatment is at best temporary, and at worst, toxic (Morgan *et al.* 1985).

PROGNOSIS

A life-table study of factors affecting survival in 124 patients with poly-myositis was published from Memphis (Medsger, Robinson & Masi 1971). Forty-three deaths were recorded, 42 occurring within seven years of diagnosis. The cumulative survival rate for the total patient series showed a relatively rapid decline to 72% after two years (Fig. 7.5) followed by a levelling off.

The worst prognostic feature was the development of pneumonitis, in which the most common aetiology was aspiration. Children had a better prognosis with a 90% cumulative survival rate over the follow-up periods and whites appeared to have a somewhat better prognosis than blacks.

These studies indicate that because the highest proportion of deaths occurs within the first two years after diagnosis, treatment should be particularly focused on this high-risk period, with special attention to the danger of aspiration pneumonia.

More recent mortality figures for the USA have also been published (Hochberg, Lopez-Acuna & Gittelsohn 1983).

REFERENCES

Adams R.D. (1975) *Diseases of Muscle*, 3rd ed. Harper & Row, London.
Askari A.D. & Huettner T.L. (1982) Cardiac abnormalities in polymyositis/dermato-

myositis. *Seminars in Arthritis and Rheumatism*, **12**, 208−219.

Barnes B.E. (1976) Dermatomyositis and malignancy. A review of the literature. *Annals of Internal Medicine*, **84**, 68.

Barwick D.D. & Walton J.N. (1963) Polymyositis. *American Journal of Medicine*, **35**, 646.

Bohan A. & Peter J.B. (1975) Polymyositis and dermatomyositis. *New England Journal of Medicine*, **292**, 344, 403.

Bohan A., Peter J.B., Bowman R.L. & Pearson C.M. (1977) A computer-assisted analysis of 153 patients with polymyositis and dermatomyositis. *Medicine*, **56**, 255.

Bernstein R.M., Morgan S.H., Chapman J., Bunn C.C., Mathews M.B., Turner-Warwick M. & Hughes G.R.V. (1984) AntiJo-1 antibody: a marker for myositis with interstitial lung disease. *British Medical Journal*, **289**, 151−153.

Callen J.P. (1982) The value of malignancy evaluation in patients with dermatomyositis. *Journal of the American Academy of Dermatology*, **6**, 235−239.

Chou S.M. & Gutmann L. (1970) Picornavirus-like structures in acute dermatomyositis. *Journal of Clinical Pathology*, **58**, 245.

Diessner G.R., Howerd F.M. Jr, Winkelmann R.K., Lambert E.H. & Mulder D.W. (1966) Laboratory tests in polymyositis. *Archives of Internal Medicine*, **117**, 757.

Dubowitz L.M.S. & Dubowitz V. (1964) Acute dermatomyositis presenting with pulmonary manifestations. *Archives of Disease in Childhood*, **39**, 293.

Dubowitz V. (1976) Treatment of dermatomyositis in childhood. *Archives of Disease in Childhood*, **51**, 494.

Feldman D., Hochberg M.C., Zizic T.M. & Stevens M.B. (1983) Cutaneous vasculitis in adult polymyositis/dermatmoyositis. *Journal of Rheumatology*, **10**, 85−89.

Hashimoto K., Robison L., Velayos E. & Niizuma K. (1971) Dermatomyositis, Electron microscopic and immunologic and tissue culture studies of paramyxovirus-like inclusions. *Archives of Dermatology*, **103**, 120.

Hochberg M.C., Lopez-Acuna D. & Gittelsohn A.M. (1983) Mortality from polymyositis and dermatomyositis in the United States 1968−1978. *Arthritis and Rheumatism*, **26**, 1467−1472.

Hughes G.R.V. (1984) Autoantibodies in lupus and its variants: experience in 1000 patients. *British Medical Journal*, **289**, 399−342.

Kagen L.J. (1971) Myoglobinaemia and myoglobinuria in patients with myositis. *Arthritis and Rheumatism*, **14**, 457.

Kalovidouris A.E. (1992) Immune aspects of myositis. *Current Opinion in Rheumatology*, **4**, 809−814.

Leddy J.P., Griggs R.C., Klemperer M.R. & Frank M.M. (1975) Hereditary complement (C2) deficiency with dermatomyositis. *American Journal of Medicine*, **58**, 83.

Mathews M.B. & Bernstein R.M. (1983) Myositis autoantibody inhibits histidyl-tRNA synthetase: a model for autoimmunity. *Nature*, **304**, 177−179.

Medsger T.A., Robinson H. & Masi A.T. (1971) Factors affecting survivorship in polymyositis. *Arthritis and Rheumatism*, **14**, 249.

Miller F.W. (1991) Humoral immunity and immunogenetics in the idiopathic inflammatory myopathies. *Current Opinion in Rheumatology*, **3**, 901−910.

Miller G., Heckmatt J.Z. & Dubowitz (1983) Drug treatment of juvenile dermatomyositis. *Archives of Disability in Children*, **58**, 455−450.

Morgan S.H., Bernstein R.M., Coppen J. & Hughes G.R.V. (1985) Total body irradiation and the course of polymyositis. *Arthritis and Rheumatism*, **28**, 831−835.

Morgan S.H., Bernstein R.M. & Hughes G.R.V. (1985) Intractable polymyositis: prolonged remission induced by total body irradiation. *Journal of the Royal Society of Medicine*, **78**, 496−497.

Nishikai M. & Reichlin M. (1977) Radioimmunoassay of serum myoglobin in polymyositis and other conditions. *Arthritis and Rheumatism*, **20**, 1514.

Nishikai M. & Reichlin M. (1979) Heterogeneity of precipitating antibody systems in polymyositis and dermatomyositis. Characterisation of the Jo-1 system. *Arthritis and Rheumatism*, **23**, 881–888.

Norton W.L., Kelayos E. & Robinson L. (1970) Endothelial inclusions in dermatomyositis (1970) *Annals of the Rheumatic Diseases*, **29**, 67.

Pearson C.M. (1966) Polymyositis. *Annual Review of Medicine*, **17**, 63.

Schochet S.S., Jr & McCormick W.F. (1973) Polymyositis with intranuclear inclusions. *Archives of Neurology*, **28**, 280.

Schwartz M.I., Mattay R.A., Sahn S.A., Stanford R.E., Marmorstein B.L. & Scheinhorn D.J. (1976) Interstitial lung disease in polymyositis and dermatomyositis. Analysis of 6 cases and review of the literature. *Medicine*, **55**, 89.

Travers R.L., Hughes G.R.V., Cambridge G. & Sewell J.R. (1977) Coxsackie B neutralisation titres in polymyositis/dermatomyositis. *Lancet*, **ii**, 1268.

Vignos P.J. & Goldwyn J. (1972) Evaluation of laboratory tests in diagnosis and management of polymyositis. *American Journal of the Medical Sciences*, **263**, 291.

Walton J.N. & Adams R.D. (1958) *Polymyositis*. Churchill Livingstone, Edinburgh.

Winkelmann R.K., Mulder D.W., Lambert E.H., Howard F.M. & Diessner G.R. (1968) Course of dermatomyositis-polymyositis: comparison of untreated and cortisone treated patients. *Mayo Clinic Proceedings*, **43**, 545.

8: *Mixed Connective Tissue Disease*

Despite the objections to the all-embracing diagnosis of 'connective tissue disease', there are undoubted cases of 'overlap syndrome' where features of two or more of the connective tissue diseases are present. This is particularly true of dermatomyositis and scleroderma, where skin and muscle abnormalities may make the differentiation difficult.

An important contribution to the differentiation of one group of patients with apparent overlap syndrome came with the description by Sharp *et al.* (1972) and by Mattioli & Reichlin (1971, 1973) of a group of patients with a definable group of symptoms and serological findings which has been called 'mixed connective tissue disease'. The increasing acceptance of this syndrome in which features of SLE, polymyositis and scleroderma coexist, is based on two important points:

1 High titres of antibody to a ribonucleoprotein antigen (RNP) are found.
2 Renal disease is mild or absent, and the prognosis is good.

Although the aetiology is uncertain, and the name of the syndrome uninviting, the possibility that a serological test — the presence of antibodies to RNP — may help to define a subgroup of patients with SLE or scleroderma as having a more favourable prognosis is important and deserves recognition.

For most clinicians, the serological feature most useful in drawing attention to the diagnosis is the finding of a 'speckled' pattern ANA test (see below).

CLINICAL FEATURES

Table 8.1, taken from the original report by Sharp *et al.* (1972), shows the comparative incidence of various clinical features of the syndrome. Although the list appears to embrace many of the features of both SLE and scleroderma renal involvement and neuropsychiatric disease were absent, and alopecia, photosensitivity, mucosal lesions, pleurisy, pericarditis, and myocarditis were not prominent. In Sharp's report, patients presented at different times with a 'scleroderma-like' diagnosis (Raynaud's, swollen hands, abnormal oesophageal motility) and at others with an 'SLE' diagnosis (arthritis, rashes, serositis, fever and leucopenia). In a few patients,

Table 8.1 Clinical characteristics of 25 patients with mixed connective tissue disease (MCTD)

Characteristic	Percentage
Arthritis/arthralgias	96
Swollen hands	88
Raynaud's	84
Abnormal oesophageal mortality	77
Myositis	72
Lymphadenopathy	68
Fever	32
Hepatomegaly	28
Serositis	24
Splenomegaly	21
Anaemia	48
Leukopenia	52
Hypergammaglobulinaemia	80
(Renal involvement)	0

features of polymyositis (eyelid oedema and rash, erythema of the knuckles, muscle weakness and pain) predominate.

The group of patients described by Dubois *et al.* (1971) may also have fallen into this category.

It was noted by Sharp *et al.* (1972) that, in addition to a good prognosis, these patients had a favourable response to steroids. This had not been entirely the case in our own patients. Although the prognosis for life does appear to be good, the morbidity may be high, as in one girl under our care who lost most of her fingertips due to severe Raynaud's phenomenon (Kitchiner *et al.* 1975).

Case report. *The patient, a housewife, presented in 1960 with joint pains and morning stiffness. The following year she developed Raynaud's phenomenon, recurrent abdominal pain and pleuritic chest pain. A year later she was observed to have active synovitis of her hands and knees and lymphadenopathy. Investigations revealed Hb 10·9%, ESR 60 mm/hour, hypergammaglobulinaemia, ANA + ve. A diagnosis of SLE was made and she was treated with chloroquine. Over the next two years the Raynaud's phenomenon became severe resulting in progressive sclerodactyly, infection, ischaemic necrosis and amputation of the tips of most of her fingers (Fig. 8.1). Bilateral cervical and later transthoracic sympathectomies were performed with only transient improvement. Apart from the severe circulatory problems, she remained well until 1974 when she was reinvestigated, complaining of fatigue. Apart from the sclerodactyly and amputation of most of her fingertips, the rest of her skin was normal. There was*

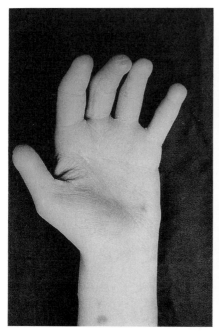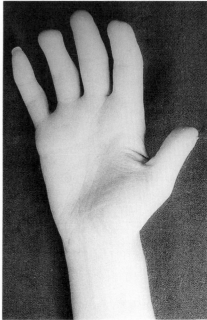

Fig. 8.1 Ischaemic necrosis and amputation of fingertips in Raynaud's phenomenon associated with MCTD. (From Kitchiner *et al.* 1975.)

moderately severe anaemia and the ESR remained high at 60 mm/hour. Muscle enzyme levels were slightly elevated. X-ray of the hands showed no soft-tissue calcification or bony erosions and chest X-rays were normal. A small hiatus hernia was present but oesophageal motility studies were normal. Renal function tests and serum complement levels were normal. DNA binding was normal but the ANA was positive at 1 in 1250 with a speckled pattern. Precipitating antibodies to ENA were present and antibodies against RNP were detectable to a serum dilution of 1 in 10 000. During recent years the patient has remained a perfectly well and active housewife.

Although present experience suggests that renal involvement is rare, cases of mixed connective tissue disease with immune-complex nephritis have been described (Rao *et al.* 1976).

A variety of cardiac manifestations may occur, including pericarditis, mitral valve prolapse, coronary artery involvement and pulmonary hypertension.

The major clinical manifestations are Raynaud's phenomenon, arthritis and arthralgia and lymphadenopathy (Table 8.2). One patient had a mild

Table 8.2 Clinical features of patients with MCTD (Bresnihan *et al.* 1977)

Characteristic	Percentage
Arthralgia/arthritis	13
Raynaud's phenomenon	13
Lymphadenopathy	13
Pulmonary disease	7/12 cases
Serositis	6
Sicca symptoms	4
Myositis	3
Oesophageal abnormality	3/7 cases
Fever	2
Nephritis	1
Splenomegaly	1
Hepatomegaly	0

focal nephritis. None had evidence of systemic sclerosis. There were 12 females and 1 male, aged between 27 and 63 years, and with a mean age of 46 years — greater than that seen in SLE. Duration of symptoms ranged between 1 and 31 years with a mean of 9·5 years, confirming the generally good prognosis associated with this disease.

Bennett & O'Connell (1980) stressed the severity of the polyarthritis and found a high incidence of neuropsychiatric disease and myositis. Twenty per cent developed glomerulonephropathy.

Our own experience has led us to regard MCTD as a serious and troublesome condition. Indeed, the morbidity seen in MCTD patients exceeds that seen in most SLE patients, largely due to severe Raynaud's, polyarthritis, and neuropsychiatric and pericardial symptoms.

The natural history of most of our MCTD patients is of a gradual loss of the serological features and a clinical progression towards scleroderma.

SEROLOGICAL FEATURES (Table 8.3)

While serological overlap with SLE occurs, the unifying feature serologically is the speckled pattern on immunofluorescence and antibody against the extractable nuclear antigen ribonucleoprotein 'RNP'. The antigen was found to be sensitive to both RNase and trypsin. One of the remarkable findings of MCTD is the finding of positive haemagglutination reactions at serum dilutions of up to 1 in 1 600 000.

Reichlin & Mattioli (1972) reported a correlation between the presence of an antiribonucleoprotein (antiRNP) and a low prevalence of nephritis in patients with SLE. In a further study (Parker 1973), it was found that

Table 8.3 Serological characteristics of 25 patients with MCTD (from Sharp *et al.* 1971)

Characteristics	Percentage
High-titre ENA antibody	100
High-titre speckled fluorescent antibody	100
Precipitating antibody to Sm antigen	0
Positive LE cell test	20
DNA antibodies (haemagglutination)	12
Normal serum complement	100

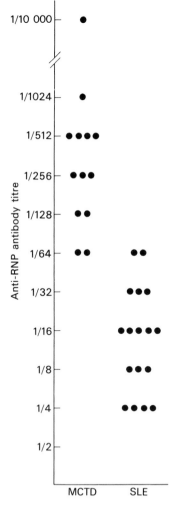

Fig. 8.2 Titration of antiRNP antibodies in patients with MCTD and SLE. (From Bresnihan *et al.* 1977.)

antiRNP antibody, where found alone, was associated with MCTD. When antibodies to other antigens such as DNA or Sm were present, other features of SLE such as nephritis and hypocomplementaemia occurred. Furthermore, antiRNP antibodies have not been found in two series of patients with classical scleroderma. Although up to 20% of SLE patients demonstrate RNP antibodies, the presence of this antibody in our patients, did not appear to identify a subgroup of lupus patients with individual clinical characteristics (Bresnihan, Grigor & Hughes 1977).

Kurata & Tan (1976) reported the use of counterimmunoelectrophoresis, in the detection of these antibodies. This method has not only the virtue of simplicity, but also distinguishes antiRNP and antiSm when both are present as separate precipitin lines, the former was abolished by RNase treatment. In our study of 172 patients with various connective tissue diseases, high-titre antiRNP antibodies (serum dilutions greater than 1:64) were seen only in the MCTD patients (Fig. 8.2). Low-titre antiRNP anti-bodies were found in 14 SLE patients (Fig. 8.2). No patients with sclero-derma demonstrated antiRNP antibodies. In seven SLE sera, both antiSm and antiRNP antibodies were detected.

The negative correlation between antiRNP antibodies and renal disease is of theoretical, as well as diagnostic, interest. The antigen is labile and theoretically poor material for the formation of immune complexes (Mattioli & Reichlin 1971).

For a description of the serological features of the extractable nuclear antigens see p. 302.

REFERENCES

Bennett R.M. & O'Connell D. (1980) Mixed connective tissue disease. A clinico-pathologic study of 20 cases. *Seminars in Arthritis and Rheumatism*, **10**, 25–51.

Bresnihan B., Bunn C., Snaith M. & Hughes G.R.V. (1977) Antiribonucleoprotein anti-bodies in connective tissue diseases. Estimation by counter immunoelectrophoresis. *British Medical Journal*, **1**, 610.

Bresnihan B., Grigor R. & Hughes G.R.V. (1977) Prospective analysis of anti RNP antibodies in systemic lupus erythematosus. *Annals of the Rheumatic Diseases*, **36**, 557.

Dubois E.L., Chandor S., Friou G.J. & Bischel M. (1971) Progressive systemic sclerosis (PSS) and localised scleroderma (morphoea) with positive LE cell test and unusual systemic manifestations compatible with systemic erythematosus (SLE). *Medicine*, **50**, 199.

Kitchiner D., Edmonds J., Bruneau C. & Hughes G.R.V. (1975) Mixed connective tissue disease with digital gangrene. *British Medical Journal*, **i**, 249.

Kurata N. & Tan E.M. (1976) Identification of antibodies to nucleic acid antigens by counterimmunoelectrophoresis. *Arthritis and Rheumatism*, **19**, 574.

Mattioli M. & Reichlin M. (1971) Characterization of a soluble nuclear ribonucleoprotein antigen reactive with SLE sera. *Journal of Immunology*, **107**, 1281.

Mattioli M. & Reichlin M. (1973) Physical association of two nuclear antigens and mutual occurrence of their antibodies: the relationship of the Sm and RNA protein (Mo) systems in SLE sera. *Journal of Immunology,* **110**, 1318.

Parker M.D. (1973) Ribonucleoprotein antibodies: frequency and clinical significance in systemic lupus erythematous/scleroderma, and mixed connective tissue disease. *Journal of Laboratory and Clinical Medicine,* **82**, 769.

Rao K.V., Berkseth R.O., Grosson J.T., Raij L. & Shapiro F.L. (1976) Immune complex nephritis in mixed connective tissue disease. *Annals of Internal Medicine,* **84**, 174.

Reichlin M. & Mattioli M. (1972) Correlation of a precipitin reaction to an RNA protein antigen and a low prevalence of nephritis in patients with systemic lupus erythematosus. *New England Journal of Medicine,* **236**, 908.

Sharp G.C., Irvin W.S., Laroque R.L., & Velez C., Daly V., Kaiser A.D. & Holman H.R. (1971) Association of autoantibodies to different nuclear antigens with clinical patterns of rheumatic disease and responsiveness to therapy. *Journal of Clinical Investigation,* **50**, 350.

Sharp G.C., Irvin W.S., Tan E.M., Gould R.G. & Holman H.R. (1972) Mixed connective tissue disease — an apparently distinct rheumatic disease syndrome associated with specific antibody to an extractable nuclear antigen (ENA). *American Journal of Medicine,* **52**, 148.

9: *Relapsing Polychondritis*

This is a rare and serious disease affecting primarily the mucopoly-saccharide component of cartilage ground substance, resulting clinically in inflammation and weakening of cartilage, particularly in the pinna of the ear, the nasal septum, larynx and trachea. Associated features are fever and malaise, synovitis, vasculitis, aortic valve disease, arterial aneurysm and ocular manifestations. Untreated there is a high mortality rate, usually from respiratory or cardiovascular complications.

Males and females are affected with equal frequency, and the disease has been reported at all ages. Polychondritis is rare; Arkin & Masi (1975) collected 132 cases from the world literature.

PATHOLOGY

The intercellular matrix of connective tissue is composed of fibrillar elements and ground substance, the latter being composed of mucopolysaccharides (also called glycosaminoglycans) and mucoproteins. The major mucopoly-saccharides of cartilage are chondroitin sulphate A and B. Chondroitin sulphate (together with hyaluronic acid) is also found in tendons, heart valves and the aorta. The chondrocytes lie in the intercellular matrix. These cells possess the properties of lysosomal enzyme release (especially proteases and collagenases) with resultant matrix degradation, and of the synthesis of new intracellular material (Hashimoto, Arkin & Kang 1977).

In polychondritis, a marked depletion of mucopolysaccharides can be demonstrated.

AETIOLOGY

Both biochemical and immunological factors are implicated in the genesis of mucopolysaccharides changes though neither has been shown to be the primary defect.

Biochemical

The possibility that excessive proteolytic enzyme activity is responsible is suggested by animal experiments. One such animal model which closely resembles relapsing polychondritis is the intravenous administration of papain into rabbits. The normally rigid ears collapse rapidly and their cartilage shows basophilia and loss of metachromasia. Involvement of the aorta also occurs in these animals (see Giroux *et al.* 1983).

Immunological

Evidence for an immunological basis for the pathogenesis of relapsing polychondritis is at best patchy. Humoral anticartilage antibodies have been demonstrated in some, but by no means all patients, using immuno-fluorescence (Hughes *et al.* 1972). Delayed hypersensitivity reactions to cartilage have also been demonstrated in some patients using macrophage-aggregation (Herman & Dennis 1973) and macrophage migration inhibition methods (Rajapakse & Bywaters 1974).

One interesting model having possible relevance to the aetiology of relapsing polychondritis is the culture of embryonic chick cartilage. Using this model, Lachmann *et al.* (1969) demonstrated that alteration of the chrondrocyte cell with subsequent lysosomal enzyme release might be achieved by antibody — complement interaction. The mechanism by which complement or one of its products achieves this effect is still unclear.

CLINICAL FEATURES

Table 9.1 lists the frequency of some of the features of 132 cases reviewed by Arkin & Masi (1975).

Ear

Although the 'classical' sign of relapsing polychondritis is a violaceous swollen and tender pinna, this is the presenting feature in only a third of cases. After frequent attacks the pinna loses its shape and firmness and may become floppy. Two frequent accompaniments are hearing impairment, and serous otitis media with eustachian tube obstruction. The inflammatory process may affect the nasopharyngeal two-thirds of the eustachian tube. Vestibular abnormalities may also occur with ataxia and vomiting. The reason for this is unclear.

Nose

Nasal cartilage inflammation ultimately results in collapse and a 'saddle nose' occurs in three-quarters of all patients.

Table 9.1 Percentage frequency of major clinical features positive at presentation and during the course of relapsing polychondritis. (From Arkin & Masi 1975).

Features	Presenting features of 113 cases (%)	Positive features during course of 132 cases (%)
Inflammation in pinna	32	86
Arthropathy	22	70
Nasal cartilage involvement	17	72
Laryngotracheal involvement	12	44
Fever	4	45
Episcleritis	10	39
Hearing impairment	—	30
Conjunctivitis	4	23
Iritis	3	19
Aortic insufficiency	—	9

Respiratory tract

One of the more serious clinical problems is involvement of the cartilage of the epiglottis and bronchial rings. Hoarseness may occur and, in extreme cases, stridor may be marked (Fig. 9.1). As cartilage is present even in the smaller bronchioles, widespread pulmonary involvement may occur, leading to dyspnoea and wheezing and to superinfection and death from pneumonia. Lung function tests show airflow obstruction without small airways disease (Gibson & Davis 1974).

Eyes (Fig. 9.2)

Episcleritis, iritis and keratitis occur in up to 60% of patients. Perhaps the least known ocular manifestation is recurrent conjunctivitis (Hughes *et al.* 1972). Other rarer manifestations include lateral rectus weakness, retinal exudates, retinal artery thrombosis and complete blindness (Barth & Berson 1968).

Heart and blood vessels

Aortic valve disease and aortic aneurysms are complications of relapsing polychondritis and are a major cause of death in this disease (Pearson *et al.* 1967; Alexander *et al.* 1971; Hughes *et al.* 1972; Hemry, Moss & Jacox 1972). In a number of patients, valve replacements have been required. Aneurysms of the ascending, thoracic and abdominal aorta have been described, and recurrent aneurysm formation may also occur.

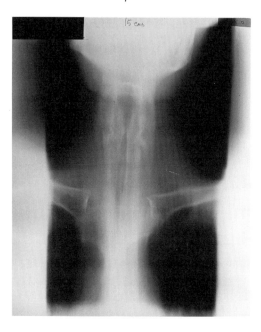

Fig. 9.1 Stridor in a patient with advanced polychondritis, showing narrowing of the tracheal cartilage involvement. (Dr David Allison, Royal Postgraduate Medical School, Hammersmith Hospital).

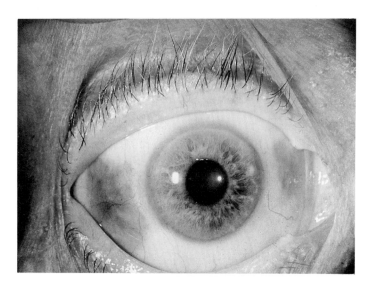

Fig. 9.2 Scleral changes in polychondritis resulting from involvement of scleral acid mucopolysaccharide. (Mr Peter Wright, Moorfield's Eye Hospital.)

Joints

Arthropathy may be transient, or persistent with secondary deformities. It tends towards a 'seronegative' or asymmetrical pattern, affecting, for example, the sternoclavicular joint and occasionally the sacroiliac joints (Pearson, Kline & Newcomber 1960; O'Hanlan *et al*. 1976). There may also be involvement of the costal cartilage, leading in rare cases to chest deformities. While rare, patients with both rheumatoid arthritis and relapsing poly-chondritis have been described and it must be realized that the joint symptoms may precede the rest of the picture by several years.

Association with other diseases

Polychondritis, like arthritis, is a disease pattern, and a number of other conditions have been described in association with polychondritis. Some of the reports reviewed by Arkin & Masi (1975) are listed in Table 9.2. In our own practice, polychondritis has been seen in association with cases of Churg-Strauss vasculitis, polyarteritis nodosa and acute onset reactive arthritis. The significance of these rare associations is unknown but hints at least that immunological features may play a role in the pathogenesis.

LABORATORY FEATURES

There is no specific test for relapsing polychondritis. The usual haemato-logical triad of high ESR, normochromic anaemia and leucocytosis common to most chronic inflammatory conditions is seen. Rheumatoid factor and ANA tests may be positive and elevations of IgG, IgM and IgA have been observed. Complement levels are normal or raised.

Table 9.2 Conditions reported in association with polychondritis

Condition	Number of cases reported
Rheumatoid arthritis	5
SLE	3
Sjøgren's syndrome	3
Vasculitis	Several
Scleroderma	1
Ulcerative colitis	3
Diabetes	2
Myxoedema	2
Malignancy	3

Estimations of urinary acid mucopolysaccharides were thought (Kay & Sones 1964) to be important in the diagnosis, but the tests are difficult to perform and possibly unreliable (Swain & Stroud 1972).

DIAGNOSIS

The clinical diagnosis is confirmed by cartilage biopsy, remembering that cartilage involvement may be patchy.

Aids to diagnosis include tomography of the trachea to detect narrowing, and pulmonary function tests, showing the pattern of bronchial involvement particularly reduced FEV_1 without diffusion abnormalities.

Other radiographic abnormalities may include calcification of the pinna, aortic aneurysms, cardiomegaly and pneumonia. Erosion and deformity of the joints are both very unusual in this condition.

The differential diagnosis includes infection of the pinna (or infectious perichondritis), Wegener's granulomatosis, rheumatoid arthritis, Reiter's syndrome and Cogan's syndrome (arteritis with interstitial keratitis, vertigo, tinnitus, ataxia and bilateral nerve deafness).

TREATMENT

Corticosteroids

These are still the drugs of choice, and are frequently life-saving in this condition. Prednisone is often effective in doses between 10 and 20 mg daily though higher starting doses such as 60 mg daily are needed in acute cases. A curious 'threshold' phenomenon is sometimes seen, the disease regularly 'flaring' at the same dose level on repeated attempts at steroid reduction. Such a case is described here.

Case report. *A 36-year-old Iranian bodyguard developed a productive cough, bronchospasm and pyrexia. He failed to respond to antibiotics and broncho-dilators and 3 months later had lost 12 kg in weight. At this point he was noted to have a tender nasal cartilage and a tender manubrio-sternal joint. There was an expiratory stridor and he was pyrexial. A diagnosis of relapsing polychondritis was made and he was started on 60 mg of prednisone with rapid improvement. During the next 6 months prednisone dosage was reduced to 15 mg daily with return of the previous symptoms. There was tenderness of the nasal and auricular cartilages which were also softened and mobile. In addition, there was tenderness of the trachea and costal cartilages and a harsh expiratory stridor and tachypnoea. Cardiovascular and locomotor systems were normal. Abnormal investigations included ESR 77 mm/hour and non-specific elevation of α_1- and*

α_2-globulins. Other investigations (including FBC, renal function tests, chest X-rays) were normal, but tomography of the upper respiratory tract showed narrowing of the entire trachea and of the major bronchi. The pattern of flow rate in respiratory function tests suggested that the obstruction was mainly in the larger bronchi and trachea. During the course of the ensuing 2 months a number of attempts were made to reduce his prednisone dosage, but at a recurrent threshold of 15 mg prednisone, his condition regularly deteriorated; 30 mg and even 40 mg of prednisone on alternate days failed to control symptoms. He was discharged apyrexial and relatively symptom free on 17·5 mg prednisone daily, but at follow-up 1 year later, there was deterioration in airway function with a halving of the FEV_1 and considerable CO_2 retention at rest, despite minimal change in his symptoms. There was no response to bronchodilators.

Cytotoxic drugs

Azathioprine (Dolan, Lemmon & Teitelbaum 1966) and methotrexate have been tried in a few cases, the former resulting in the need for less steroid. Cyclosporin may prove effective in some cases.

Other treatments

Aspirin and non-steroidal antiinflammatory drugs are regularly used for lesser manifestations, but are disappointing in this disease.

Surgery may be needed for aortic aneurysms and tracheostomy for tracheal collapse.

PROGNOSIS

Of the 132 cases reviewed by Arkin & Masi (1975), 29 patients died, with a mean survival of 5¼ years from onset. The commonest causes of death were pneumonia and aortic aneurysm rupture.

Many patients maintain a relatively low grade course over many years, and, as encouragement to those unfortunate patients, a number have recovered or maintained almost complete control of their symptoms (Dolan et al. 1966; Thurston & Curtis 1966).

REFERENCES

Alexander C.S., Deer R.F. *et al.* (1971) Abnormal amino acid and lipid composition of aortic valve in relapsing polychondritis. *American Journal of Cardiology,* 28, 337.

Arkin T. & Masi A. (1975) Relapsing polychondritis: Review of current status and case report. *Seminars in Arthritis and Rheumatism,* 5, 41.

Barth W.F. & Berson E.L. (1968) Relapsing polychondritis, rheumatoid arthritis and blindness. *American Journal of Ophthalmology*, **66**, 890.

Dolan D.L., Lemmon G.B. & Teitelbaum S.L. (1966) Relapsing polychondritis. *American Journal of Medicine*, **41**, 285.

Gibson G.J. & Davis P. (1974) Respiratory complications of relapsing polychondritis. *Thorax*, **29**, 726.

Giroux L., Paquin F., Guerard-Desjardins M. & Lefaivre A. (1983) Relapsing polychondritis. *Seminars in Arthritis and Rheumatism*, **13**, 182–187.

Hashimoto K., Arkin C.R. & Kang A.H. (1977) Relapsing polychondritis. An ultrastructural study. *Arthritis and Rheumatism*, **20**, 91.

Hemry D.A., Moss A.J. & Jacox R.F. (1972) Relapsing polychondritis, a 'floppy' mitral valve, and migratory polytendinitis. *Annals of Internal Medicine*, **77**, 576.

Herman J.H. & Dennis M.V. (1973) Immunopathologic studies in relapsing polychondritis. *Journal of Clinical Investigation*, **52**, 549.

Hughes R.A.C., Berry C.L., Seifert M. & Lessof M.H. (1972) Relapsing polychondritis. *Quarterly Journal of Medicine*, **163**, 363.

Kay R.L. & Sones D.A. (1964) Relapsing polychondritis. *Annals of Internal Medicine*, **60**, 653.

Lachmann P.J., Coombes R.R.A., Fell H.B. *et al.* (1969) The breakdown of embryonic (chick) cartilage and bone cultivated in the presence of complement sufficient antiserum. III. Immunological analysis. *International Archives of Allergy*, **36**, 469.

O'Hanlan M., McAdam L.P., Bluestone R. & Pearson C.M. (1976) The arthropathy of relapsing polychondritis. *Arthritis and Rheumatism*, **19**, 191.

Pearson C.M., Kline H.M. & Newcomber V.D. (1960) Relapsing polychondritis. *New England Journal of Medicine*, **263**, 51.

Pearson C.M., Kraening R., Verity M.A. *et al.* (1967) Aortic insufficiency and aortic aneurysm in relapsing polychondritis. *Transcripts of the Association of American Physicians*, **80**, 71.

Rajapakse D.A. & Bywaters E.G.L. (1974) Cell mediated immunity to cartilage proteoglycan in relapsing polychondritis. *Clinical and Experimental Immunology*, **16**, 497.

Swain R.E. & Stroud M.H. (1972) Relapsing polychondritis. *Laryngoscope*, **82**, 891.

Thurston C.S. & Curtis A.C. (1966) Relapsing polychondritis. *Archives of Dermatology*, **93**, 664.

10: *Vasculitis*

INTRODUCTION

During the past few years there have been three notable developments in the area of vasculitis. Firstly, the American College of Rheumatology has provided a comprehensive classification of vasculitis. Secondly, newer tests such as antibodies against neutrophil cytoplasmic antigen (ANCA) and anti-endothelial cell antibodies have at least provided some help in diagnosis. Thirdly, and possibly the most important, recognition of milder forms of vasculitis (especially in limited forms of Wegener's granulomatosis) may have been instrumental in the rapid increase of cases of vasculitis now being reported and treated.

A whole issue of *Arthritis and Rheumatism* was devoted to the multiple papers resulting from the American College of Rheumatology's work on classification (see Hunder *et al.* 1990, *et seq.*).

From data collected from 48 centres, the committee identified classification (but not diagnostic) criteria for seven vaculitides (reviewed by Michel 1992).

The seven main groups (plus an eighth unspecified group), female ratio and age at onset are shown in Table 10.1.

POLYARTERITIS NODOSA (PAN)

PAN is a rare and grave disease, characterized pathologically by intense inflammation involving all three layers of the small and medium-sized arteries leading to multiple aneurysm formation, thromboses and infarctions. Its clinical manifestations are protean, with fever and leucocytosis being regular features, together with arthritis, muscle pain, abdominal pain, neuropathy, hypertension and renal disease, pulmonary and cerebral involvement presenting together or singly, and each leading to wide possibilities for differential diagnosis.

Lightfoot *et al.* (1990) developed criteria for the classification of PAN by comparing 118 patients with 689 control patients with other forces of vasculitides. With this classification, a patient is said to have PAN if at least three of the ten criteria are met (Table 10.2).

215

Table 10.1 ACR 1990 Vasculitis classes

Category	Age at onset	Women (%)
Polyarteritis nodosa	48	38
Churg−Strauss	50	37
Wegener's	45	36
Hypersensitivity vasculitis	47	54
Henoch−Schönlein	17	46
Giant cell arteritis	69	75
Takayasu	26	86
Others (unspecified)	44	55

Table 10.2 ACR classification criteria for PAN (from Lightfoot *et al*. 1990, with permission)

Weight loss >4 kg
Livedo reticulosis
Testicular pain
Myalgia or leg tenderness
Mono or poly neuropathy
Diastolic BP > 90 mmHg
BUN 40 mg/dl or creatinine > 1.5 mg/dl
Hepatitis B virus
Arteriographic abnormality
Biopsy positive

PATHOLOGY

The acute illness is characterized by swelling of the muscle fibres of the media of medium-sized arteries, with intimal oedema and narrowing of the vascular lumen. This is followed by fibrinoid change, and by an intense infiltration by polymorphs and occasionally by eosinophils. The infiltrate may extend through to the adventitia and intimal layers (Fig. 10.2), hence the alternative title 'periarteritis' is unsatisfactory. While fibrinoid is an important finding in PAN, it is not universally present.

In more chronic stages the infiltrate becomes mononuclear, the formation of granulation tissue may result in further weakening of the wall of the blood vessel. Giant cells are usually absent.

The process ends in multiple aneurysm formation ('nodosa'), in total occlusion with or without recanalization, or in scar formation.

The extent of arterial involvement is variable, ranging from short segments of inflammation perhaps involving only one part of the vessel circumference, to massive acute inflammation and necrosis. Veins and the vasa nervora of the nerves are frequently involved in this process.

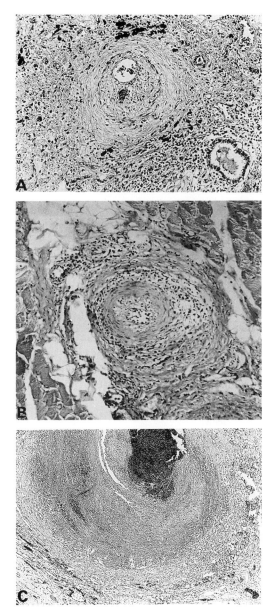

Fig. 10.1 Arteries from (A) lung and (B) muscle in PAN, showing intense panarteritis. (C) Intralobular renal artery with thrombus in the lumen, and aneurysmal dilatation (H & E ×54). (Dr Shirley Amin, University Hospital of the West Indies.)

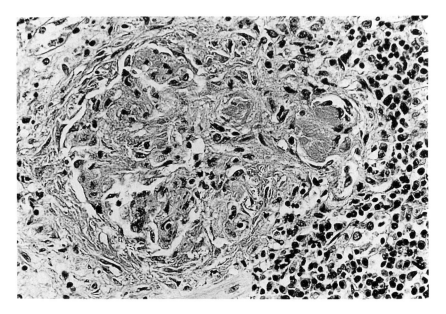

Fig. 10.2 Kidney in PAN (H & E ×340). Fibrin thrombus in afferent arteriole. Fibrinoid change in vessel wall with adjacent interstitial inflammation.

During periods of disease activity, different phases of inflammation and healing may be seen in the same region, thus a characteristic finding is of both fresh and healing lesions in the same biopsy.

The arteritic process may involve any part of the body, though arteritis and infarcts are particularly common in kidney, muscles, brain, nerves, heart, liver, gall bladder and gastrointestinal tract.

AETIOLOGY

Hepatitis B antigen

In 1970, Gocke *et al.* reported four patients with polyarteritis nodosa and circulating hepatitis B antigenaemia. This finding proved to be an important discovery, in that it provided the first direct association of a virus — virus antibody immune complex in the pathogenesis of one of the connective tissue diseases.

This association has now been confirmed in several other centres — indeed it has turned out to be a surprisingly strong association — some 25 to 40% of all patients with generalized necrotizing vasculitis carrying the hepatitis B antigen (Lockshin & Sergent 1976).

These patients have a number of features in common: the disease often starts with skin rash and myalgia, and progresses to severe and often fatal polyarteritis nodosa, with fever, neuropathy, abdominal pain and hypertension (Table 10.3).

Histologically, there was typical inflammatory angiitis with arterial wall necrosis and pan-arteritis. A spectrum of pathological severity has been seen and, for this reason, some authors have preferred the more general term 'necrotizing vasculitis' to PAN. Two clinical features are of note in this group — pulmonary disease has not been prominent and the hepatitis appeared to be mild: though in a follow-up of nine such cases, chronic liver disease was the cause of death in one patient 6 years after the acute syndrome. Three died of complications of vasculitis. Five patients survived, though only one has completely recovered from the effects of the vasculitis. The acute stage has usually been short-lived, lasting from 3 to 12 months, and no patient has had a recurrence of vasculitis.

Is PAN an immune complex disease?

Most of these patients had transiently reduced complement levels during the acute phase of their disease. Gocke *et al.* (1970) showed localization of hepatitis B antigen, IgM and C_3 in the blood vessel wall by immunofluorescence, and Almeida & Waterson (1969) used the electron microscope to demonstrate circulating aggregates of hepatitis B antigen and antibody with complement. However, serological methods such as density gradient studies, C_{1q} precipitation and anticomplementary testing have failed consistently to demonstrate complexes (Prince & Trepo 1971).

Table 10.3 Major clinical manifestations in nine patients with PAN and Australia antigenaemia (from Lockshin & Sergent 1976)

Symptom or sign	No. of patients	Percentage
Arthritis/myalgia	9	100
Mononeuritis	7	78
Fever	6	67
Abdominal pain	5	56
Hypertension	5	56
Renal disease	4	44
Cerebrovascular disease	3	33
Skin rash	1	12

Other infections

A number of vasculitic syndromes have been associated with HIV infection (reviewed by Mader & Keystone 1992). Hepatitis C infection, now known to be strongly associated with mixed cryoglobulinaemia, is not apparently linked with PAN.

Hypersensitivity

The hypothesis that hypersensitivity reactions might play a part in the pathogenesis of PAN is based on both experimental and clinical observations. The injection of foreign protein into the rabbit produces many of the lesions of PAN (Germuth 1953). In man, Rich (1942) showed that arteritis was a sequel to serum sickness following both foreign serum and sulphonamides. Sulphonamides (usually in high doses) have long been implicated in occasional cases of PAN. Other drugs reported as causing an arteritis include penicillin, thiouracil, iodides, organic arsenicals, oestrogens and hydantoins. In the majority of these cases, however, the lesion described has been hypersensitivity angiitis rather than full-blown PAN.

A number of drug addicts have been noted to develop polyarteritis nodosa (Citron *et al.* 1970). Most of these addicts were taking a variety of drugs in addition to methamphetamine and heroin, and the precise agent responsible (hepatitis B antigen remains a possibility in some) is unclear. A number of patients infected with viral hepatitis develop serum sickness-like illnesses (reviewed by Duffy *et al.* 1976) again suggesting a hypersensitivity mechanism in some cases.

CLINICAL FEATURES (see Travers, Allison & Hughes 1979; Lightfoot *et al.* 1990; Michael 1992)

The main clinical features of PAN are listed in Table 10.4. As distinct from the other connective tissue diseases, PAN is commoner in males, the male : female ratio being approximately 4 : 1. Any age group may be affected.

In general, the onset of PAN is more acute than that of SLE and the course more malignant. Despite the protean manifestations, a number of clinically useful pointers are found, and Shulman & Harvey (1972) make the point that a number of different presenting clinical patterns are recognizable:
1 PUO and weight loss.
2 Nephritis.
3 Hypertension (rapidly developing).
4 Acute abdomen.

Table 10.4 Clinical features of PAN

General	Renal
Malaise	Acute glomerulonephritis
Fever	Hypertension
Arthralgias	Nephrotic syndrome
Arthritis	
Weight loss	*Alimentary tract*
Myalgia	Acute abdomen
Testicular pain	Malabsorption syndrome
Deafness	Hepatic failure
	Bowel and gall bladder infarction
Circulatory system	
Digital gangrene	*Nervous system*
Intermittent claudication	Peripheral neuropathy
Livedo reticularis	Mononeuritis multiplex
	Organic psychosis
Heart	Hemiplegia
Tachycardia	Brainstem lesions
Cardiac infarction	Cranial nerve lesions
Heart failure	Ocular lesions
Pericarditis	
Arrhythmias	*Respiratory*
	Infiltrates
Skin	Loeffler's pneumonia
Nodules, purpura, livedo, rashes	Haemorrhage

5 Asthma or focal pulmonary infiltrates.
6 Myocardial infarction.
7 Muscle pain, tenderness and wasting.
8 Peripheral neuropathy (predominantly motor).

The fever is variable and may precede other manifestations by weeks. Weight loss and muscle wasting are frequent accompaniments and both may be profound (Sack, Cassidy & Bole 1975).

Muscle pain, especially in the legs, is often marked and exacerbated by exercise. It may be difficult to distinguish the lower limb muscle pain from true intermittent claudication due to major vessel involvement. In rare cases the disease may be localised to this site (Golding 1970).

Case report. *A 50-year-old gynaecologist developed a widespread erythematous urticarial rash. This lasted for a week and was followed by the development of lower limb muscle pains. Over the ensuing 2 months he complained of pain or weakness in the leg muscles, exacerbated by exercise. He was investigated for intermittent claudication by a vascular surgeon who noted in addition a persistent pyrexia, a raised ESR and a neutrophil leukocytosis. Muscle biopsy showed the changes of an acute necrotizing polyarteritis with a predominantly polymorph infiltrate. His serum was positive for hepatitis B antigen and in addition large circulating complexes of hepatitis B antigen and antibody and complement were seen using electron microscopy (see Fig. 15.5).*

Other general features of the disease include arthralgias (rarely arthritis) (Rose & Spencer 1957), testicular pain, sore throat, headaches and fatigue. Nasal symptoms (stuffiness, rhinorrhoea or epistaxis, crusting) occur in up to 25% of cases (Ford & Siekert 1965) lending support to the contention that Wegener's granulomatosis is one variant of PAN.

Alopecia is rarely seen in PAN, an important distinguishing feature from SLE.

Skin (Table 10.5)

As in SLE a wide variety of cutaneous manifestations are seen (Lyell & Church 1954). The nodules, first described by Kussmaul & Maier (1866) and to which the disease owes its name, are the clinical exception rather than the rule. They vary in size from 1 to 2 mm to aneurysms of several centimetres. They characteristically occur in crops or linearly along the course of blood vessels.

A variety of rashes occur of which an urticarial rash may be one of the earliest to appear suggesting, as it does, a hypersensitive mechanism. Purpura is occasionally a recurrent feature and may become chronic.

As in SLE a useful guide to cutaneous vasculitis in some patients is the presence of livedo reticularis.

A strong case has been made (Borrie 1972) for the separation of cutaneous PAN as an entity. In his series, 13 patients were found to have PAN (necrotizing vasculitis involving small arteries lying in the subcutis) affecting the skin. The severity of the arteritis in this series varied from fibrinoid necrosis to complete destruction of the vessel wall with polymorph infiltration.

Table 10.5 Cutaneous manifestations of PAN

Nodules
Rashes
Urticaria
Erythema multiforme
Purpura
Infarcts
Livedo reticularis

There was, however, little correlation between the severity of the microscopic lesion and that either of the individual cutaneous lesion or the disease as a whole. Other features apart from skin involvement were fever, peripheral neuropathy and myositis. The overall prognosis was good, and it was noted that of 102 cases of PAN in this series, only 13 had histological evidence of specific cutaneous lesions and in these the overall prognosis was excellent.

A rare type of vasculitic nodule is seen in Mondor's disease, in which thickened inflamed arteries become palpable on the chest wall (Hatteland & Kluge 1965).

Peripheral circulatory system

Perhaps surprisingly, Raynaud's phenomenon is not a major feature of PAN. Equally, it is somewhat the exception for PAN to present as peripheral gangrene (Keech & Puro 1965). However, as in other vasculitides, localized small digital infarcts may be seen. Cryoglobulinaemia has been described in association with Raynaud's phenomenon and gangrene (Butler & Palmer 1955) but is rare, as are other overt immunological disturbances in PAN. Involvement of the veins may present as multiple episodes of thrombophlebitis.

Heart

Tachycardia, disproportionate to any fever present, may be an early feature of the disease and is of serious prognostic significance. Cardiac involvement occurs in up to 80% of patients with PAN and is second only to renal disease as a cause of death in this condition (Holsinger, Osmundson & Edwards 1962). In this review of the cardiac pathology observed in PAN, the major manifestations were coronary arteritis (62%), myocardial infarction (62%) and acute pericarditis (33%). While arrhythmias were described in only 9%, tachycardia was seen in two-thirds of the patients, the latter possibly related to involvement of the cardiac conduction system (James & Birk 1966).

Congestive cardiac failure results either from direct cardiac involvement or secondary to renal hypertension.

Kidney

Renal disease is the commonest cause of death in PAN, the prognosis of the disease depending largely on the extent of involvement of these organs. In classical PAN, the incidence of renal involvement is over 75% (Ralston

& Krale 1949; Patalano & Sommers 1961). In one series of 300 cases (Wilson & Alexander 1945) 60% had proteinuria and 40% haematuria. The recognition of milder forms of the disease, and the difficulties of classifying the arteritides makes the estimation of absolute percentages difficult at present.

A variety of pathological pictures is seen, ranging from aneurysmal involvement of the main renal artery to a widespread glomerulitis. The most characteristic distribution is seen in the arcuate and interlobar arteries (Fig. 10.3). Gross infarcts are seen in 40–70%, the high figure occurring in those in whom larger arteries are affected. Scars of differing ages may be seen, and there may be reduction of parenchyma brought about by hypertension. Prominent inflamed and thrombosed arcuate vessels may be seen at the corticomedullary junction. A glomerulonephritis or glomerulitis is seen in up to 82% of patients (Patalano & Sommers 1961), though this high figure includes many cases showing necrotic or scarred glomeruli.

The full, though limited, spectrum of renal clinical response to injury may be seen, from haematuria or proteinuria to acute rapidly progressive glomerulonephritis and renal failure. In others, there may be attacks of renal pain associated with haematuria due to infarction. A particularly difficult clinical problem is hypertension which occurs in up to 60% of cases of PAN. Its onset may be sudden and the level of blood pressure difficult to control if accompanied by other systemic features such as muscle pain, fever or leucocytosis. In such cases, renal arteriography should be an early investigation (Bron, Stilley & Shapiro 1971).

Alimentary tract

Abdominal pain is a major complaint in PAN, occurring in two-thirds of

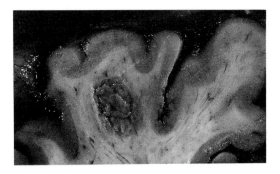

Fig. 10.3 Localized area of cerebral infarction in fatal PAN.

cases. Presentation of PAN as an 'acute abdomen' (Table 15.6) is well recognized in surgical departments. In a 10-year survey in one centre, three-quarters of all PAN patients were initially referred as surgical emergencies (Cotton & Butler 1967).

The vasculitis may result in massive infarcts or haemorrhages in all the abdominal viscera, including the pancreas, liver and gall bladder (Cotton & Butler 1967). Complications which have been described in PAN embrace almost the whole diagnostic spectrum of the acute abdomen (Table 10.6) (Pugh & Stringer 1956).

Gastric ulceration and appendicitis secondary to occlusion of the appendicular artery may occur, as may intestinal obstruction. Subacute occlusion of the superior mesenteric artery may lead to steatorrhoea and weight loss (Carron & Douglas 1965). A more serious manifestation of mesenteric arteritis is bloody diarrhoea, associated with abdominal pain. Barium studies in this situation may show 'thumb printing' of the small intestinal mucosa suggestive of ischaemia. Gastrointestinal haemorrhage and ulceration accounted for the majority of surgical complications in one large series of PAN patients (Matolo & Albo 1971). Myocardial infarction, due to coronary arteritis or secondary to hypertension, may present as abdominal pain.

PAN is one of the few causes of hepatic artery occlusion, and massive hepatic necrosis, or infarction of the gall bladder, is an occasional terminal event in this disease (Cotton & Butler 1967).

Nervous system involvement

CNS disease. While mononeuritis multiplex is the best known neurological manifestations of PAN, central nervous system involvement is common and, as in SLE, may present in many guises.

Table 10.6 The acute abdomen in PAN

Gastrointestinal haemorrhage
Intussusception
Infarction of the gall bladder
Hepatic infarction
Superior mesenteric artery occlusion
Gastric ulceration
Jejunal and ileal ulceration
Pancreatitis
Peritonitis
(Intrathoracic pathology)

In a survey of 114 cases of PAN, Ford and Siekert (1965) found symptoms and signs of CNS or cranial nerve involvement in 46% and peripheral neuropathy in 68%. As in the case of SLE, the most common cerebral manifestation was of mental derangement, usually an organic psychosis or confusional state. The most common abnormalities on examination were retinopathy, hemiparesis, cranial nerve and brainstem lesions.

CSF examination is, in general, unhelpful. In the majority of cases the pathological lesion is found to be vasculitis with cerebral infarction (Fig. 10.4), though subarachnoid haemorrhages are also seen.

Peripheral neuropathy (Table 10.7). This occurs in one-half to two-thirds of all patients with the disease (Ford & Siekert 1965) and may be the presenting manifestation. Two distinct types are seen — mononeuropathy and multiple mononeuropathy (mononeuritis multiplex) — the successive involvement of distinct peripheral nerves is related to arteritis of the vasa nervorum. The polyneuritis of PAN is predominantly motor in type. It is usually more prominent in the legs and may be asymmetrical.

Ocular changes

A variety of ocular and fundal changes occur which are related either directly to ophthalmic arteritis or are secondary to hypertension (Boeck 1956; Duguid 1954; Ford & Siekert 1965; Kimbrell & Wheliss 1967).

Table 10.7 Peripheral neuropathy in PAN (from Ford & Siekert 1965)

Overall incidence in 114 cases	68%
Mononeuropathy or multiple mononeuropathy (mononeuritis multiplex)	58%
Mixed mono- and polyneuritis	23%
Polyneuritis	18%

Table 10.8 Ocular changes in PAN

Haemorrhage and exudates
Papilloedema
Hypertensive arteriolar changes
Uveitis, keratitis, iritis choroiditis
Field defects
Primary optic atrophy
Scleritis
Conjunctivitis
Conjunctival oedema
Corneal ulceration

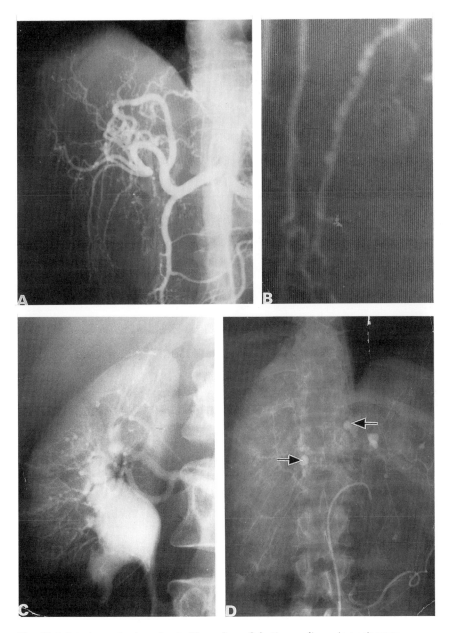

Fig. 10.4 Arteriography in polyarteritis nodosa. Selective coeliac axis angiogram showing small aneurysms in the hepatic arteries (A). The multiple nature of the changes is well seen on a magnification study (B). In many patients the aneurysms are most readily demonstrated in the renal vascular bed (C). Late films in such renal series commonly show nephrographic defects due to multiple infarcts. The aneurysms depicted in (A), (B) and (C) are fairly typical in size; however, occasionally larger lesions may be seen (D). (Professor David Allison, Royal Postgraduate Medical School, Hammersmith Hospital.)

The commonest changes are those secondary to hypertension though exudates in the absence of hypertension (cytoid bodies) and related to vasculitis are an important diagnostic aid. They occur more frequently in PAN than in other vasculitides.

Other manifestations of ocular vasculitis include sudden unilateral visual loss, transient and permanent field defects and amaurosis fugax (Ford & Siekert 1965).

Pulmonary involvement

The incidence of pulmonary involvement, as in the case of cutaneous vasculitis, depends largely on which classification is used. In an early major review of 300 cases of polyarteritis, Wilson & Alexander (1945) found that 18% had asthma. In this group, 94% had eosinophilia, and in most pulmonary manifestations preceded other evidence of systemic vasculitis. In another study of 72 cases of systemic 'allergic' vasculitis (McCoombs 1965) haemoptysis, cough and dyspnoea were evident in nearly one-third of cases, and in most of these pulmonary infiltrates were demonstrable on X-ray. Rose & Spencer (1957), in their study of III cases of PAN, chose to separate cases with lung involvement into a separate group, this group being characterized by granuloma formation, eosinophilia and a predominantly respiratory illness. It is probable that some of these cases were Wegener's granulomatosis. Thus although granulomatous angiitis, Loeffler's pneumonia, hypersensitivity angiitis and PAN overlap, in practice pulmonary involvement appears to be relatively rare in classical PAN.

LABORATORY TESTS

The ESR is raised in most cases, though frequently the figure is in the 30–60 mm/h range. Non-specific elevations of IgG, IgM and IgA may be seen (Sairanen & Wasastjerna 1972) and ANA and RF tests, when positive are in low titre. It is perhaps more important to point out that in differential diagnosis, a notable *absence* of immunological abnormalities is more a feature of PAN than of the usual differential diagnoses. Although eosino-philia is reported in up to one-third of cases, this feature is strongly associated with pulmonary involvement (Sack *et al.* 1975) and is rare in cases without lung infiltrates. The most important feature in diagnosis is neutrophilia, sometimes in excess of 30000; the change in absolute neutrophil count may provide the only yardstick for monitoring disease activity. Another useful test is the C-reactive protein — high in active PAN and conspicuously low in uncomplicated SLE.

ANCA testing is positive in a number of patients with PAN, though with a much lower frequency than in Wegener's granulomatosis (see Chapter 11). For example, in the review by Cross *et al.* (1991) C-ANCA positivity was found in 14 of 49 cases of PAN, as opposed to 295 of 383 cases of Wegener's.

POLYARTERITIS IN CHILDREN

Roberts and Fetterman in 1963 drew attention to the frequency and clinical features of PAN in infancy. In describing 2 cases and reviewing reports of 18 further cases, they concluded that a distinctive clinical pattern emerged in such infants, including a transient macular exanthema, transient conjunctivitis, prolonged pyrexia, cardiomegaly, congestive heart failure, ECG changes and abnormal urinary sediment. Particularly prominent was coronary artery involvement in this and in other series (Roberts & Fetterman 1963; Benyo & Perrin 1968). Tang and Segal (1971) described a 22-month-old baby boy who died following a number of Stokes−Adams attacks and was found at postmortem to have multiple aneurysms of the coronary tree. Leff, Harver and Bayliss (1971) reported two brothers who died of PAN at the age of 30 months and 4 years. In both, the disease was characterized by rashes, anaemia, raised sedimentation rates, fever and hypertension. Autopsy findings in the two children were remarkably similar with ruptured cerebral aneurysms as well as widespread aneurysms and thromboses. Of interest was the observation that the mother had been diagnosed as having SLE and a material aunt and uncle had rheumatic fever. There was a marked family history of allergy to drugs and to natural allergens.

Many of these cases would now be classified as Kawasaki's syndrome (see p. 259).

DIAGNOSIS

The patterns of disease presentation mentioned earlier usually lead to an early diagnosis in classical PAN. Important laboratory findings are neutrophilia, the presence of ANCA and the usual lack of markers of immunological diseases such as strongly positive ANA and latex fixation tests. Indeed, a normal or low polymorph count should raise doubts about the diagnosis, as in the following case:

Case report. *A 29-year-old driver was referred with a 6-month history of weight loss, malaise, muscle pains, 'nodules' in the calf muscles and a mild mixed neuropathy. A muscle biopsy in the region of a nodule showed an intense vasculitis, the predominant cells being (apparently) polymorphs. He responded initially to steroids, but developed transient cerebral localizing signs when attempts at steroid withdrawal were made. A puzzling feature of his illness was a persistent leucopenia (3500 with normal differential count) and the finding of a palpable spleen. Further biopsy of a vasculitic nodule showed that the vascular infiltrate was malignant — histiocytic medullary reticulosis — and although the patient made an initial improvement on antimitotic drugs, he subsequently died of widespread lymphoma. A feature of this tumour is its marked sensitivity to corticosteroids in its early stages.*

While ideally biopsy should include a purpuric lesion, or part of a clearly involved organ, in practice this usually means a 'blind' muscle biopsy — a diagnostic procedure which has proved less than satisfactory. If no tender muscle is available for biopsy, a site in a major girdle muscle well clear of previous sites is chosen. The diagnostic yield from such a procedure is small: Maxeiner, McDonald & Kirklin (1952) obtained positive results in only 13% of 136 muscle biopsies in 106 patients suspected of having polyarteritis. In 26 patients subsequently proven to have PAN at autopsy, positive muscle biopsies had been obtained in only 9. The positive yield in the series of Sack, Cassidy & Bole (1975) was higher at 56%.

An alternative site for biopsy which has been suggested is the testis but this procedure has not achieved widespread use (Dahl, Baggenstoss & Deweerd 1968).

Of increasing importance is the use of angiography as a diagnostic aid (Fig. 10.4) and many reports testify to its value in PAN (Halpern & Citron 1971; McLain, Bookstein & Kelsch 1972; Sack *et al.* 1975). Biopsies of the liver and kidneys have obvious added risks in suspected PAN, and angiography should be a routine procedure prior to such attempts.

In the study by Halpern & Citron (1971), necrotizing angiitis and polyarteritis nodosa were found in 30 patients who had histories of flagrant drug abuse. Arteriographic evidence of angiitis was obtained in 13, and included a number of features (Table 10.9). Arteriographic findings of multiple aneurysms of the same or varying sizes in medium and small calibre visceral and peripheral arteries are considered to be almost pathognomonic of PAN. Arteriography may also occasionally demonstrate regression of aneurysms, and in a number of cases has resulted in a diagnosis of PAN being made where muscle biopsy was unhelpful.

Table 10.9 Arteriographic pattern of angiitis (from Halpern & Citron 1971)

Microaneurysms (especially at bifurcations)
Indistinct vessel outlines
Stenotic segments
Obliteration and thrombosis of vessels

The use of angiography in PAN has been reviewed by Allison, Travers and Hughes (1979).

MANAGEMENT

One of the most compelling arguments for 'splitters' as opposed to 'lumpers' of disease syndromes is that prognosis and thus management may be more precisely assessed. Nowhere is the need for careful classification more pressing than in arteritis.

Classical PAN is now known to be a 'one shot' disease. For example, of the 17 patients described in our paper of 1979 (Travers, Allison & Hughes 1979), all but one death occurred during the initial months of the disease. Of the 12 survivors not one at follow-up has had a second attack (all have residual hypertension). This is an entirely different disease pattern from that of some of the allergic and granulomatous vasculitides (see later).

By implication, it follows that early, aggressive, therapy is the rule. Most clinicians now regard the combination of corticosteroids and immuno-suppressives as the choice of treatment.

Our own therapy, in acute PAN, is the combination of pulse methyl-prednisolone (1000 mg i.v.) then oral prednisolone 60 mg daily, with pulse cyclophosphamide 500–1000 mg i.v. repeated weekly as the WBC allows.

Plasmapheresis has not been of value. Hypertension may prove extremely difficult to manage.

As the disease responds therapy can be tailed. None of our 1979 patients is now on specific treatment.

PROGNOSIS

The prognosis depends in large part on the intensity and type of vasculitis and on the organs involved. In a small series of 10 patients with PAN, a 70% five-year survival and 50% 10-year survival were observed (Sairanen & Wasastjerna 1972). Twenty-five to 30% of all patients with PAN die of renal failure (Ralston & Krale 1949; Griffith & Vural 1951; Rose & Spencer 1957). In the small group of 9 patients with Australia antigenaemia and vasculitis, reported by Lockshin & Sergent (1976), 3 died during the acute phase of vasculitis and 1 died subsequently of liver disease. Of 5 survivors 4 had residual abnormalities — neuropathy, hypertension, uraemia and residue of cerebrovascular accidents. The authors also comment that the syndrome appeared to be a 'one-shot' illness, and that none of the patients who achieved a prolonged remission had had any recurrence of vasculitis despite withdrawal of therapy.

There is broad agreement that corticosteroid therapy has contributed to an improvement in prognosis. Two large prognostic studies — from the Mayo Clinic (Frohnert & Sheps 1967) and the Medical Research Council (1960) — report a three-year survival in treated patients of 52% and 62% respectively.

These figures are confirmed in the study of Sack *et al.* (1975) where a five-year survival of 57% was obtained. In this study two important points were made: firstly, that hypertension did not invariably affect the prognosis adversely, presumably because of more effective antihypertensive therapy, and secondly that the first 3 months were the most critical to survival.

Thus if the patient can be sustained over the acute phase of the disease it is probable that even in classical PAN the overall prognosis may be improved. The devastating nature of the acute disease has been personally recorded by a young nurse (MacConachie 1972).

Case report. A nurse working in a renal dialysis unit in Boston complained of tiredness and irritability. She was referred to a psychiatrist and subsequently developed flitting arthralgia and joint swelling and diarrhoea. The following day she developed a maculo-papular rash, muscle stiffness and ankle swelling. On admission she was febrile and was found to have hepatitis B antigenaemia and raised liver enzymes. She became semi-comatose and was treated successfully with prednisone. However, following gradual prednisone withdrawal, she developed fever and hypertension, headaches, a grand-mal seizure and become unconscious. In addition, she developed a painful peripheral neuropathy. Over the ensuing months she was treated with prednisone, azathioprine, antihypertensives, diuretics and chlorpromazine. Two years after her original illness, she was able to reduce the various medications and once again was able to start leading a normal life, working part-time as a medical receptionist. She subsequently married and had a healthy child.

REFERENCES

Allison D., Travers R. & Hughes G.R.V. (1979) The use of visceral angiography in the diagnosis of PAN. *European Journal of Rheumatology*, **3**, 120–124.

Almeida J.D. & Waterson A.P. (1969) Immune complexes in hepatitis. *Lancet*, **ii**, 983.

Benyo R.B. & Perrin E.V. (1968) Periarteritis nodosa in infancy. *American Journal of Diseases of Children*, **116**, 539.

Boeck J. (1956) Ocular changes in periarteritis nodosa. *American Journal of Ophthalmology*, **42**, 567.

Borrie P. (1972) Cutaneous polyarteritis nodosa. *British Journal of Dermatology*, **87**, 87.

Bron K.M., Stilley J.W. & Shapiro A.P. (1971) Renal arteriography enhanced by tolazine: value in the diagnosis of polyarteritis nodosa complicated by perinephric haematoma. *Diagnostic Radiology*, **99**, 295.

Butler K.R. & Palmer J.A. (1955) Cryoglobulinaemia in polyarteritis nodosa with gangrene of extremities. *Canadian Medical Association Journal*, **72**, 686.

Carron D.B. & Douglas A.P. (1965) Steatorrhoea in vascular insufficiency of the small intestine. Five cases of polyarteritis nodosa and allied disorders. *Quarterly Journal of Medicine*, **34**, 331.

Citron B.P., Halpern M., McCarron M., Lundberg G.D., McCormick R., Pincus I., Tatler D. & Haverback B.J. (1970) Necrotising angiitis associated with drug abuse. *New England Journal of Medicine*, **283**, 1003.

Cotton C.L. & Butler T.J. (1967) The surgical problem of polyarteritis nodosa. *British Journal of Surgery*, **54**, 393.

Dahl E.V., Baggenstoss A.H. & Deweerd J.H. (1968) Testicular lesions of periarteritis nodosa with special reference to diagnosis. *American Journal of Medicine*, **282**, 22.

Duffy J., Lidsky M.D., Sharp J.S., Davis J.S., Person D.A., Hollinger F.B. & Mink W. (1976) Polyarthritis, polyarteritis and hepatitis B. *Medicine*, **55**, 19−37.

Duguid J.B. (1954) Periarteritis nodosa. *Transcripts of the Ophthalmological Society, UK*, **74**, 25.

Ford R.G. & Siekert R.G. (1965) Central nervous system manifestations of periarteritis nodosa. *Neurology*, **15**, 124.

Frohnert P.P. & Sheps S.G. (1967) Long term follow-up study of periarteritis nodosa. *American Journal of Medicine*, **43**, 8.

Germuth F.G., Jr (1953) A comparative histologic and immunologic study in rabbits of induced hypersensitivity of the serum sickness type. *Journal of Experimental Medicine*, **97**, 257.

Gocke D.J., Hsu K., Morgan G., Bombardieri S., Lockshin M. & Christian C.L. (1970) Association between polyarteritis and Australian antigen. *Lancet*, **ii**, 1149.

Golding D.N. (1970) Polyarteritis presenting with leg pains. *British Medical Journal*, **i**, 277.

Griffith G.C. & Vural I.L. (1951) Polyarteritis nodosa: a correlation of clinical and post-mortem findings in 17 cases. *Circulation*, **3**, 481.

Gross W.L. (1991) Antineutrophil cytoplasmic autoantibody associated with diseases: a rheumatologist's perspective. *American Journal of Kidney Disease*, **2**, 175−179.

Halpern M. & Citron B.P. (1971) Necrotising angiitis associated with drug abuse. *American Journal of Roentgenology*, **III**, 663.

Hatteland K. & Kluge T. (1965) Mondor's disease. A subcutaneous form of periarteritis nodosa. *Acta Chirurgica Scandinavica*, **129**, 67.

Holsinger D.R., Osmundson P.J. & Edwards J.E. (1962) The heart in pericarditis nodosa. *Circulation*, **25**, 610.

Hunder G.G., Arend W.P., Bloch D.A. *et al.* (1990) The American College of Rheumatology 1990 criteria for the classification of vasculitis: introduction. *Arthritis and Rheumatism*, **33**, 1065−1067.

James T.N. & Birk R.E. (1966) Pathology of the cardiac conduction system in polyarteritis nodosa. *Archives of Internal Medicine*, **117**, 561.

Kimbrell O.G., Jr & Wheliss J.A. (1967) Polyarteritis nodosa complicated by bilateral optic neuropathy. *Journal of the American Medical Society*, **201**, 61.

Keech M.K. & Puro H.E. (1965) Fatal polyarteritis presenting as asymmetrical peripheral gangrene. *Annals of the Rheumatic Diseases*, **24**, 549.

Kussmaul A. & Maier R. (1866) A previously undescribed arterial disease (periarteritis nodosa) with kidney disease and rapidly progressive muscle weakness (Ger). *Deutsches Archiv für Klinische Medizin*, **1**, 484.

Leff R., Harver W.V. & Bayliss C. (1971) Polyarteritis nodosa in two siblings. *American Journal of Diseases of Children*, **121**, 67.

Lightfoot R.W. (1990) The American College of Rheumatology 1990 criteria for the classification of polyarteritis nodosa. *Arthritis and Rheumatism*, **33**, 1088–1093.

Lockshin M.D. & Sergent J.S. (1976) Necrotising vasculitis and HB antigen. In: *Modern Topics in Rheumatology*, Ed: G.R.V. Hughes. Heinemann, London.

Lyell A. & Church R. (1954) The cutaneous manifestations of polyarteritis nodosa. *British Journal of Dermatology*, **66**, 335.

MacConachie E. (1972) Serum hepatitis with polyarteritis nodosa — a personal account. *Nursing Times*, August 24th, 1070.

McCoombs R.P. (1965) Systemic 'allergic' vasculitis. Clinical and pathological relationships. *Journal of the American Medical Association*, **194**, 1059.

McLain L.G., Bookstein J.J. & Kelsch R.C. (1972) Polyarteritis nodosa diagnosed by renal arteriography. *Journal of Paediatrics*, **80**, 1032.

Medical Research Council (1960) Treatment of polyarteritis nodosa with cortisone: Results after 3 years. *British Medical Journal*, **1**, 1399.

Mader R. & Keystone E.C. (1992) Infections that cause vasculitis. *Current Opinion in Rheumatology*, **4**, 35–38.

Matolo N.M. & Albo D. (1971) Gastrointestinal complications of collagen vascular diseases. Surgical implications. *American Journal of Surgery*, **122**, 678.

Maxeiner S.J., Jr, McDonald J.R. & Kirklin J.W. (1952) Muscle biopsy in the diagnosis of periarteritis nodosa. An evaluation. *Surgical Clinics of North America*, **32**, 1225.

Michel B.A. (1992) Classification of vasculitis. *Current Opinion in Rheumatology*, **4**, 3–8.

Patalano V.J. & Sommers S.C. (1961) Biopsy diagnosis of periarteritis nodosa: Glomerulonephritis and renal arteriolitis as aids. *Archives of Pathology*, **72**, 1.

Prince A.M. & Trepo C. (1971) Role of immune complexes involving SH antigen in the pathogenesis of chronic active hepatitis and polyarteritis nodosa. *Lancet*, **i**, 1309.

Pugh J.I. & Stringer P. (1956) Abdominal periarteritis nodosa. *British Journal of Surgery*, **44**, 302.

Ralston D.E. & Krale W.F. (1949) The renal lesions of periarteritis nodosa. *Proceedings of the Mayo Clinic*, **24**, 18.

Rich A.R. (1942) The role of hypersensitivity in periarteritis nodosa: As indicated by 7 cases developing during serum sickness and sulphonamide therapy. *Bulletin of the Johns Hopkins Hospital*, **71**, 123.

Roberts F.B. & Fetterman G.H. (1963) Polyarteritis nodosa in infancy. *Journal of Paediatrics*, **63**, 519.

Rose G.A. & Spencer H. (1957) Polyarteritis nodosa. *Quarterly Journal of Medicine*, **26**, 43.

Sack M., Cassidy J.T. & Bole G.G. (1975) Prognostic factors in polyarteritis. *Journal of Rheumatology*, **2**, 411.

Sairanen E. & Wasastjerna C. (1972) Periarteritis nodosa. A 10 year follow up of ten cases. *Acta medica Scandinavica*, **191**, 501.

Shulman L. & Harvey H. (1972) Polyarteritis nodosa. In: *Arthritis and Allied Conditions*, p. 918, Ed: J. Hollander. Lea & Febiger, Philadelphia.

Tang P.H.L. & Segal A.J. (1971) Polyarteritis nodosa of infancy. *Journal of the American Medical Association*, **217**, 1666.

Travers R.L., Allison D. & Hughes G.R.V. (1979) Polyarteritis nodosa: A clinical and angiographic analysis of 17 cases. *Seminars in Arthritis and Rheumatism*, **8**, 184.

Wilson K.S. & Alexander H.L. (1945) *Journal of Laboratory and Clinical Medicine*, **30**, 195.

11: *Wegener's Granulomatosis*

Wegener's granulomatosis was once considered a rare disease. Recently, the diagnosis of milder cases has resulted in a rapid increase in prevalence. It consists of necrotizing vasculitis of the upper and lower respiratory tract, associated with granuloma formation and with glomerulonephritis. Although granuloma formation is an important feature of the disease, the major pathology consists of vasculitis and the disease is considered by most to be a variant of polyarteritis nodosa. As with PAN, males are affected more frequently than females and any age group may contract the disease, though 40–50-year-olds predominate. Untreated, the course is malignant, 82% of patients dying within 1 year and with a mean survival of 5 months (Walton 1958). During recent years, however, the grim prognosis of this disease has been improved dramatically, by the use of the immunosuppressive drugs cyclophosphamide and azathioprine.

In 1990 Leavitt and colleagues participating in the American College of Rheumatology vasculitis study group developed criteria for the classification of Wegener's granulomatosis by comparing 85 WG patients with 722 control patients with other forms of vasculitis. The four classification criteria were: nasal or oral inflammation, abnormal chest X-ray, abnormal urinary sediment and granulomatous inflammation on biopsy. Although the ANCA test is proving useful in diagnosis, its accuracy could not be assessed by Leavitt *et al*. because it was not then widely available.

PATHOLOGY

Godman & Churg (1954) reviewed the pathology of Wegener's granulomatosis and listed three principal pathological criteria:
1 Necrotizing granulomas of the respiratory tract.
2 Generalized necrotizing angiitis.
3 Necrotizing glomerulitis.
Microscopically, the granulomata, which are not a feature of true PAN, resemble tuberculous granulomata in which areas of necrosis are prominent. At the edges of the necrotic infarcted tissue, giant cells, together with varying numbers of acute and chronic inflammatory cells, are seen.

These lesions may be found throughout the whole extent of the air passages as well as in the lung parenchyma. Necrotizing granulomata may also be found in the paranasal sinuses and nasal septum, nasopharynx, maxillary, ethmoid, frontal and sphenoid sinuses. Secondary effects of ulceration and invasion include saddle-nose deformity, pulmonary infarction, orbital compression and proptosis and intracranial spread. In addition to granuloma formation, widespread vasculitis may occur, resulting in infarctions in lung, heart, spleen and other organs, and a clinical and pathological picture identical to that of PAN. The kidney may show (in addition to necrotizing vasculitis) a focal necrotizing glomerulitis similar to that seen in subacute bacterial endocarditis, with fibrinoid necrosis and destruction of one or more glomerular capillary loops (Godman & Churg 1954). Granulomas and vasculitis may be seen in the skin (Hu, O'Loughlin & Winkelmann 1977).

AETIOLOGY

The aetiology is unknown. Hypersensitivity, as in the case of PAN, is thought to play a part, and while the prominent respiratory tract involvement suggests an airborne allergen, no aetiological agent has been incriminated.

Case report. A 51-year-old shop owner received an influenza vaccination. One week later he developed arthralgias. After a further week he developed widespread vasculitis, pulmonary and sinus shadowing and renal failure.

An association with HLA DR1 has been reported (Papiha *et al.* 1992).

CLINICAL FEATURES
(see Leavitt & Fauci 1992; D'Cruz & Hughes 1992)

Table 11.1 shows the clinical and pathological features of 21 patients, reviewed at the NIH in 1974 (Wolff *et al.* 1974)

The commonest presentation is with nasopharyngeal symptoms including sinusitis, local discomfort and rhinorrhoea. The diagnosis is most frequently made by nasopharyngeal biopsy where granulomata with or without vasculitis are seen. Thickening of the mucosa of the maxillary antrum especially in the absence of a fluid level, is said to be suggestive of Wegener's granulomatosis (Fauci & Wolff 1973). Later stages include spread to the orbital fossa, secondary infection, and erosion of the nasal cartilage leading to saddle-nose deformity. Serous or purulent otitis media and hearing loss occur. Although upper respiratory tract involvement may apparently occur in isolation, in the majority pulmonary involvement is

Table 11.1 Typical clinicopathological features of 21 patients with Wegener's granulomatosis

	Patients(%)	Typical features
Lungs	100	Bilateral nodular and cavitary infiltrates
		Necrotizing granulomatous vasculitis
Paranasal sinuses	95	Sinusitis
		Necrotizing granulomas. Secondary infection
Nasopharynx	91	Mucosal ulceration. Saddle nose
Kidneys	81	Focal nephritis. Fulminant nephritis
Joints	57	Fleeting polyarthralgia
Skin	48	Ulceration secondary to vasculitis
Eyes	43	Granulomatous sclero-uveitis
Ears	38	Serous otitis media
Heart	29	Coronary vasculitis. Pericarditis
Nervous system	24	Mononeuritis multiplex
		Cranial neuritis
Fever	39	(Excluding infection)

From Wolff *et al.* (1974). (Reproduced by permission of the authors and editor of the *Annals of Internal Medicine*.)

detectable at an early stage, even though some pulmonary infiltrates are fleeting.

Lungs

A variety of chest X-ray appearances is seen, including solitary and multiple nodules (Fig. 11.1), infiltrates and cavitation (Rogers & Roberto 1956; McGregor & Sandler 1964; Felson 1959). Focal areas of atelectasis and pleural effusions may rarely occur. An important point of differentiation from sarcoidosis is that hilar lymph node enlargement is rare (Kornblum & Fienberg 1955). Chest infections are common (Pinching *et al.* 1983). Pulmonary features may be subtle.

Case report. *A young woman with Wegener's granulomatosis and in clinical remission on decreasing therapy, developed a cough and slight haemoptysis. Chest X-ray was normal. At bronchoscopy, a roughened patch of one of the lower lobe bronchi was biopsied and revealed the characteristic histology of active Wegener's granulomatosis.*

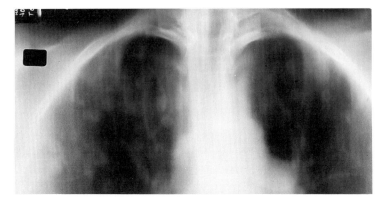

Fig. 11.1 Tomogram from patient with Wegener's granulomatosis showing multiple cavitating lesions. (Dr David Allison, Royal Postgraduate Medical School, Hammersmith Hospital.)

Kidneys

Unlike lung involvement, which may be transient, renal disease, when it appears, is usually fulminant if untreated. In Walton's series (1958) the mean survival time from the onset of clinically apparent renal disease was 5 months. The usual presentation is with acute nephritis, though early in the disease the only abnormality may be proteinuria or an abnormal sediment (Fauci & Wolff 1973). Hypertension is rare — an important point of differentiation from PAN (Fahey *et al.* 1954; Pinching *et al.* 1983; Leavitt & Fauci 1992).

Joints

Transient arthralgia or synovitis occur in over one-half of the patients. Chronic arthritis is not a feature of the disease, though a case of Wegener's granulomatosis occurring in a patient with pre-existing rheumatoid arthritis has been reported (Sturrock 1974).

Skin

As in PAN, a variety of changes is seen, including papules, nodules and ulceration, secondary to necrotizing angiitis of the dermal vessels (Reed, Jensen & Konwaler 1963; Fauci & Wolff 1973; Hu O'Laughlin & Winkelmann 1977). The elbow is a frequent site of vasculitic lesions.

Eyes

Ocular lesions include conjunctivitis, episcleritis and retinal vasculitis (Pinching *et al.* 1983). In Straatsma's series (1957) 19 of 44 cases and in Fauci & Wolff's (1973) 7 of 39 had eye symptoms. The wide variety of manifestations includes conjunctivitis, granulomatous keratitis, sclero-uveitis, scleromalacia performans, pseudotumour of the orbit and prop-tosis. Coutu *et al.* (1975) describe a patient in whom bilateral uveitis was the initial manifestation of a limited form of Wegener's granulomatosis. Despite regression of pulmonary lesions with treatment, the ocular lesion progressed to blindness.

Heart

Cardiac lesions include myocardial granulomas, coronary vasculitis, peri-carditis and pancarditis (Godman & Churg 1954; Walton 1958; McCrea & Childers 1964). Death may result from intractable arrhythmias. Arrhyth-mias are common (Pinching *et al.* 1983).

Nervous system

One-quarter to one-half of all patients develop neurological involvement (Wolff *et al.* 1974; Drachman 1963). Direct granulomatous invasion of the cranial vault as well as local intracerebral granuloma formation may occur. Both cerebral vasculitis and peripheral mononeuritis multiplex are des-cribed (Drachman 1963; Sahn & Sahn 1976; Pinching *et al.* 1983).

Other manifestations

Systemic features such as fever are common, as is superinfection. Involve-ment of the gingivae, breast, prostate and larynx have all been reported. Less frequent features of the condition have been reviewed by Leavitt & Fanci (1992).

MINIMAL WEGENER'S

It has always been recognized that limited forms of Wegener's granuloma-tosis exist, particular forms confined to the ear, nose and throat. During the past few years, we have run a weekly vasculitis clinic at St Thomas' Hospital, and have been increasingly impressed by the prevalence of mild, subacute or limited forms. Furthermore, it was apparent that a number of our patients had histories of chronic ear, nose and throat (ENT) symptoms going back as long as 20 years, and had attended ENT and rheumatology clinics without a firm diagnosis being made (D'Cruz *et al.* 1989). Our observations have led us to suggest that a possibly distinct syndrome occurs, attributable to vasculitis, but with recurrent, non-life-threatening features — the syndrome of joint pains, sinusitis, wheezing and mild vasculitis (Hughes & D'Cruz 1991) (Table 11.2).

Table 11.2 The syndrome of joint pains, sinusitis, wheezing and mild vasculitis (from Hughes & D'Cruz 1991)

Recurrent sinusitis — sometimes bloodstained
Arthritis or arthralgia
Wheezing or mild asthma
Red eye (usually episcleritis)
Digital vasculitis
Mild neutropenia

LABORATORY (Table 11.3)

An important point in diagnosis is that whereas textbooks talk about histological diagnosis, in practice this may be difficult. Dr Margaret Turner-Warwick, for example, makes the point that lung biopsy material is often necrotic — indeed this in itself, in the right clinical setting, may be more suggestive of Wegener's granulomatosis than, say, of malignancy.

If the clinical suspicion of Wegener's granulomatosis is strong, treatment should not be delayed pending histology.

There are few laboratory guides to disease activity, the best being leucocytosis.

Anaemia and raised ESR are usual. Raised polymorph counts are the rule (though possibly not as marked as in PAN) by eosinophilia is rare (Fauci & Wolff 1973). Cryoproteins, ANA tests and LE cells are usually negative. IgG levels are not grossly raised.

Table 11.3 Wegener's laboratory findings in 18 cases (from Pinching *et al.* 1983)

Neutrophilia	17 (mean 13 000/mm^3)
Eosinophilia	6
Raised ESR	18 (mean 112 mm/h)
Raised CRP	5
Raised gammaglobulin	5
C1q binding	11
Rheumatoid factor	12

ANCA

Antibodies directed against cytoplasmic antigens are now recognized as being useful markers for Wegener's granulomatosis (reviewed by Jennette & Falk 1992). Two patterns are seen on immunofluorescence, cytoplasmic (C-ANCA) and perinuclear (P-ANCA). The latter are not specific for the condition, being found in a variety of rheumatological disorders. C-ANCA, directed against serine-proteinase (proteinase 3) is found in over three-quarters of all patients with Wegener's granulomatosis. It is therefore a useful test in confirming the diagnosis; in management, however, variations in titre are less useful — certainly in the author's experience.

DIAGNOSIS

Although Wegener's granulomatosis in its widespread form is unmistakble, early or 'limited' forms may present diagnostic difficulty. The main differential diagnoses are of other causes of pulmonary shadows, other granulomatous diseases such as sarcoidosis and mid-line granuloma (Walton 1959) and other arteritides. Table 11.4 summarizes some of the more clinical pointers to differential diagnosis.

TREATMENT

One of the most potent arguments for the efficacy of immunosuppressive drugs in the connective tissue diseases is the dramatic change their

Table 11.4 Differential diagnosis of Wegener's granulomatosis

Condition	Comment
Sarcoid	Renal involvement rare. Granulomas not necrotizing Kveim tests negative in Wegener's
Midline granuloma	Localized
Goodpasture's syndrome	No antiGBM antibodies in Wegener's Glomerular deposits linear in Goodpasturer's, granular in Wegener's
Malignancy	Histology
PAN	Smaller vessels in Wegener's Granulomata rare in PAN Hypertension rare in Wegener's. Pulmonary involvement uncommon in PAN. Eosinophilia uncommon in Wegener's
Hypersensitivity angiitis	Granulomata absent. Smaller vessels

introduction has made to the course of Wegener's granulomatosis. Corticosteroids alone had little effect on the outcome (Hollander & Manning 1967).
Since 1954, an increasing number of reports of successful therapy with
alkylating agents, purine antimetabolites and folic acid antagonists have
been reported.

Wolff *et al.* (1974) reviewed experience with cytotoxic agents in 21
patients. Seventeen of these received cyclophosphamide at a dose of
1–2 mg/kg body weight, with increases of 25 mg if deterioration had
occurred.

With the exception of three patients with very advanced renal disease
at the start of therapy, the outcome was a complete remission in all but
two — both in those with renal involvement and those with limited forms
of the disease. Though relapses do occur in some patients on withdrawal
of cyclophosphamide, in the majority, the remission appears complete. In
a report of 10 patients treated with cyclophosphamide and followed up for
periods of up to seven years, Reza *et al.* (1975) found that in all, remissions
were sustained.

Figure 11.2 shows one such example in whom corticosteroids alone
were ineffective. The mean duration of remission was 38 months (to date)
and two have been disease-free for seven years. Only one patient relapsed
and she responded to a second course of cyclophosphamide.

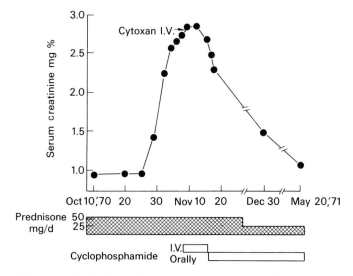

Fig. 11.2 Effect of cyclophosphamide on progressive uraemia. Following therapy, serum
creatinine has been less than 1·0 mg% with a creatinine clearance of 120 ml per minute.
(From Reza *et al.* 1975.)

The importance of combined treatment cannot be emphasized too strongly.

In our vasculitis clinic we have attempted to study the use of 'low dose' pulse cyclophosphamide — a regimen usually consisting of three weekly i.v. pulses of 500 g cyclophosphamide, always combined with MESNA to reduce the risk of cystitis. Subsequent treatment is with further pulses (usually 3–6 successive monthly pulses), or with oral cyclophosphamide or azathioprine. Details of our recipes and results have been published by Haga *et al.* (1992).

Case report. A 25-year-old woman diagnosed as having Wegener's granulomatosis was treated successfully with prednisolone 60 mg daily. Clinical evidence of vasculitis disappeared. Two months later, still on 40 mg prednisolone, she developed multiple pulmonary shadows and the bridge of her nose collapsed. The chest shadows resolved following the addition of cyclophosphamide.

PROGNOSIS

What was once one of the worst diseases to afflict man now appears to be largely curable. The long-term hazards of immunosuppressive therapy and the incidence of late recurrence have yet to be learnt (Fauci *et al.* 1983).

MIDLINE GRANULOMA

Midline granuloma (non-healing granuloma of the nose and upper respiratory tract) is a 'relentlessly progressive, localized, destructive inflammatory

Table 11.5 Clinicopathologic criteria that distinguish midline granuloma from Wegener's granulomatosis

Midline granuloma	Wegener's granulomatosis
Destructive upper airway lesions with characteristic extension through palate	Inflammatory upper airway disease predominantly of sinuses and nasal mucosa. Rarely, if ever, erodes through palate and face
Lungs not involved	Characteristic pulmonary infiltrates. Histopathology shows no necrotizing granulomatous vasculitis
Kidneys not involved	Characteristic early focal glomerulitis, progressing to fulminant glomerulonephritis
Disseminated vasculitis very rarely, if ever, occurs	Characteristic disseminated small vessel vasculitis

process that predominantly involves the nose, paranasal sinuses and palate, with erosion through contiguous structures, particularly the face' (Fauci, Johnson & Wolff 1976). Death is due to haemorrhage, sepsis or meningitis.

It presents a number of important differences from Wegener's granulomatosis, summarized in Table 11.5 (from Fauci, Johnson & Wolff 1976).

Encouraging therapeutic results have been achieved by Fauci, Johnson and Wolff at Bethesda (1976) using high-dose deep local irradiation. During a 15-year period, 10 patients were so treated with a long-term remission (>7 years) in 7 patients. Subsets of this granulomatous syndrome have been described (Toscos, Fauci & Costa 1982).

REFERENCES

Coutu R.E., Klein M., Lessell S., Friedman E. & Snider G.L. (1975) Limited form of Wegener's granulomatosis. Eye involvement as a major sign. *Journal of the American Medical Association*, **233**, 868.

D'Cruz D. & Hughes G.R.V. (1992) Systemic vasculitis. New treatments, new tests. *British Medical Journal*, **304**, 269.

D'Cruz D., Baguley E., Asherson R.A. & Hughes G.R.V. (1989) Ear nose and throat symptoms in subacute Wegener's granulomatosis. *British Medical Journal*, **299**, 419–422.

Drachman D.A. (1963) Neurological complications of Wegener's granulomatosis. *Archives of Neurology*, **8**, 145.

Fahey J., Leonard E., Churg J. & Godman G. (1954) Wegener's granulomatosis. *American Journal of Medicine*, **17**, 168.

Fauci A.S., Haynes B.F., Katz P. & Wolff S.M. (1983) Wegener's granulomatosis: prospective clinical and therapeutic experience with 85 patients for 21 years. *Annals of Internal Medicine*, **98**, 78–85.

Fauci A.S. & Wolff S.M. (1973) Wegener's granulomatosis. *Medicine*, **52**, 535.

Fauci A.S., Wolff S.M. & Johnson J.S. (1971) Effect of cyclophosphamide upon the immune response in Wegener's granulomatosis. *New England Journal of Medicine*, **285**, 1493.

Fauci A.S., Johnson R.E. & Wolff S.M. (1976) Radiation therapy of mid-line granuloma. *Annals of Internal Medicine*, **84**, 140.

Felson B. (1959) Less familiar roentgen patterns of pulmonary granulomas. *American Journal of Roentgenology, Radium Therapy and Nuclear Medicine*, **81**, 211.

Godman G.C. & Churg J. (1954) Wegener's granulomatosis: pathology and review of the literature. *Archives of Pathology*, **58**, 533.

Haga H., D'Cruz D., Asherson R. & Hughes G.R.V. (1992) The short term effect of IV pulse cyclophosphamide in the treatment of connective tissue diseases. *Annals of the Rheumatic Diseases*, **51**, 885–888.

Hollander D. & Manning R.T. (1967) The use of alkylating agents in the treatment of Wegener's granulomatosis. *Annals of Internal Medicine*, **67**, 393.

Hu C.-H., O'Loughlin S. & Winkelmann R.V. (1977) Cutaneous manifestations of Wegener's granulomatosis. *Archives of Dermatology*, **113**, 175.

Hughes G.R.V. & D'Cruz D. (1991) Joint pains, sinusitis, wheezing and mild vasculitis —

a distinct syndrome. *Journal of Rheumatology,* **18** (4), 495−496.

Jennette J.C. & Falk R.J. (1992) Disease associations and pathogenic role of antineutrophil antibodies in vasculitis. *Current Opinion in Rheumatology,* **4**, 9−15.

Kornblum D. & Fienberg R. (1955) Roentgen manifestations of necrotizing granulomatosis and angiitis of the lungs. *American Journal of Roentgenology, Radium Therapy, and Nuclear Medicine,* **74**, 587.

Leavitt R.Y. & Fauci A.S. (1992) Less common manifestations and presentations of Wegener's granulomatosis. *Current Opinion in Rheumatology,* **4**, 16−22.

Leavitt R.Y. (1990). The American College of Rheumatology criteria for the classification of Wegener's granulomatosis. *Arthritis and Rheumatism,* **33**, 1101−1107.

McCrea P.C. & Childers R.W. (1964) Two unusual cases of giant cell arteritis myocarditis associated with mitral stenosis with Wegener's syndrome. *British Heart Journal,* **26**, 490.

McGregor M.B. & Sandler G. (1964) Wegener's granulomatosis. A clinical and radiological survey. *British Journal of Radiology,* **37**, 430.

Papiha S.S., Murty G.E., Ad Hia A., Mains B.T. & Venning M. (1992) Association of Wegener's granulomatosis with HLA antigens and other genetic markers. *Annals of the Rheumatic Diseases,* **51**, 246−248.

Pinching A.J., Lockwood C.M., Pussell B.A., Rees A.J., Sweny P., Evans D.J., Bowley N. & Peters D.K. (1983) Wegener's granulomatosis: observations on 18 patients with severe renal disease. *Quarterly Journal of Medicine,* **52**, 435−460.

Reed W.B., Jensen A.K. & Konwaler (1963) The cutaneous manifestations of Wegener's granulomatosis. *Acta Dermatologica Venereologica (Stockholm),* **43**, 250.

Reza M.J., Dornfield L., Goldberg L.S., Bluestone R. & Pearson C.M. (1975) Wegener's granulomatosis. Long term follow up of patients treated with cyclophosphamide. *Arthritis and Rheumatism,* **18**, 501.

Rogers J.V., Jr & Roberto A.E. (1956) Circumscribed pulmonary lesions in periarteritis nodosa and Wegener's granulomatosis. *American Journal of Roentgenology,* **76**, 88.

Sahn E.E. & Sahn S.A. (1976) Wegener's granulomatosis with aphasia. *Archives of Internal Medicine,* **136**, 87.

Straatsma B.R. (1957) Ocular complications of Wegener's granulomatosis. *American Journal of Ophthalmology,* **44**, 789.

Sturrock R.D. (1974) Wegener's granulomatosis occurring in a patient with pre-existing rheumatoid arthritis. *British Journal of Clinical Practice,* **28**, 183.

Toscos M., Fauci A.S. & Costa J. (1982) Idiopathic midline destructive disease. A subgroup of patients with the 'midline granuloma' syndrome. *American Journal of Clinical Pathology,* **77**, 162−168.

Walton E.W. (1958) Giant cell granuloma of the respiratory tract (Wegener's granulomatosis). *British Medical Journal,* **2**, 265.

Walton E.W. (1959) Non healing granulomata of the nose. *Journal of Laryngology and Otolaryngology,* **73**, 242.

Wolff S.M., Fauci A.S., Horn R.G. & Dale D.C. (1974) Wegener's granulomatosis (NIH Conference). *Annals of Internal Medicine,* **81**, 513.

12: *Takayasu's Arteritis*

As in so many eponymous diseases, the syndrome of aortic arch aortitis with its characteristic pattern of pulse abnormalities was described long before 1908, when Takayasu, a Tokyo ophthalmologist, described 'a case of peculiar changes of the central retinal vessels'. Furthermore, it was Onishi, a colleague of Takayasu, who in the discussion following the case presentation correctly ascribed the ocular changes to major artery disease in reporting a similar case in whom 'no radial pulses were felt, no matter how hard we tried' (quoted by Judge *et al.* 1962).

Since that time, a distinctive syndrome has become recognized, predominantly affecting young women, and characterized by malaise and inflammatory involvement of the thoracic aorta and proximal ends of its major branches. While the syndrome is becoming increasingly recognized in Western countries most of the major studies have come from Japan and the Far East (Fraga *et al.* 1972; Deutsch, Wexler & Deutsch 1974).

Confusion has arisen over the term 'pulseless disease' which is a generic term covering many aetiologies (Table 12.1). These have been reviewed by Ross & McKusick (1953) on whose series of 100 cases much of Table 12.1 is based. While differentiation in some cases of giant cell arteritis involving the aortic arch may be difficult (Klein *et al.* 1975) there appears to be little doubt that Takayasu's arteritis is a distinct entity.

In 1992, Arend and colleagues in the American College of Rheumatology published criteria for this classification of Takayasu's arteritis.

PATHOLOGY

Figure 12.1 shows the frequency of patterns of involvement in 31 cases based on an angiographic study by Sano, Tadashi & Saito (1970). The pathology consists essentially of a stenosing inflammatory process of the thoracic aorta and the proximal segments of the large branches. There is sparing of the distal portions of the vessels, as well as the cerebral, coronary and other muscular arteries. Macroscopically there is extensive intimal irregularity, narrowing or aneurysmal dilatation.

Histologically, late cases are characterized by diffuse loss of muscular and elastic tissue with extensive fibrosis of the media and destruction of

Table 12.1 Causes of aortic arch syndromes (diminished or absent pulses in arteries arising from the aortic arch)

Atheromatous aneurysm
Syphilitic aortitis (with or without aneurysm)
Trauma
Congenital anomalies
Chronic dissection of the aorta
Thrombocytosis
Thrombotic disorders (including the antiphospholipid syndrome)

Arteritides
Takayasu's syndrome
Giant cell arteritis
Buerger's disease
Polyarteritis nodosa
SLE
Seronegative arthritides
Polychondritis
Behçet's syndrome

---

the elastic lamina. Some areas, particularly those more recently involved, show in growths of new capillaries resembling granulomata. Giant cells are occasionally seen, but are smaller and less frequent than in giant cell (temporal) arteritis (Chopra *et al.* 1983).

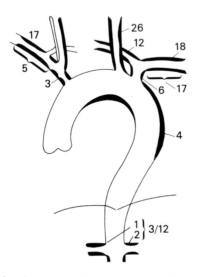

Fig. 12.1 Frequency of occlusion in each main branch of the aorta in pulseless disease. (From Sano, Tadashi & Saito 1970.) Based on 31 cases.

AETIOLOGY

The aetiology is obscure. The geographical preponderance of cases in Asia does not appear to be solely due to differences in diagnostic criteria and may represent genetic factors. The predominantly female distribution, together with the systemic features, erythema nodosum, and mild hyperglobulinaemia have led to suggestions that the disease has an immunological basis. However, apart from the occasional low titre positive antinuclear antibody, evidence for a specific immunological defect has been lacking. Antiaorta antibodies have been described but their specificity is doubtful (Lessof & Glynn 1959; Nakao *et al.* 1967; Asherson, Asherson & Schrire 1968). HLA studies have suggested a relationship with HLA Bw 52 (Numaro *et al.* 1983). Another suggestion is that the disease might, in some cases, be a coagulopathy (Kanaida, Takeshita & Nakamura 1982).

CLINICAL FEATURES

The disease predominantly affects young women in their teenage years and twenties (Nakao *et al.* 1967; Fraga *et al.* 1972). The 'classical' course consists of two stages; firstly, a generalized illness, often acute, which may include fever, polymyalgia rheumatica (indistinguishable from that associated in older patients with temporal arteritis), palpitations, syncope and joint pains. The degree of synovitis may initially suggest a diagnosis of rheumatoid arthritis (Sandring & Wellin 1961). A few cases have been associated with erythema nodosum (Nakao *et al.* 1967).

The prominence of this early 'systemic' phase emphasized by Strachan (1974) and Fraga *et al.* (1972) is not often appreciated. This systemic phase is followed after a period of weeks or months by the more well-known vascular manifestations of the disease — occasionally presenting with bruits or local tenderness, but more usually with upper limb claudication or absent pulses. The frequency with which the upper limb pulses are affected in association with normal lower limb pulses has led to the use of the term 'reversed coarctation' in this condition.

Table 12.2 (from Fraga *et al.* 1972) shows the frequency of various pulse alterations in 22 patients.

In addition to the lack of arterial pulsations, variable systemic manifestations may occur at this time, including headaches, tiredness, paraesthesiae, dizziness, exertional dyspnoea and weight loss. Raynaud's phenomenon is surprisingly rare (Fraga *et al.* 1972).

Coronary artery involvement (either direct or secondary to decreased perfusion) (Schrine & Asherson 1965) though rare may proceed to myocardial infarction (Fraga *et al.* 1972).

Table 12.2 Pulse abnormalities in 22 patients (from Fraga *et al.* 1972)

Arteries	Absent	Diminished
Ulnar	14	3
Radial	11	6
Brachial	10	5
Axillary	3	0
Carotid	1	1
Innominate	3	0
Femoral	4	4
Tibial	1	0
Popliteal	1	0
Total	48	19

Aortic incompetence, while described, is noticeably rare — a distinguishing feature from syphilitic aortitis and dissecting aneurysms. Patients studied by aortography not infrequently demonstrate subclavian-steal syndromes. Pulmonary artery involvement may be more frequent than earlier studies suggested (Deutsch, Wexler & Deutsch 1974). A number of cases develop hypertension — a complication now known to be secondary to renal artery involvement (Deutsch 1974). The central nervous system and ocular manifestations have been particularly emphasized by the Japanese and include transient visual disturbances, cataracts, iris atrophy, retinal haemorrhages, and hyperaemia of the conjunctiva and sclera (Shimizu 1951; Ostler 1957).

DIAGNOSIS

The few abnormal laboratory findings include a moderate neutrophil leucocytosis, a raised ESR (occasionally over 100 mm/h), moderate increases in IgG, IgM and IgA, and occasionally, as in other arteritides, a transient mild eosinophilia. Angiography is essential for confirmation of the diagnosis (Gotsman, Beck & Schrire 1967; Fraga *et al.* 1972).

MANAGEMENT AND PROGNOSIS

In 1972, Fraga *et al.* observed that of 135 patients reported, three-quarters had died within two years of diagnosis. In their own series of 22 patients only 5 died, the improved outlook being attributed to corticosteroid therapy. Their experience suggested that an initial dose of 30 mg/day of prednisone for 9 weeks followed by a maintenance dose of 5–10 mg/day resulted in the disappearance of systemic symptoms, a fall in ESR, and, in 7 cases, return of arterial pulses.

Other forms of treatment include anticoagulants (Spittal & Siekert 1957; Judge *et al*. 1962) and arterial surgery (Warren & Triedman 1957).

A longer-term outlook, including the possibility of normal pregnancy, is now being reported (Wong, Wang & Tse 1983).

REFERENCES

Arend W.P. (1990) The American College of Rheumatology 1990 criteria for the classification of Takayasu's arteritis. *Arthritis and Rheumatism*, **33**, 1129–1134.

Asherson R.A., Asherson G.L. & Schrire V. (1968) Immunological studies in arteritis of the aorta and great vessels. *British Medical Journal*, **iii**, 589.

Chopra P., Datta R.K., Dasgupta A. *et al*. (1983) Non-specific aorto-arteritis (Takayasu's disease): an immunologic and autopsy study. *Japanese Heart Journal*, **24**, 549–556.

Deutsch V., Wexler L. & Deutsch H. (1974) Takayasu's arteritis. *American Journal of Roentgenology, Radium Therapy and Nuclear Medicine*, **122**, 13.

Fraga A., Mintz G., Valle L. & Flores-Izquierdo G. (1972) Takayasu's arteritis: frequency of systemic manifestations (study of 22 patients) and favourable response to maintenance steroid therapy with adrenocorticosteroids (12 patients). *Arthritis and Rheumatism*, **15**, 617.

Gotsman M.S., Beck W. & Schrire V. (1967) Selective angiography in arteritis of the aorta and its major branches. *Radiology*, **88**, 232.

Judge D.R., Currier D.R., Gracie A.W. & Figley M.M. (1962) Takayasu's arteritis and aortic arch syndrome. *American Journal of Medicine*, **32**, 379.

Kanaida H., Takeshita A. & Nakamura M. (1982) Etiologic aspects of coagulopathy in Takayasu's aortitis. *American Heart Journal*, **104**, 1039–1045.

Klein R.G., Hunder G.G., Stanson T.W. & Sheps S.G. (1975) Large artery involvement in giant cell (temporal) arteritis. *Annals of Internal Medicine*, **83**, 806.

Lessof M.H. & Glynn L.E. (1959) The pulseless syndrome. *Lancet*, **i**, 806.

Nakao K., Ikesa M., Kimata H. *et al*. (1967) Takayasu's arteritis. Clinical report of 84 cases and immunological studies of 7 cases. *Circulation*, **35**, 1141.

Numano F., Ishohisa I., Egami M., Ohta N. & Sasazuki T. (1983) HLA-DR MT and MB antigens in Takayasu's disease. *Tissue Antigens*, **21**, 208.

Ostler H.B. (1957) Pulseless disease. *American Journal of Ophthalmology*, **43**, 583.

Ross R.S. & McKusick V.A. (1953) Aortic arch syndromes. *Archives of Internal Medicine*, **92**, 701.

Sandring H. & Wellin G. (1961) Aortic arch syndrome with special reference to rheumatoid arthritis. *Acta Medica Scandinavica*, **170**, 1.

Sano K., Tadashi A. & Saito I. (1970) Angiography in pulseless disease. *Radiology*, **94**, 69.

Schrine A. & Asherson R.A. (1965) Arteritis of the aorta and its major branches. *Quarterly Journal of Medicine*, **33**, 439.

Shimizu K. (1951) Pulseless disease. *Journal of the American Medical Association*, **145**, 1095.

Spittal J.A. & Siekert G. (1957) Anticoagulant therapy of patients with aortic arch syndrome. *Mayo Clinic Proceedings*, **32**, 723.

Strachan R.W. (1974) Natural history of Takayasu's arteriopathy. *Quarterly Journal of Medicine*, **33**, 57.

Warren R. & Triedman L.J. (1957) Pulseless and carotid artery thrombosis. Surgical considerations. *New England Journal of Medicine*, **257**, 685.

Wong V.C.W., Wang R.Y.C. & Tse T.F. (1983) Pregnancy and Takayasu's arteritis. *American Journal of Medicine*, **75**, 597–601.

13: *Other Vasculitides*

As mentioned in earlier chapters, many of the vasculitides overlap both clinically and histologically. Attempts at clinical separation, while difficult, have some practical value, if only for prognostic purposes, and while some of the conditions discussed below overlap with polyarteritis nodosa, present knowledge dictates that they probably deserve their present separate labels.

HYPERSENSITIVITY ANGIITIS

In the studies of Zeek (1953) hypersensitivity angiitis was distinguished by its predilection for smaller-sized vessels, and by the finding that all lesions were at approximately the same stage in evolution — unlike the situation in PAN, though some clinicians investigating patients with these disorders interchange the labels (McCombs 1965; Sergent *et al.* 1976). The majority of virus-induced arteritides in animals conform more to the pattern of hypersensitivity angiitis than to full-blown PAN. The subject has been reviewed by Calabrese *et al.* (1990) and Michael (1992).

CHURG–STRAUSS VASCULITIS
(Lanham *et al.* 1984; Masi *et al.* 1990)

Like Wegener's granulomatosis, Churg–Strauss vasculitis is characterized by prominent granuloma formation. This condition links the eosinophilic syndromes with the vasculitides. Characteristically, the patient has a long history of asthma (and/or allergic rhinitis), then develops a vasculitis accompanied by eosinophilia (often extreme) and (often) raised IgE levels. Figures 13.1 and 13.2 (from Lanham *et al.* 1984)) outline the relationships between eosinophilia, asthma and vasculitis. Criteria for the classification of Churg–Strauss syndrome have been proposed by Masi *et al.* (1990).

Tables 13.1 and 13.2 give the clinical and laboratory features of 16 cases reviewed by our group (Lanham *et al.* 1984) together with a comparison with figures previously published.

Eosinophil counts can rise to over 12 000/ml and IgE may be high. Skin lesions are often highlighted by large, necrotic purplish ulcers on the elbows (Finan & Winkelman 1983; Lanham *et al.* 1984).

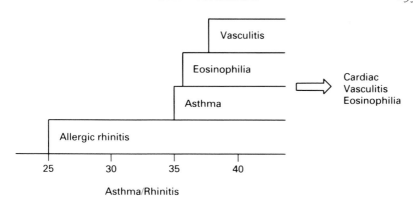

Fig. 13.1 Churg—Strauss syndrome.

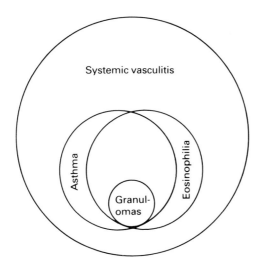

Fig. 13.2 Schematic representation of the relationship of asthma and granulomatous disease in systemic vasculitis (from Lanham *et al.* 1984).

Perhaps the most striking clinical point of difference from other vasculitides is the high morbidity and mortality from cardiac disease (Table 13.2).

Interestingly, the vasculitis occasionally follows desensitization 'shots'.

Case report. *A 23-year-old Saudi female had suffered from mild-to-moderate asthma for many years. Two weeks after a series of desensitization injections, she developed arthritis, fever and abdominal pain. She was found to have an ESR of 150, a WBC of 30 000 and an eosinophil count of 18 000.*

Chapter 13

Table 13.1 Clinical features of Churg–Strauss syndrome in 16 patients (from Lanham *et al.* 1984)

	Clinical features	No. of cases
Asthma	Past history	16
	Exacerbation during vasculitic phase	5
Pulmonary disease	Loffler prodrome	5
	Infiltrates	10
	Pleural effusion	4
	Recurrent infections	7
Upper respiratory tract	Allergic rhinitis	12
	Surgical procedure(s)	9
Cardiovascular disease	Hypertension	12
	Cardiac failure	4
	Pericarditis	2
	Abnormal electrocardiogram	8
Gastrointestinal disease	Abdominal pain	7
	Diarrhoea	5
	Bleeding	4
Renal disease	Mild	14
	Renal failure	1
	Nephrotic syndrome	3
Cutaneous disease	Nodules	2
	Purpura	9
	Erythema/urticaria	9
Muscoloskeletal disease	Arthritis/arthralgia	11
	Myalgia	11
Nervous system disease	CNS	4
	Mononeuritis multiplex	12

Table 13.2 Causes of death in 50 cases of Churg–Strauss syndrome

	No.	Percentage
Congestive cardiac failure/myocardial infarction	24	48
Cerebral haemorrhage	8	16
Renal failure	9	18
Gastrointestinal tract Perforation or haemorrhage	4	8
Status asthmaticus	4	8
Respiratory failure	1	2

Her hospital course was stormy. She developed multiple bowel infarcts requiring surgery. She developed severe congestive cardiac failure and a large anterior myocardial infarct.

She gradually improved on prednisone and cyclophosphamide but cardiac function remained severely impaired.

Renal disease is characteristically mild but hypertension may be severe. Although the disease may respond to steroids alone, combined steroid and immunosuppressive therapy is recommended.

CUTANEOUS VASCULITIS
(Figs 13.3, 13.4)

Dermatologists and physicians dealing with connective tissue diseases recognize that cutaneous vasculitides account for significant and chronic

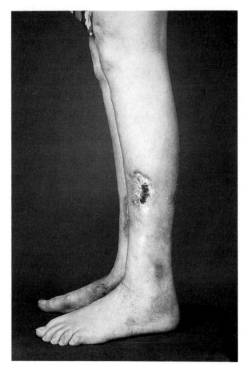

Fig. 13.3 Chronic leg ulceration in a patient with cutaneous vasculitis. Despite corticosteroids and many other forms of therapy, complete healing of the ulcers did not occur.

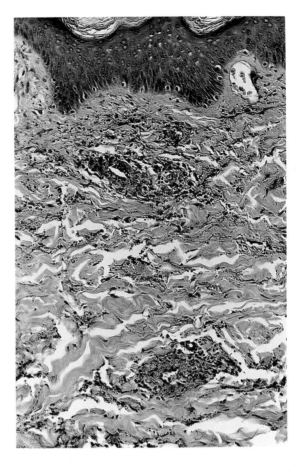

Fig. 13.4 Cutaneous vasculitis. Skin biopsy showing fibrinoid necrosis of vessel wall with extravasation of red blood cells and inflammation of surrounding tissue. (Dr Shirley Amin, University Hospital of the West Indies.)

morbidity in a sizeable group of patients. Cutaneous vasculitis encompasses a range of disorders (Cunliffe 1976) which includes nodular vasculitis, Behçet's syndrome (O'Duffy, Carney & Deodhar 1971), Henoch–Schönlein purpura and necrotizing vasculitis. The term cutaneous angiitis is reserved by some for cases where veins rather than arteries or arterioles are involved (Copeman 1975).

It appears likely from the parallels in animal diseases, referred to earlier, that immune complex mechanisms play a role in the pathogenesis of some of these cases. Cream (1972) reported mixed cryoglobulins in cutaneous vasculitis and in a 1973 study of 32 patients with cutaneous vasculitis noted 11 with anticomplementary activity. In 5 of these, immune complexes in the form of mixed cryoglobulins were detected.

Despite its lack of emphasis, chronic cutaneous vasculitis is an unpleasant, troublesome condition which is often resistant to treatment. These patients often come to haunt outpatient departments. The immunological abnormalities such as the very high C1q binding values of these patients (note the difference from the acute, fulminant PAN where immunological abnormalities are few) suggest that plasma exchange and immunosuppression might prove effective. In our experience, the results to date are only partly successful.

ESSENTIAL MIXED CRYOGLOBULINAEMIA
(The 'purpura–myalgia–cryoglobulinaemia syndrome')

It has been recognized for over a decade that some cases of vasculitis were associated with cryoglobulinaemia, and that the cryoprecipitate contained 19S and 7S proteins.

In 1966 Meltzer *et al*. described a group of 11 patients with a distinctive clinical pattern, which has come to be known as essential mixed cryoglobulinaemia, or the purpura–myalgia–cryoglobulinaemia syndrome.

The cryoglobulinaemia is of the mixed type, i.e. at least two different immunoglobulin classes. In most cases one of the immunoglobulins is IgM, with rheumatoid factor (antiIgG) activity. In some cases circulating high molecular weight (22S) complexes have been found on ultracentrifugation of serum at 37°C (Klein *et al*. 1968; MacKenzie *et al*. 1968).

In an elegant study, Gharavi took the cryoprecipitate from a patient with mixed essential cryoglobulinaemia, separated the rheumatoid factor, raised an anti-idiotype to it, and used this preparation to demonstrate the cells in a bone marrow preparation responsible for the synthesis of the rheumatoid factor (Gharavi *et al*. 1984).

The clinical features of these cases are sufficiently similar to form a distinct syndrome, with purpura (in particular gravitational purpura exacerbated by exercise), arthralgias, myalgias, and muscle weakness, anaemia and hypergammaglobulinaemia. Additional features are hepatomegaly, splenomegaly, Sjøgren's syndrome (see Chapter 4), thyroiditis and cutaneous vasculitis. Other features which have occasionally been observed are thrombocytopenia, epistaxis (Golde & Epstein 1968), Raynaud's phenomenon (Feizi & Gitlin 1969), digital gangrene (Goldberg & Barnett 1970), leg ulceration (Mathison *et al*. 1971), intestinal vasculitis (Reza *et al*. 1974) and peripheral neuropathy (Logothetis *et al*. 1968; Cream *et al*. 1974). Central nervous involvement has been reported with encephalopathy, cranial nerve palsies, pyramidal tract signs and myelitis (Abramsky & Slavin 1974).

Case report. A 62-year-old man presented with lower limb purpura and heavy proteinuria. Serum contained a heavy mixed crypoprotein. He was mildly demented and periodically demonstrated persistent choreoathetotic movements. These cerebral abnormalities disappeared rapidly with institution of therapy.

Chronic active hepatitis and cirrhosis have also been associated with this condition (Feizi & Gitlin 1969; Jori & Buonanno 1972).

The most important complication is nephritis, sometimes ending in acute renal failure (Meltzer *et al.* 1966). Histologically, the renal lesion is one of diffuse glomerulitis, with fibrinoid necrosis in small to medium-sized vessels and granular basement membrane deposits of IgM and IgG.

Skin biopsies may show vasculitis — thus mixed cryglobulinaemia may be alternatively classified as one of the causes of cutaneous vasculitis.

While the disease generally involves smaller vessels, occasional cases with major visceral involvement (see above) are seen, and one case ending in polyarteritis nodosa has been described (Schimmer & Bloch 1975).

An association with hepatitis B virus has been observed, with virus particles demonstrable on electron microscopy of the cryoprecipitate (Levo *et al.* 1977), though this association is unusual. More important is the association with hepatitis C virus infection (Bambara *et al.* 1991; Mader & Keystone 1992).

Treatment of severe cases including those with nephritis is most frequently with corticosteroids and cyclophosphamide (Mathison *et al.* 1971), together with plasmapheresis.

At present, the clinical differentiation of the cutaneous and purpuric vasculitides is at best sketchy.

Cream (1976) has attempted an alternative method of classification based on immunological findings, in particular on analysis of cryoglobulins (Table 13.3).

NECROTIZING VASCULITIS AFTER ACUTE SEROUS OTITIS

Sergent & Christian reported seven patients with necrotizing vasculitis developing after serous otitis media. There was no pulmonary or histological evidence of Wegener's granulomatosis, or episcleritis to suggest Cogan's syndrome (deafness, interstitial keratitis and occasionally vasculitis) (Cody & Williams 1960). The patients did not develop eosinophilia or asthma, and hepatitis B antigen was not found. Other viral studies were negative,

Table 13.3 Classification of the cutaneous vasculitides (Cream 1976)

Evidence of circulating immune complexes:
Immune complex cryoglobulins
Intermediate complexes
Anticomplementary serum
Hypocomplementaemia
IgA mesangiopathy (including cases of Henoch–Shönlein purpura)
Low serum IgM
Single component cryoglobulin
Negative findings

but the clustering of cases seen by these physicians led to speculation regarding an infective aetiology (reviewed by Lockshin & Sergent 1976).

ISOLATED ANGIITIS OF THE CNS

This extremely rare condition is characterized by headaches, altered mental function and focal neurological defects (Cupps, Moore & Fauci 1983).

MUCOCUTANEOUS LYMPH NODE SYNDROME OF INFANTS (Kawasaki's disease)

Japanese workers have described a disease of unknown aetiology, affecting most frequently infants and children under the age of 5 years, having some similarity to the Stevens–Johnson syndrome, and characterized by fever, conjunctival congestion, redness and fissuring of the tongue and reddening of the pharyngeal mucosa.

In the peripheries, there is reddening of the palms and soles, exanthematous rash, and cervical lymphadenopathy. More serious is the development of carditis or pericarditis, leading to sudden death in 1–2%. The aetiology of this condition is unknown (*Lancet* editorial 1982).

Between 1968 and 1978 over 18 000 cases have been reported in Japan (Hamashima 1980). Of the 184 deaths (1·8%) the majority were from multiple aneurysm formation or coronary disease. Hamashima, in his review (1980), lists six main features:

1 Fever (lasting over 5 days).
2 Fingertip oedema and shinyness, with a scarlet fever-like exfoliation at the same site.
3 An irregular widespread skin eruption.
4 Conjunctival hyperaemia.
5 Red dry lips and strawberry tongue.
6 Lymphadenopathy (often unilateral).

ARTERITIS AND HAIRY CELL LEUKAEMIA
(Hughes 1983)

In 1979, we reported a new syndrome, linking arteritis with chronic hairy cell leukaemia (Hughes *et al.* 1979; Elkon *et al.* 1979).

Histologically, the vasculitis has been characterized by arterial wall necrosis, and on angiography, aneurysms have been demonstrated.

Hairy cell leukaemia, putatively of B cell origin, is a chronic leukaemia, often responding to splenomegaly and therapy including interferon. Studies of reticuleondothelial function in this condition have, as expected, shown grossly impaired clearance. Thus this syndrome, as well as linking reticuleondothelial system malignancy with vasculitis, may provide clues to immune-complex and other pathogenetic mechanisms in some forms of arteritis (Hughes 1983).

Recent reviews of the association with hairy cell leukaemia, as well as with other malignancies are by Greek *et al.* (1988) and Mertz and Conn (1992).

ADULT ONSET STILL'S DISEASE
(Elkon *et al.* 1982)

In many ways this is the most dramatic, and often poorly diagnosed, disease in rheumatology.

Clinical features

The main trial consists of arthritis, high fevers and a rash. Other clinical pointers are lymphadenopathy, recurrent sore throat and leucocytoses. As in childhood Still's disease, occasional cases have gone on to amyloidosis.

Fever. This is the most striking feature. It may go on for weeks or even months on end, and attacks may recur over periods of many years. The temperature is often extreme, rising to over 104°F daily. The temperature chart is sometimes 'saw tooth' with, for example, a high temperature each evening and a normal temperature in the morning. During the fever, there may be drenching sweats.

Rash. This is classically morbilliform and transient. Draw a circle round one of the lesions on one day and the distribution will be seen to be different the next.

The histological picture is one of a leucocytoclastic small vessel vasculitis. Other skin rashes include wheals and dermatographia. The rash is usually prominent at the time of the high fever. Fever may, however, persist without the appearance of the rash.

Arthritis. This is often severe. It has particular propensity for the wrists and ultimately leads to erosion, damage and even fusion of the wrists. Any other joints may be affected, but as in childhood Still's disease, the neck, distal interphalangeal joints and feet are often inflamed.

Aetiology

The aetiology is unknown. HLA studies have been inconclusive because of the rarity of the disease.

Diagnosis

Look at the wrists. Get the patient to place his or her hands in a prayer position and extend both wrists together. There are few diseases (rheumatoid arthritis and psoriasis) which cause bilateral permanent wrist inflammation and damage.

There is *no* other disease where the physician is called to the bedside of a patient with a five-year history of fever, rashes and erosive arthritis.

Most patients with adult Still's disease have, not unnaturally, undergone previous intensive therapy for tuberculosis, lymphomas etc. As always, hindsight helps, and clearly, infection must be excluded as best possible.

Usually, all immunological tests (ANA, rheumatoid factor, etc.) are negative. Indeed, the only abnormal findings in this clinically dramatic condition are leucocytosis (occasionally over $30\,000/mm^3$), a raised ESR and C-reactive protein, and non-specific liver enzyme rises.

Treatment and prognoses

The initial treatment is full dose salicylates. My own preference has been for benorylate (a salicylate-paracetamol ester). Some patients have responded moderately well to NSAIDs. However, in our retrospective studies of adult Still's disease, treatment in the long term had *not* proved highly successful. Some patients (but not others) had responded to gold and some to penicillamine. Unfortunately, a number of patients had ended up on steroids, though even here, response had been variable. Perhaps most promising has been the clinical improvement recently reported with the use of methotrexate.

REFERENCES

Abramsky O. & Salvin S. (1974) Neurologic manifestations in patients with mixed cryoglobulinaemia. *Neurology*, **24**, 245.

Bambara C.M. (1991) Cryoglobulinaemia and hepatitis C virus infection. *Clinical and Experimental Rheumatology*, **9**, 96–97.

Calabrese L.H., Michel B.A., Bloch D.A. *et al.* (1990) The American College of Rheumatology 1990 classification of hypersensitivity vasculitis. *Arthritis and Rheumatism*, **33**, 1108–1113.

Cody D.T. & Williams H.L. (1960) Cogan's syndrome. *Laryngoscope*, **70**, 447.

Copeman P.W.M. (1975) Cutaneous angiitis. *Journal of the Royal College of Physicians*, **9**, 103.

Cream J.J. (1972) Cryoglobulins in vasculitis. *Clinical and Experimental Immunology*, **10**, 117.

Cream J.J. (1973) Anticomplementary sera in cutaneous vasculitis. *British Journal of Dermatology*, **89**, 555.

Cream J.J. (1976) Clinical and immunological aspects of cutaneous vasculitis. *Quarterly Journal of Medicine*, **45**, 255.

Cream J.J., Hern J.E., Hughes R.A. *et al.* (1974) Mixed or immune complex cryoglobulinaemia and neuropathy. *Journal of Neurology, Neurosurgery and Psychiatry*, **37**, 82.

Cunliffe W.J. (1976) Fibrinolysis and vasculitis. *Clinical and Experimental Dermatology*, **1**, 1.

Cupps T.R., Moore P.M. & Fanci A.S. (1983) Isolated angiitis of the central nervous system. *American Journal of Medicine*, **74**, 97–105.

Elkon K.B., Hughes G.R.V., Catovsky D., Cleavel J.P., Dumont J., Seligmann M., Tannenbaum H. & Esdaile J. (1979) Hairy cell leukaemia with polyarteritis nodosa. *Lancet*, **ii**, 280.

Elkon K.B., Hughes G.R.V., Bywaters E.G.L., Ryan P., Inman R.D., Bowky N.B., James M.P. & Eady R. (1982) Adult onset Still's disease. Twenty year follow up and further studies of patients with active disease. *Arthritis and Rheumatism*, **25** (6), 647–654.

Feizi T. & Gitlin N. (1976) Immune complex disease of the kidney associated with chronic hepatitis and cryoglobulinaemia. *Lancet*, **ii**, 873.

Finan M.C. & Winkelman R.K. (1983) The cutaneous extravascular necrotizing granuloma (Churg–Strauss granuloma) and sytemic disease: a review of 27 cases. *Medicine*, **62**, 142–158.

Gharavi A.E., Elkon K., Hughes G.R.V. *et al.* (1984) Use of anti-idiotypic antibodies to antibodies to demonstrate rheumatoid-factor producing bone marrow cells in essential mixed cryoglobulinaemia. *Annals of the Rheumatic Diseases*, **43**, 651–652.

Goldberg L.S. & Barnett E.V. (1970) Essential cryoglobulinaemia. Immunologic studies before and after penicillamine therapy. *Archives of Internal Medicine*, **125**, 145.

Golde D. & Epstein W. (1968) Mixed cryoglobulins and glomerulonephritis. *Annals of Internal Medicine*, **69**, 1221.

Greer J.M., Longley S., Edwards N.L. *et al.* (1988) Vasculitis associated with malignancy. *Medicine*, **67**, 220–230.

Hamashima Y. (1980) Kawasaki's disease. In: *Clinics in Rheumatic Diseases*, Vol. 6 (2), Ed: D. Alarcon-Segovia. Saunders, Philadelphia.

Hughes G.R.V. (1983) Hairy cell leukaemia and arteritis. *Clinical and Experimental Rheumatology*, **1**, 9.

Hughes G.R.V., Elkon K.B., Spiller R., Catovsky D. & Jamieson I. (1979) Polyarteritis nodosa and hairy cell leukaemia. *Lancet*, **i**, 678.

Jori G.P. & Buonanno G. (1972) Chronic hepatitis and cirrhosis of the liver in cryoglobuli-naemia. *Gut*, **13**, 610.

Klein F., Van Rood J.J., Van Furth R. *et al.* (1968) IgM—IgG cryoglobulinaemia with IgM paraprotein component. *Clinical and Experimental Immunology*, **3**, 703.

Lancet (1982) Kawasaki's — might it be? (Editorial). *Lancet*, **ii**, 1441—1442.

Lanham J.G., Elkon K.B., Pusey C.D. & Hughes G.R.V. (1984) Systemic vasculitis with asthma and eosinophilia: a clinical approach to the Churg—Strauss syndrome. *Medicine*, **63**, 65—81.

Levo Y., Gorevic P.D., Kassab H.J. *et al.* (1977) Association between hepatitis B virus and essential mixed cryoglobulinaemia. *New England Journal of Medicine*, **296**, 1501.

Lockshin M. & Sergent J.S. (1976) Necrotising vasculitis and HB antigen. In: *Modern Topics in Rheumatology*. Ed: G.R.V. Hughes. Heinemann, London.

Logothetis J., Kennedy W., Ellington A. *et al.* (1968) Cryoglobulinaemic neuropathy. Incidence and clinical characteristics. *Archives of Neurology*, **19**, 389.

MacKenzie M.R., Goldberg L.S., Barnett E.V. *et al.* (1968) Serological heterogeneity of the IgM components of mixed (monoclonal IgM polyclonal IgG) cryoglobulins. *Clinical and Experimental Immunology*, **3**, 931.

Mader R. & Keystone E.C. (1992) Infections that cause vasculitis. *Current Opinion in Rheumatology*, **4**, 35—38.

Masi A.T., Hunder G.G., Lie J.T. *et al.* (1990) The American College of Rheumatology criteria for the classification of Churg—Strauss syndrome. *Arthritis and Rheumatism*, **33**, 1094—1100.

Mathison D.A., Condemi J.J., Leddy J.P. *et al.* (1971) Purpura, arthralgia and IgM—IgG cryoglobulinaemia with rheumatoid factor activity. Response to cyclophosphamide and splenectomy. *Annals of Internal Medicine*, **74**, 383.

McCombs R.P. (1965) Systemic 'allergic' vasculitis. *Journal of the American Medical Association*, **194**, 1059.

Meltzer M., Franklin E.C., Eilias K. *et al.* (1966) Cryoglobulinaemia — a clinical and laboratory study. II. Cryoglobulin with rheumatoid factor activity. *American Journal of Medicine*, **40**, 837.

Mertz L.E. & Conn D.L. (1992) Vasculitis associated with malignancy. *Current Opinion in Rheumatology*, **4**, 39—46.

Michel B.A. (1992) Classification of vasculitis. *Current Opinion in Rheumatology*, **4**, 3—8.

O'Duffy J.D., Carney J.A. & Deodhar S. (1971) Behçet's disease. *Annals of Internal Medicine*, **75**, 56.

Reza M.J., Roth B.E., Pops M.R. *et al.* (1974) Intestinal vasculitis in essential mixed cryoglobulinaemia. *Annals of Internal Medicine*, **81**, 632.

Schimmer B.M. & Bloch K.J. (1975) Mixed IgM—IgG cryoglobulinaemia terminating in polyarteritis nodosa. *Journal of Rheumatology*, **2**, 241.

Sergent J.S., Lockshin M.D., Christian C.L. & Gocke D.J. (1976) Vasculitis with hepatitis B antigenaemia. *Medicine*, **55**, 1.

Zeek P.M. (1953) Periarteritis nodosa and other forms of necrotising angiitis. *New England Journal of Medicine*, **248**, 764.

14: *Polymyalgia Rheumatica and Giant Cell Arteritis*

It is often surprising in retrospect that a syndrome such as polymyalgia rheumatica and giant cell (or temporal) arteritis with such distinctive features should have been widely recognized only in recent years. The recognition of an association between these two conditions has proved a major contribution to clinical medicine.

It is somewhat artificial to separate giant cell arteritis from polymyalgia rheumatica as many of the features described below are seen in the former condition, which may be a widespread disease in some patients.

Temporal arteritis (or more correctly 'giant cell' or 'cranial' arteritis, as the disease affects an area far greater than the temporal arteries alone) was first clearly described by Jonathan Hutchinson at The London Hospital in 1890.

The 'elderly father of a well remembered beadle of the London Hospital' was described as having 'red streaks' on his head, which were found to lie over the temporal arteries which were inflamed and swollen on both sides and which prevented him from wearing his hat. Hutchinson referred to the condition as 'a peculiar form of thrombotic arteritis of the aged'.

Polymyalgia rheumatica (PMR) was possibly first described by Bruce in 1888, who entitled it 'senile rheumatic gout'. Since then, a wide variety of names have been applied to the syndrome, some unpronounceable. Barber in 1957 described the clinical features in detail. In 1960 Paulley & Hughes first drew attention to the association between PMR and giant cell arteritis. A useful (though not totally exact) working definition was provided by Healey, Parker & Wilke (1971) — 'Polymyalgia rheumatica, a syndrome of older patients, is characterized by pain and stiffness of the shoulder or pelvic girdle muscles, without weakness or atrophy; these symptoms persist for at least a month, with a sedimentation rate of greater than 50 mm/hr, and dramatic relief of symptoms with the use of steroids.'

The syndrome of polymyalgia in some cases may be a manifestation of early RA, or of underlying malignancy, in particular multiple myeloma. However, in the majority of cases no such association is found, and the main hazard to the patient is the danger of giant cell arteritis and of blindness. The two conditions will be described together.

PATHOLOGY
(reviewed by Nordborg *et al.* 1991, 1992)

Giant cell arteritis affects both large and medium-sized arteries. The vessels are enlarged and the lumen narrowed. 'Skip lesions' are common and a normal biopsy is possible even in an inflamed vessel. The adventitia contains a mononuclear cell infiltrate, often around the vasa vasorum. The infiltrating lymphocytes are mainly T cells (Anderson *et al.* 1987). In the media (and less commonly in the adventitia) large multinucleate giant cells are seen. Acute inflammatory lesions and fibrinoid necrosis are both rare. The internal elastic lamina is swollen and fragmented and portions are phagocytosed by the giant cells. The arteritis may be widespread, and in a postmortem examination of 12 patients who died with active giant cell arteritis, Wilkinson and Russell (1972) observed a high incidence of involvement of the superficial temporal, vertebral, ophthalmic and posterior ciliary arteries, with less frequent involvement of the internal and external carotid and central retinal arteries. Giant cell arteritis is also one of the conditions occasionally causing aortic arch syndrome (Klein *et al.* 1975).

The distribution of arteritis corresponds broadly with the amount of elastic tissue within the vessels. Pulmonary and renal vessels are usually not involved. Also of interest is the observation that although lesions of the arteries of the head and neck predominate, intracranial vessels (which have little elastic tissue) are seldom involved.

In PMR there is little to find on muscle biopsy, even histochemically. Muscle enzymes and EMG examinations are normal.

EPIDEMIOLOGY
(see Chuang *et al.* 1982; Smith *et al.* 1983; Nordborg *et al.* 1992)

The temporal arteries of all adults dying in one year in Malmö (Sweden) were examined and evidence of previous arteritis was found in 1% (Ostberg 1971). While this incidence figure has not been reached clinically, it is now recognized that polymyalgia, at least, is a relatively common disease of the aged. While most patients are over the age of 60 years, in one series (Mowat & Hazleman 1974) 35% of patients were under 60 years. All series agree that the disease is commoner in women, and the condition appears to be rare in blacks (Bell & Klinefelter 1967; Smith *et al.* 1983).

There is an impression that the disease is more prevalent in northern countries than further south. For example, in a recent study from Italy, Salvorini (1991) showed a low incidence of polymyalgia rheumatica and giant cell arteritis (for the latter, 6·9 cases per 100 000 individuals over 50 years), differing strikingly from a study from Göteborg, Sweden, with an incidence rate of 18·3 cases per 100 000 inhabitants over 50 years of age (Nordborg & Bengtsson 1990).

Of considerable interest have been reports of familial aggregation of PMR. In some of these cases the onset of the illness began in two members of a family within 12 months of each other (Barber 1957; Hamrin 1972; Wadman & Werner 1972).

AETIOLOGY
(reviewed by Nordborg *et al.* 1992)

Infective

There appears to be a seasonal variation in the disease, and an association with upper respiratory infections has been reported (Bell & Klinefelter 1967), though to date no respiratory viral studies have been positive.

Bacon, Doherty & Zuckerman (1975) reported hepatitis-B surface antibody in 9 out of 12 patients tested prior to therapy. Hepatitis-B antigen was not detected. This finding has not been confirmed by others.

In another study, it was seen that in a group of 28 patients with PMR, 15 had had significant contact with birds, especially parakeets (Healey, Parker & Wilke 1971), though this has not been substantiated.

Although infection as an aetiology is not proven on present evidence, a combination of infective and genetic actors is still conceivable.

Immunological

Evidence for an immunological mechanism is weak. The transformation response of peripheral blood lymphocytes to human muscle antigen and to arterial antigen *in vitro* has been found to be increased in PMR (Hazleman, MacLennan & Esiri 1975). It has been suggested by these workers that the arterial antigen in question might be elastin — a theory which would fit in with the distribution of the disease, and with the distribution of immuno-globulins in the vessel walls (Liang, Simkin & Mannik 1974). Other findings have been the occasional reports of ANCA — possibly an epiphenomenon (Bosch *et al.* 1991), and inflammatory flags such as raised IL-6 levels (Dasgupta and Panayi 1990).

CLINICAL FEATURES

Myalgic features

The classical features of PMR are severe stiffness, and in some a feeling of pain in the muscles. Muscle tenderness is usually mild. The stiffness is worst around the neck and shoulders, and less prominently around the pelvic girdle. Symptoms are worse in the mornings and the patient may have to be lifted out of bed. In subacute cases the patient finds it hard to pinpoint symptoms, but may 'feel 100 years old' or complain only of 'rheumatics'. It is often only when the patient is diagnosed and treated that the severity and duration of the disease are recognized. True synovitis may be prominent in the early stages of the disease (Bruk 1967) and may cause difficulties in differentiation from early rheumatoid arthritis. Joint scanning often shows hot joints.

There may be marked localized tenderness over the C7 spinal process and a common differential diagnosis is cervical spondylosis, with stiffness and pain referred to both shoulders. The ESR in this situation is an important test. Peripheral muscle stiffness, weakness and pain are not seen as prominently in cervical spondylosis.

Systemic features

An acute 'flu-like' illness may be the presenting feature, and malignancy is often the main differential diagnosis. Weight loss, low-grade pyrexia, synovitis, normochromic normocytic anaemia are all frequent features. In one study (Whitaker, Hagedorn & Pease 1966) a significant normochromic normocytic anaemia was seen in 60% of 64 cases with 'temporal arteritis', and the leukocyte count was normal in 72%. A typical example of the diagnostic difficulties of cases presenting with systemic features is shown here.

Case report. *A 68-year-old woman was admitted to New York Hospital with a six-month history of general malaise and weight loss of over 14 lb. She was found to be anaemic (Hb 11−12 g) and to be running a low grade pyrexia to 99 F. A mobile lump was found in the left breast and liver function tests were marginally abnormal. The sedimentation rate was 61 mm/h. A diagnosis of carcinoma of the breast was made with possible liver metastases. The lump was removed and found to be benign. Liver scan was normal. A survey for malignancy including gynaecological examination under anaesthetic, barium meal and enema, and bone scans were normal. Three weeks after admission the patient complained of a slight increase in her shoulder aches, which she had had for some months. At this point a diagnosis of polymyalgia rheumatica was made. A temporal artery biopsy was negative. It was decided to try the effect of 30 mg steroids daily. Within 24 hours the patient was markedly improved and realized retrospectively how much muscle stiffness she had been tolerating. Over the following two years, with two recurrences of polymyalgia on withdrawal of prednisone, the patient improved and was seen at follow-up four years after the original illness, perfectly well.*

Abnormalities of liver function (Glick 1972) and of thyroid function (Thomas & Croft 1974) have been described in PMR. Perversely, the ESR may occasionally remain normal (Norborg *et al.* 1992).

Giant cell arteritis

The obvious acute temporal arteritis in giant cell arteritis (GCA) is easily diagnosed and hardly requires biopsy proof. The whole of the length of the artery is tender, swollen and sometimes nodular. There may be over-lying redness and oedema. In milder cases tenderness is minimal, and a common complaint is of hypersensitivity of the scalp on combing the hair. There may be tenderness and swelling of the facial artery at the jaw.

Involvement of other cranial arteries may present as jaw claudication — pain in the masseter muscles on chewing — one of the most important symptoms. Tongue pain on eating may be another sign suggesting wide-spread cranial arteritis.

Eye involvement

Blindness, due to involvement of branches of the ophthalmic artery, is the most devastating complication of cranial arteritis. Some evidence suggests that 40–50% of patients with giant cell arteritis develop ocular compli-cations (Hunder, Disney & Ward 1969; Hamilton, Shelley & Tumulty 1971). Visual loss is often sudden but in many patients warning episodes of visual blurring occur. A frequent problem in patients already receiving steroids is the distinguishing of mild pain due to raised intraocular pressure from recurrent ophthalmic artery arteritis, and close collaboration with ophthalmologists is needed. Horven (1970) suggested that the ocular pulse pressure is damped in patients with eye involvement, while in other patients visual field defects may occur. Ocular bruits are rare.

The incidence of blindness in temporal arteritis is unknown. Hunder, Disney & Ward (1969) who have extensively studied this condition at the Mayo Clinic suggest that the figure is 10%, though with increased diag-nostic awareness and a more aggressive approach to temporal artery biopsy, this figure may be lower.

Other features suggestive of intracranial involvement are occipital (as opposed to monocular) blindness, brainstem ischaemia and, rarely, cerebral hemisphere ischaemia.

One of the more subtle signs of cerebral arteritis, as with most other generalized arteritides, is mental disturbance, particularly depression.

Case report. *An 80-year-old woman had, over a period of several months, become increasingly depressed. She had been found by the psychiatrist to have an ESR of over 100 mm/h, and a mild anaemia. After neurological investigation was negative and a search for malignancy had failed to reveal a lesion, a diagnosis of giant cell arteritis was made. Temporal artery biopsy was positive despite the absence of tenderness and the patient made a dramatic response to steroids, returning to her normal, very active life.*

Periorbital pain and diplopia, possibly resulting from ischaemia of the extraocular muscles, are seen occasionally. Headaches, perhaps surprisingly, are not very common, though, in some individuals, the presence of head-aches correlates closely with the sedimentation rate and other evidence of disease activity.

Large artery involvement

It has been recognized for years that more widespread extracranial arterial involvement may occur in giant cell arteritis. Klein *et al.* (1976) in reviewing 248 patients with giant cell arteritis seen at the Mayo Clinic noted that 34 had evidence of disease involvement of the aorta or its major branches. Symptoms suggestive of large artery involvement were intermittent claudication, paraesthesia and Raynaud's phenomenon. Angiography and the discovery of urinary casts were helpful in differentiating arteritis from atheroma in such patients. In the author's opinion, peripheral vessel involvement is still underrecognized.

INTERRELATIONSHIP OF PMR AND GCA

Following the recognition of the association between these two conditions, the pendulum swung so far that some observers considered that all cases of polymyalgia were due to a giant cell arteritis (Hamrin 1972) (Fig. 14.1). The high incidence of ocular involvement in the latter condition makes corticosteroid therapy mandatory. Thus, logically, all cases of PMR might be expected to require the same treatment. Clearly the widespread use of high-dosage corticosteroids in elderly people is not satisfactory.

Fauchald, Rygvold and Oystese (1972) studied 94 biopsies from patients with PMR and/or GCA. Positive temporal artery biopsies were obtained in 61. Of those with myalgia alone, 40% had a positive biopsy, and of those with a proven arteritis, only 11 did not have myalgia (Fig. 14.2). This study apart, the larger series have shown that, in general, the vast majority of patients presenting with polymyalgia alone will have negative temporal artery biopsies (Dixon *et al*, 1966; Hunder, Disney & Ward 1969; Horwitz *et al.* 1977).

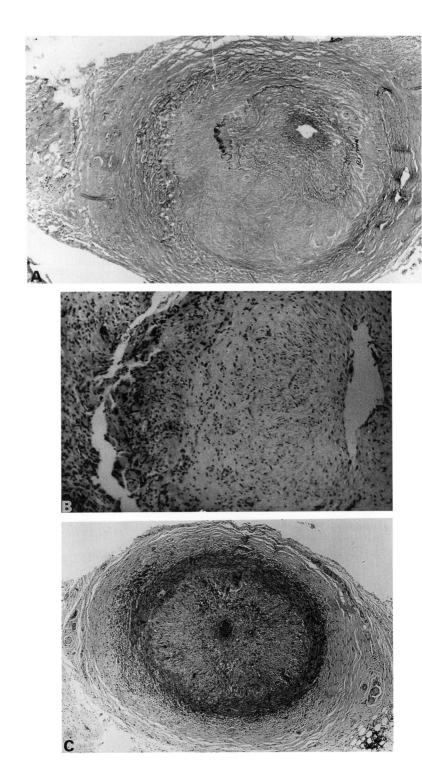

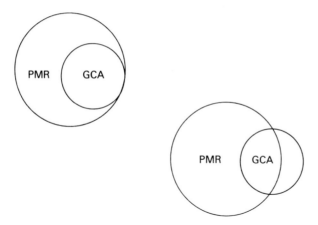

Fig. 14.2 Polymyalgia and GCA interrelationships.

DIAGNOSIS

Temporal artery biopsy is performed under local anaesthetic. Ideally at least 2 cm of artery should be studied and multiple sections should be examined. The chief significance of temporal artery biopsy has been in assessing the risk of visual impairment. In one study, in the absence of evidence of arteritis, this risk was low (15%) whereas 53% of those patients with demonstrable arteritis developed visual disturbances (Fernandez-Herlihy 1971).

The concern over missed lesions on biopsy still remains. Klein *et al.* (1976), in a careful histologic survey, found skip lesions in 28% of patients with temporal arteritis. Gillander, Strachan and Blair (1969) found that temporal arteriography provided an additional diagnostic tool in assisting with the selection of the optimal site for biopsy, though in our own hands this investigation has not been so helpful, and both 'false-positive' and 'false-negative' angiographs have been obtained (Sewell *et al.* 1980). Similar negative results have been demonstrated by Horwitz *et al.* (1977).

TREATMENT

Giant cell arteritis requires corticosteroids. PMR in the absence of clinical features of giant cell arteritis and with a normal artery biopsy may be treated with non-steroidal antiinflammatory drugs. The natural history of

Fig. 14.1 (*facing page*) Histology of active giant cell arteritis. (Dr David Tarrin, Hammersmith Hospital.)

PMR is for the disease to remit after 6 months to 2 years though occasional cases persist for 5−6 years. Relapses are common and the patient should be observed periodically after the steroid therapy has been stopped. In acute giant cell arteritis, the usual starting dose is prednisone 60 mg daily, tailoring the dose by the sedimentation rate and clinical signs. In polymyalgia most cases respond to 15−20 mg prednisolone daily, usually allowing rapid reduction to 7·5−10 mg daily. Many patients will respond to non-steroidal antiinflammatory agents, or alternatively, antimalarials such as hydroxychloroquine, but here there is an ever present (if small) risk of an underlying giant cell arteritis being missed. Alternate-day steroid therapy in the acute phase has been found wanting (Hunder *et al.* 1974). It was interesting to note that double dose prednisone on alternate days did not control the ESR as well as daily prednisone in the equivalent dose.

After the initial phase of treatment, compromise may be required in steroid dosage. The asymptomatic patient whose ESR persists into the thirties and forties can probably be weaned off all therapy, though very rarely, episodes of severe giant cell arteritis still occur in such situations, and these patients should still be observed.

Throughout this discussion the value of the ESR has been stressed. Rarely, however, this investigation lets the clinician down, and the following case history illustrates an example of giant cell arteritis with a number of interesting features, including a normal ESR during active disease.

Case report. *A 73-year-old senior hospital administrator had complained of girdle aches and pains for three months. For the week prior to his first outpatient visit, he had complained of headaches and occasional transient 'flashing' visual disturbances. On examination he was found to have slight girdle muscle tenderness, and moderate tenderness over both temporal arteries. A diagnosis of giant cell arteritis was made and arrangements were made for admission to hospital the following day. The next morning, prior to his admission, he was exercising his dog when a 'veil of darkness' crossed both eyes, and in a period of 10−15 min vision was down to several feet. On admission to the ward some 2 h later vision was reduced to 3 feet. There was bilateral temporal tenderness. The ESR was 95. Steroids were instituted intravenously as well as orally, the patient receiving the equivalent of 80 mg prednisone within the first 6 h of admission. Within 12 h vision had returned to near normal. A temporal biopsy performed 48 h later was entirely normal but a repeat biopsy taken on the opposite (and less tender) side showed active giant cell arteritis. The patient was discharged with normal vision and free from PMR on 40 mg prednisone. Over the following 12 months, attempts at steroid reduction because of the symptomatic (but long-standing) duodenal ulcer were hampered by polymyalgic symptoms. Twelve months later steroids were stopped, the patient was symptom-*

free and the ESR was below 20 min/h. Six months later the patient noticed a recurrence of temporal artery tenderness. There were minor myalgic symptoms. The ESR was normal and no treatment was given. Two weeks later the patient complained of a recurrence of visual symptoms, but still the temporal artery tenderness was minimal. Again the ESR was normal but on this occasion it was decided to rebiopsy. The specimen obtained showed active arteritis with fragmentation of elastin, multiple giant cells and a mixed chronic and acute inflammatory infiltrate. Prednisone was reinstituted, with rapid reversal of symptoms.

REFERENCES

Andersson R., Jonsson R., Tarkowski A., Bengtsson B.A. & Malmvall B.E. (1987) T cell subsets and expression of immunological activation markers in the arterial walls of patients with giant cell arteritis. *Annals of the Rheumatic Diseases*, **46**, 915–923.

Bacon P.A., Doherty S.M. & Zuckerman A.J. (1975) Hepatitis-B antibody in polymyalgic rheumatica. *Lancet*, **ii**, 476.

Barber H.S. (1957) Myalgic syndrome with constitutional effects. Polymyalgia rheumatica. *Annals of the Rheumatic Diseases*, **16**, 230.

Bell W.R. & Klinefelter H.F. (1967) Polymyalgia rheumatica. *Johns Hopkins Medical Journal*, **121**, 175.

Bosch X. (1991) Anti neutrophil cytoplasmic antibodies in giant cell arteritis. *Journal of Rheumatology*, **18**, 787–788.

Bruce W. (1888) Senile rheumatic gout. *British Medical Journal*, **ii**, 811.

Bruk M.I. (1967) Articular and vascular manifestations of polymyalgia. *Annals of the Rheumatic Diseases*, **26**, 103.

Chuang T.Y., Hunder G.G., Ilstrup D.M. & Kurland L.T. (1982) Polymyalgia rheumatica: a 10-year epidemiologic and clinical study. *Annals of Internal Medicine*, **97**, 672–680.

Dasgupta B. & Panayi G. (1990) Interleukin-6 in serum in patients with polymyalgic and giant cell arteritis. *Journal of Rheumatology*, **29**, 456–458.

Dixon A.J., Beardwell K.A., Wanka J. & Wong Y.T. (1966) Polymyalgia, rheumatica and temporal arteritis. *Annals of the Rheumatic Diseases*, **25**, 203.

Fauchald P., Rygvold O. & Oystese B. (1972) Temporal arteritis and polymyalgia rheumatica. Clinical and biopsy findings. *Annals of Internal Medicine*, **77**, 845.

Fernandez-Herlihy L. (1971) Polymyalgia rheumatica. *Seminars in Arthritis and Rheumatism*, **3**, 236.

Gillander L.A., Strachan R.W. & Blair D.W. (1969) Temporal arteriography: a new technique for the investigation of giant cell arteritis and polymyalgia rheumatica. *Annals of the Rheumatic Diseases*, **28**, 267.

Glick E.N. (1972) Raised serum alkaline phosphatase levels in polymyalgia rheumatica. *Lancet*, **ii**, 328.

Hamilton C.R., Shelley W.M. & Tumulty P.A. (1971) Giant cell arteritis including temporal arteritis and polymyalgia rheumatica. *Medicine*, **50**, 1.

Hamrin B. (1972) Polymyalgia arteritica. *Acta Medica Scandinavica (Suppl.)*, **533**, 62.

Hazleman B.L., MacLennan I.C.M. & Esiri M.M. (1975) Lymphocyte proliferation to artery antigen as a positive diagnostic test in polymyalgia rheumatica. *Annals of the Rheumatic Diseases*, **34**, 122.

Healey L.A., Parker F. & Wilke K.R. (1971) Polymyalgia rheumatica and giant cell arteritis. *Arthritis and Rheumatism*, **14**, 138.

Horven I. (1970) Dynamic tonometry (iv). The corneal indentation pulse in giant cell arteritis. *Acta Ophthalmologica*, **48**, 710.

Horwitz H.M., Pepe P.F., Johnsrude I.S., McCoy R.C., Jackson D.C. & Farmer J.C. (1977) Temporal arteriography and immunofluorescence as diagnostic tools in temporal arteritis. *Journal of Rheumatology*, **4**, 77.

Hunder C.G., Disney T.F. & Ward L.E. (1969) Polymyalgia rheumatica. *Mayo Clinic Proceedings*. **44**, 849.

Hunder C.G., Sheps S.G., Allen G.L. & Joyce J.W. (1974) Alternate day corticosteroid therapy in giant cell arteritis. *VI Pan American Congress on Rheumatic Diseases*.

Klein R.G., Cambell R.J., Hunder C.G. & Carney J.A. (1976) Skip lesions in temporal arteritis. *Mayo Clinic Proceedings*, **51**, 504.

Klein R.G., Hunder C.G., Stanson A.W. & Sheps S.G. (1975) Large artery involvement in giant cell (temporal) arteritis. *Annals of Internal Medicine*, **83**, 806.

Liang G.C., Simkin P.A. & Mannik M. (1974) Immunoglobulins in temporal arteries: An immunofluorescent study. *Annals of Internal Medicine*, **81**, 20.

Mowat A.G. & Hazleman B.L. (1974) Polymyalgia rheumatica: a clinical study with particular reference to arterial disease. *Journal of Rheumatology*, **1**, 190.

Nordberg E. & Bengtsson B.A. (1990) Epidemiology of biopsy-prone giant cell arteritis. *Journal of International Medicine*, **227**, 233–236.

Nordberg E., Bengtsson B.A. & Nordberg C. (1991) Temporal artery morphology and morphometry in giant cell arteritis. *Acta Pathologica Microbiologica Immunologica Scandinavica*, **99**, 1013–1023.

Nordberg E., Nordberg C. & Bengtsson B.E. (1992) Giant cell arteritis. *Current Opinion in Rheumatology*, **4**, 23–30.

Ostberg G. (1971) Temporal arteritis in a large necropsy series. *Annals of the Rheumatic Diseases*, **30**, 224.

Paulley J.W. & Hughes J.P. (1960) Giant cell arteritis or arteritis of the aged. *British Medical Journal*, **2**, 1562.

Salvarini C. (1991) Epidemiologic and immunogenetic aspects of PMR and GCA in northern Italy. *Arthritis and Rheumatism*, **34**, 351–356.

Sewell J.R., Allison D., Tamin D. & Hughes G.R.V. (1980) Combined temporal arteriography and selective biopsy in suspected giant cell arteritis. *Annals of the Rheumatic Diseases*, **39**, 124.

Smith C.A., Fidler W.J. & Pinals R.S. (1983) The epidemiology of giant cell arteritis. *Arthritis and Rheumatism*, **26**, 1214–1219.

Thomas R.D. & Croft D.N. (1974) Thyrotoxicosis and giant cell arteritis. *British Medical Journal*, **ii**, 408.

Wadman B. & Werner I. (1972) Observations on temporal arteritis. *Acta Medica Scandinavica*, **192**, 377.

Wilkinson I.M.S. & Russell R.W.R. (1972) Arteries of the head and neck in giant cell arteritis. *Archives of Neurology*, **27**, 378.

Whitaker J.J., Hagedorn A.B. & Pease G.L. (1966) Anaemia in temporal arteritis. *Postgraduate Medical Journal*, **40**, 35.

15: *Immune Complex Disease and the Complement System*

Many of the pathological features of SLE, rheumatoid arthritis and vasculitis are thought to be mediated by immune complex formation and deposition. Because the concept of immune complex disease is so widely referred to in these chapters, a short review of the subject is given here.

Under certain conditions the interaction of antigen and antibody occurs in the circulation. If complement is taken up or 'fixed' by this reaction, a potentially pathogenic immune complex forms. The majority of immune complexes are removed by the reticuloendothelial system (RES) but if localization occurs in blood vessels, skin, glomeruli or certain other sites, inflammation results due in large part to the action of complement breakdown products.

Early experiments on serum sickness in experimental animals by Dixon and his colleagues (Dixon, Feldman & Vasquez 1961) and by Germuth (1953) showed that when a non-immune animal is repeatedly injected with foreign antigen, a slowly increasing proportion is complexed with antibody. As antibody formation increases, the rate of disappearance of antigen from the circulation becomes more rapid. At this point, when immune complexes of antibody and antigen are circulating, some animals develop arteritis, glomerulitis and arthritis. Indirect evidence that these circulating complexes may be pathogenetic is the presence of granular deposits of immunoglobulins and complement detectable in the lesions by immunofluorescence. Such deposits may be accompanied by an inflammatory infiltrate. Fibrinoid necrosis may occur. In acute experiments, these deposited complexes are removed rapidly by phagocytic cells and healing of the lesions occurs. In more chronic experiments, however, the end result is different. If rabbits are injected daily with heterologous serum proteins, some develop chronic nephritis within about five weeks. Both in man and experimental animals, abundant evidence for the involvement of immune complexes in disease processes now exists. However, there has, if anything, been a tendency to overemphasize and oversimplify the concept.

The finding of circulating immune complexes does not imply *per se* their participation in tissue damage. Conversely, the demonstration of coexistent tissue deposits of immunoglobulin and complement provides only indirect evidence of immune complex deposition.

Some of the factors influencing immune complex deposition are discussed below. For a clinical overview, the reader is referred to Williams (1981) and Inman (1982).

FACTORS INFLUENCING IMMUNE COMPLEX DEPOSITION

Size of complex

The size of the complex is critical in determining whether it is removed or continues to circulate. Large complexes tend to activate the complement system but are also rapidly removed by the RES. Small complexes (less than 19S) persist in the circulation for larger periods but in general fix complement poorly and are less of a threat. Intermediate sized complexes are thus the most potentially pathogenetic (Fig. 15.1).

The size of an immune complex is largely defined by the ratio of antigen to antibody, complexes tending to be larger in antibody excess. In the chronic immune complex disease experiments of Dixon *et al.* (1961), glomerulonephritis developed in those animals in which a state of *antigen excess* ('soluble complexes') was achieved after each injection and in whom antibody production was poor. Thus the lattice size of the complex is dependent on antigen−antibody ratio and on certain characteristics of both the antigen and antibody.

Quality of antigen

Almost any antigen may participate in immune complex formation, increasing in size from experimentally produced hapten−protein conjugates, through viruses (in the case of a number of animal diseases) to bacteria (e.g. in bacterial endocarditis nephritis). An antigen may be unable to participate in immune complex formation because it has a small number of antigenic determinants available for lattice formation or because it is tolerogenic and few of its antigenic determinants are recognized as foreign by the host.

Quality of antibody

Lattice formation with antigen is obviously limited if the valency of the antibody is low. Thus a univalent antibody is unsuitable for immune complex formation. Christian *et al.* (1969, 1970) first drew attention to the possibility that qualitative attributes of antibody other than class or valency might affect complex formation. In a series of experiments where rabbits

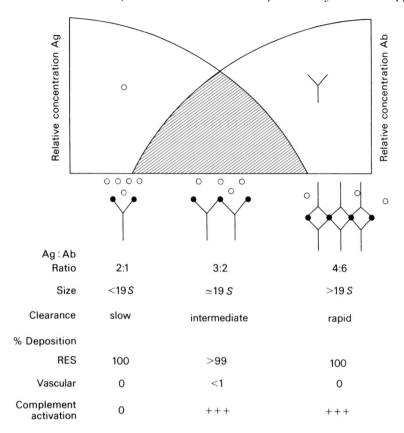

Ag : Ab Ratio	2:1	3:2	4:6
Size	<19 S	≃19 S	>19 S
Clearance	slow	intermediate	rapid
% Deposition			
RES	100	>99	100
Vascular	0	<1	0
Complement activation	0	+++	+++

Fig. 15.1 Immune complex variables.

were injected daily with antigen, one-half of the animals produced large amounts of antibody which readily precipitated the antigen, about one-third failed to respond immunologically, and 10–20% produced poorly precipitating (possible low affinity) antibody (Fig. 15.2). The small group of animals which produced the poorly precipitating antibody failed to remove antibody quickly, and complexes persisted in the circulation for a longer period. This group of rabbits developed chronic nephritis after 14–18 weeks.

Local factors

Circulating complexes are either phagocytosed by the RES or are deposited in blood vessels and other tissues. In the experimental animal, intra-venously injected complexes are almost entirely removed from the circu-

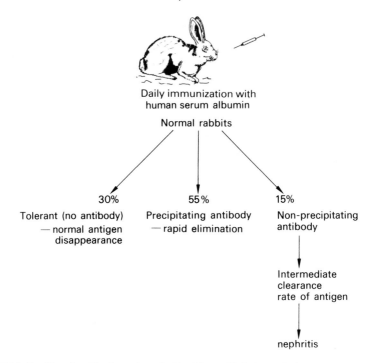

Daily immunization with
human serum albumin

Normal rabbits

30%	55%	15%
Tolerant (no antibody) — normal antigen disappearance	Precipitating antibody — rapid elimination	Non-precipitating antibody

Intermediate
clearance
rate of antigen

nephritis

Fig. 15.2 Quality of antibody and nephritis. (From Christian 1969.)

lation within 24 hours. Fatigue or saturation of the RES cells results in impairment of clearance. For example, saturation of the kidney mesangial cells may allow a greater number of complexes to be trapped in the glomerular basement membrane (Wilson & Dixon 1971). Measurement of RES function by the clearance of autologous heat-damaged red cells has shown that in SLE and rheumatoid arthritis, the titre of circulating complexes broadly relates to poor RES function, suggesting that the RES is saturated with complexes and unable adequately to clear the excess. That local factors are important is suggested by the observation that complexes localize at sites of arterial damage. Similarly the infusion of agents that increase vascular permeability or liberate vasoactive amines facilitates vascular deposition of circulating complexes. It is now known that histamine and a number of other vasoactive amines are released locally under the stimulus of certain complement breakdown products and that they facilitate vascular deposition of circulating complexes (Cochrane 1971). In experimental acute immune complex disease, antagonists of vasoactive amines, given at the time immune complexes appear in the circulation largely prevents the deposition of immune complexes in arteries and glomeruli.

The role of platelets

A major reservoir of vasoactive amines is the platelet population, and in the experiments described above, the removal of platelets decreased the severity of the vascular lesions.

The role of complement

The important role of complement in immune complex disease is reflected in the frequent depletion of serum complement levels and deposition of complement in tissue lesions in these conditions.

The complement system consists of a group of globulins, which react in a sequential manner (loosely likened to the blood coagulation system), the end point being its action on cell membranes.

The critical stage of the reaction, the conversion of C3 to C3a and C3b, and the subsequent end stage, C5–9, is reached via one of the two main pathways — the 'classical' pathway (C1q.r.s–C4–C2–C3) and the 'alter-

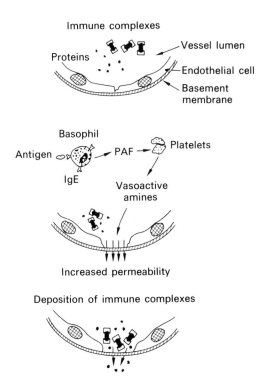

Fig. 15.3 Summary of mechanisms of immune complex deposition in rabbits. (From Cochrane & Koffler 1974.)

native' pathway (−properdin, Factor B, Factor D−C3). The classical pathway is activated by complexes containing IgM or IgG. The alternative pathway may be activated by immune complexes containing IgA, or directly by bacterial lipopolysaccharides.

The classical sequence of complement activation is shown in Fig. 15.4. The biological properties of complement are shown in simplified form in Table 15.1 (Schur 1975). The important breakdown products of complement, notably C3a and C5a, have anaphylatoxic properties and, together with the trimolecular complex $C\overline{567}$ have been shown to be chemotactic for neutrophils, eosinophils and mononuclear cells. Furthermore, C3b-containing complexes bind to polymorphs and other phagocytic cells (promoting phagocytosis and lysosomal enzyme release) and to platelets (in certain species only).

It was mentioned in earlier chapters that isolated inherited defects of complement have been associated with the development of diseases usually

Table 15.1 Properties of complement

Potentially beneficial
Lysis and phagocytosis of bacteria and viruses coated with antibody
Immune response to tumours
Initiation of inflammatory reaction
Contribution to clearance of complexes by the RES

Inflammatory
Smooth muscle contraction ('anaphylotoxins')	
Histamine release	
Platelet aggregation	C3a + C5a
Intravascular coagulation	
Chemotaxis	

Attraction of neutrophils and macrophages	C3b
Release of lysosomal enzymes	C5,6,7

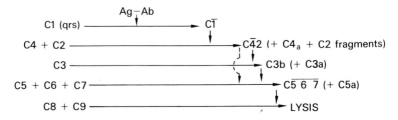

Fig. 15.4 The five-stage reaction sequence of the classical pathway. (From Lachmann 1975.)

thought to have an immune complex mechanism, in particular nephritis, vasculitis and SLE (Day *et al*. 1973; Schur 1975; Osterland *et al*. 1975) (reviewed by Agnello 1978; Rynes 1982).

Deficiency of the early components appears in particular to increase the tendency to develop SLE and other immune complex-mediated diseases. The reasons for the association are not clear, though an increased tendency to infection has been noted in these patients (Schur 1975). Of particular interest in this respect is the finding of low levels of Factor B (of the alternative pathway of complement activation) in C_2-deficient patients with infections. We observed low factor B levels in almost one-third of a group of Jamaican patients with homozygous sickle-cell disease (Wilson, Hughes & Lachmann 1976) — a condition with a known propensity both to infection and to nephritis. We have also reported patients with associated sickle-cell disease and LE (Wilson *et al*. 1976).

METHODS FOR THE DETECTION OF IMMUNE COMPLEXES (for review see Lambert *et al*. 1978; Plotz 1982)

Immunofluorescence

Indirect evidence of immune complex deposition comes from immuno-fluorescent studies of biopsy material, in particular renal and skin biopsy. Granular or lumpy deposits of immunoglobulins with similar distribution of complement (detected using fluoresceinated antiIg or $antiC_3$ antisera) are readily demonstrable in most immune complex diseases, though demonstration of the antigen usually proves more difficult. For example, in human SLE, where DNA−antiDNA complexes are the major patho-genetic complex, the convincing demonstration of DNA in tissue lesions is difficult (McCluskey 1971).

Serum complement levels

With the exception of those cases with genetic complement deficiencies, reduction of serum complement levels provides strong indirect evidence of circulating immune complexes and, by inference, of potential renal disease. In SLE, for example, depression of serum complement is a good correlate of active renal disease (Schur 1975).

Electron microscopy (EM)

The most direct methods for demonstrating immune complexes are by EM though this is possible only where the antigen is known, and recognizable on EM. Using the pellet obtained from centrifuged serum, some sera from patients with polyarteritis nodosa demonstrate Hepatitis B antigen—antibody complexes (Almeida & Waterson 1967) (Fig. 15.5).

Density gradient studies

The finding of immunoglobulins in heavier fractions of sucrose density gradient samples provides evidence that immunoglobulin is complexed to an antigen. Analytical ultracentrifugation, the best method of immune complex determination, has limited clinical use because of its expense and time-consuming nature.

Cryoprecipitins

For the clinician, cryoprecipitation of serum provides the best and easiest demonstration of immune complexes (Fig. 15.6). Care is essential in the taking of blood at 37°C and allowing it to clot at that temperature. The serum is then stored at 4°C for 3 days. Dilution of the serum increases the sensitivity of the method, and has proved vastly superior in our experience (Mola *et al.* 1983).

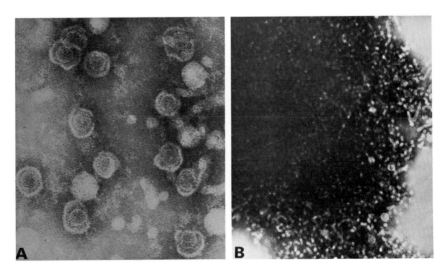

Fig. 15.5 Australia antigen (hepatitis B 'Dane' particles. A) and complexes, B, seen on electron microscopy in the serum of a patient with polyarteritis nodosa. Some of the circulating complexes were up to 7 μm in diameter. (Dr J. Almeida, Wellcome Laboratories.)

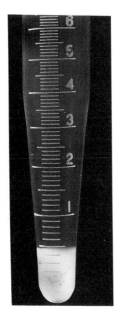

Fig. 15.6 Cryoprecipitate obtained after 72 h at 4°C from a patient with SLE.

Anticomplementary activity

Sera containing immune complexes are frequently anticomplementary, and in many laboratories measurement of anticomplementary activity is a routine clinical investigation. A variety of methods is available, but all depend essentially on inhibition of lysis of sheep RBCs normally obtained by complement, using a complement titration curve (Johnson, Mowbray & Porter 1975).

C1q precipitation and C1q binding

It was noted by Agnello *et al.* (1971) that sera containing complexes precipitated with C1q in agarose (under strict conditions of low ionic strength and pH). This method, while relatively simple, results in a number of 'false' positives and negatives and is not now widely used.

An improved and more sensitive method consists of the quantitation by binding to radiolabelled C1q (Nydegger *et al.* 1974). The use of polyethylene glycol to concentrate the complexes enhances the value of this method.

Other methods

Over twenty methods for measurement of immune complexes have been described, including the platelet aggregation, conglutinin binding, solid-phase radioassay, inhibition of complement-dependent lymphocyte formation, C1q deviation and radiobioassay using macrophages.

Each method has different sensitivity and specificity, all have technical problems and none has achieved widespread clinical usefulness as yet. Their description is beyond the scope of this book. For further technical details see *Annals of the Rheumatic Diseases*, **36** (supplement 1) (1977) on the detection and measurement of circulating complexes.

A WHO collaborative group compared 18 methods for detection of immune complexes in serum in different disease states. While there was no overall 'best buy', the study underlined the usefulness of the C1q binding assay and again clearly demonstrated that some methods seem to detect preferentially certain types of immune complexes occurring in certain diseases (Lambert *et al.* 1978).

ANIMAL IMMUNE COMPLEX DISEASES

A number of veterinary diseases, characterized by nephritis and vasculitis, are now known to be associated with an immune complex pathogenesis (Table 15.2). These have been reviewed in detail elsewhere (*Journal of*

Table 15.2 Some virus immune complex diseases in animals

Mouse
Lymphocytic choriomeningitis (LCM)
Lactic dehydrogenase virus (LDV)
Moloney sarcoma virus
Coxsackie B
Raucher, Friend, Gross virus infections

Mink
Aleutian disease

Horse
Equine anaemia

Pig
Hog cholera

Dog
SLE

Experimental Medicine Supplement (1971), **134**, pp. 7s—74s), and are mentioned because they demonstrate the pathogenetic potential of virus—antibody complexes. In man it is now certain that virus—antibody complexes are formed in a wide variety of infections.

New Zealand mouse

The mating of the New Zealand white (NZW) mouse with the haemolytic anaemia-prone NZ black mouse produces an offspring (NZB/W hybrid) (Fig. 15.7) which develops LE cells, ANF antiDNA antibodies, Coombs' antibodies, haemolytic anaemia, Sjøgren's syndrome and proteinuria (Talal 1975). Within 2 years most animals have died of classical immune complex nephritis. The immunoglobulin eluted from the kidneys shows activity against nucleoprotein and Gross virus (Dixon, Oldstone & Tonietti 1971). These animals have proved extremely useful in delineating some of the relationships between genetic and viral factors in the production of immune complex disease (Whaley, Webb & Hughes 1976) (see Chapter 2).

HUMAN IMMUNE COMPLEX DISEASE

Systemic lupus erythematosus (SLE)

SLE is the prototype of immune complex disease; the evidence for immune complex pathogenesis is as follows.

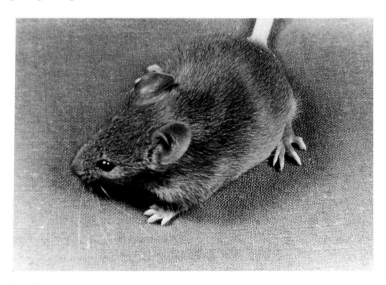

Fig. 15.7 New Zealand black/white F_1 hybrid mouse.

1   The clinical features of the disease — rash, urticaria, arthritis, protein-uria, and vasculitis — resemble those of serum sickness.

2   Immunofluorescence of renal, vascular, and skin lesions reveals 'lumpy' deposits of IgG, IgM and complement in similar distribution. Components of both the classical and alternative pathway of complement activation are demonstrable both in skin ·and kidney (Schrager & Rothfield 1976). Of more importance is that quantitative studies performed with eluted anti-nuclear antibodies indicate that those antibodies are present in significantly higher concentrations per milligram of gammaglobulin than antinuclear antibodies found in serum (Koffler *et al.* 1971).

3   Depression of serum complement levels correlates well with renal disease activity.

4   The predominant antigen involved, double-stranded DNA, is sometimes demonstrable in the serum at the same time as antibody (Tan *et al.* 1966; Hughes *et al.* 1971).

5   DNA antigens (both single- and double-stranded) and nucleoprotein are found in the glomerular deposits.

6   All the available serum tests for circulating complexes may be positive in SLE. No direct demonstration of circulating complexes by electron microscopy has been made.

7   Cryoprecipitates in SLE appear to be concentrates of immune complexes, and up to 100-fold 'enrichment' of antiDNA antibody may be seen in such precipitates (Fig. 15.8).

8   Comparisons with animal models, particularly to the NZB/W mouse, are close, and again point to an immune complex mechanism.

Rheumatoid arthritis (RA)

At first sight, there is little to suggest a major role for circulating immune complexes in most RA patients. Within the joint, however, as well as in some of the vascular lesions, immune complex mechanisms clearly play an important role. The subject has been fully reviewed by Zvaifler (1973), the main points being listed here:

1   Synovial fluid complement, in particular C_4, is reduced in most cases of active RA (Ruddy & Austen 1970).

2   There is also evidence of activation of the alternative pathway of complement in RA synovial fluid (Gotze, Zvaifler & Müller-Eberhard 1972).

3   RA synovial fluid may show anticomplementary activity.

4   Granulocytes from RA synovial fluid contain intracytoplasmic complexes of immunoglobulins, complement and rheumatoid factors.

5   Immunofluorescence of synovial membranes may reveal similar patterns of immunoglobulin and complement (Peltier 1975).

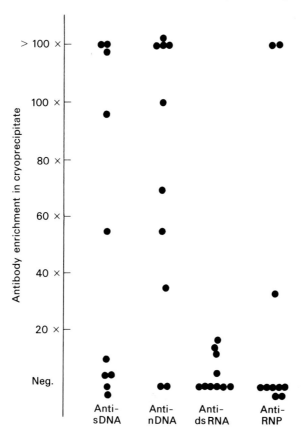

Fig. 15.8 Enrichment of various antinuclear antibodies in SLE cryoprecipitates. Up to 100-fold concentration of antibody is seen in the cryoprecipitate compared with serum levels. (From Winfield, Koffler & Kunkel (1975) by permission of the authors and editor of *Journal of Clinical Investigation*.)

6 Gammaglobulin complexes in synovial fluid have been characterised by Winchester, Agnello & Kunkel (1970) to consist of IgG—antiIgG. These complexes precipitate with C1q even in the absence of IgM rheumatoid factor. Winchester, Agnello & Kunkel (1970) found that the complexes exist as a continuum, ranging from 9S to 30S.

7 The larger complexes react with C1q but smaller ones react only with monoclonal rheumatoid factor.

8 Cryoprecipitates are demonstrable in most RA synovial fluids, and, in small amounts, in approximately one-third of RA sera — the latter cases being associated with a tendency to vasculitis (Weisman & Zvaifler 1975).

9 Complexes other than immunoglobulin complexes, such as those containing pepsin agglutinator and Fab_2 fragments, as well as DNA, may play a lesser role.

Vasculitis

Evidence for immune complex mechanisms in some cases of PAN is discussed in Chapter 10. While arterial deposition of immunoglobulin is demonstrable in other vasculitides (such as juvenile polymyositis, see Chapter 6) immune complex pathogenetic mechanisms are not convincingly seen in the majority of other vasculitides at the present time, with the exception of the demonstration of cryoglobulinaemia in some cases of cutaneous vasculitis (Cream & Turk 1971).

Other diseases

In almost any disease in which vasculitis, or proliferative nephritis, occurs, immune complex mechanisms have been postulated. The antigens implicated include bacteria (e.g. bacterial endocarditis nephritis, meningococcaemia), protozoa (malarial nephropathy), spirochaetes (syphilitic nephrosis), mycoplasma (pneumonia), tissue antigens (e.g. sickle-cell nephrosis, tumour associated nephrosis) drugs (e.g. penicillamine-induced nephrotic syndrome), and even in relatives of patients with certain connective tissue diseases (Elkon *et al.* 1983).

REFERENCES

Agnello V. (1978) Association of systemic lupus erythematosus and SLE-like syndromes with hereditary and acquired complement deficiency states. *Arthritis and Rheumatism.* **21**, S146 (Suppl.).

Agnello V., Koffler D., Eisenberg J.W., Winchester R.J. & Kunkel H.G. (1971) C1q precipitins in the sera of patients with SLE and other hypocomplementaemic states: characterisation of high and low molecular weight types. *Journal of Experimental Medicine*, **134**, 228S.

Almeida J.D. & Waterson A.P. (1967) Immune complexes in hepatitis. *Lancet*, **ii**, 983.

Christian C.L. (1969) Immune complex disease. *New England Journal of Medicine*, **280**, 878.

Christian C.L. (1970) Character of non precipitating antibodies. *Immunology*, **18**, 457.

Cochrane G.C. (1971) Mechanisms involved in the deposition of immune complexes in tissues. *Journal of Experimental Medicine*, **134**, 75S.

Cochrane G.C. & Koffler D. (1974) Immune complex disease in experimental animals and man. *Advances in Immunology*, **16**, 185.

Cream J.J. & Turk J.L. (1971) A review of the evidence for immune complex deposition as a cause of skin disease in man. *Clinical Allergy*, **1**, 235.

Day N.K., Geiger H., McLean R., Michael A. & Good R.A. (1973) C2 deficiency development of lupus erythematosus. *Journal of Clinical Investigation*, **52**, 1601.

Dixon F.J., Feldman J.D. & Vasquez J. (1961) Experimental glomerulonephritis. The pathogenesis of a laboratory model resembling the spectrum of human glomerulonephritis. *Journal of Experimental Medicine*, **113**, 899.

Dixon F.J., Oldstone M.B.A. & Tonietti G. (1971) Pathogenesis of immune complex glomerulonephritis of New Zealand mice. *Journal of Experimental Medicine*, **134**, 65S.

Elkon K.B., Walport M.J., Rynes R.I., Black C.M., Batchelor J.R. & Hughes G.R.V. (1983) Circulating C1q binding immune complexes in relatives of patients with SLE. *Arthritis and Rheumatism*, **26**, 921–924.

Germuth F.G. (1953) A comparative and immunologic study of induced hypersensitivity of the serum sickness type. *Journal of Experimental Medicine*, **97**, 257.

Gotze O., Zvaifler N.J. & Müller-Eberhard H.J. (1972) Evidence for complement activation by the C3 activator system in rheumatoid arthritis. *Arthritis and Rheumatism*, **15**, 111.

Hughes G.R.V., Cohen S.A., Lightfoot R.W., Meltzer J.I. & Christian C.L. (1971) The release of DNA into serum and synovial fluid. *Arthritis and Rheumatism*, **14**, 259.

Inman R.D. (1982) Immune complexes in SLE. In: *Clinics in Rheumatic Diseases*, Vol. 8, pp. 1–315. Ed: G.R.V. Hughes. Saunders, Philadelphia.

Johnson A.H., Mowbray J.F. & Porter K.A. (1975) Detection of circulating immune complexes in pathological human sera. *Lancet*, **i**, 762.

Koffler D., Agnello V., Thoburn R. & Kunkel H.G. (1971) Systemic lupus erythematosus: prototype of immune complex nephritis in man. *Journal of Experimental Medicine*, **134**, 169S.

Lachmann P.J. (1975) Complement. In: *Clinical Aspects of Immunology*, 3rd edn. Eds: P.G.H. Gell, R.P.A. Coombs & P.J. Lachmann. Blackwell Scientific Publications, Oxford.

Lambert P.H. (1978) A WHO collaborative study for the evaluation of 18 methods for detecting immune complex in serum. *Journal of Clinical and Laboratory Immunology*, **1**, 1.

McCluskey R.T. (1971) The value of immunofluorescence in the study of renal disease. *Journal of Experimental Medicine*, **134**, 242S.

Mola E., Gharavi A.E. & Hughes G.R.V. (1983) Enhancement of cryoprecipitation from hypotonic serum: a comparative study in normals and patients with connective tissue disease. *Clinical and Experimental Rheumatology*, **1**, 35–40.

Nydegger U.E., Lambert P.H., Gerber H. & Miescher P.A. (1974) Circulating immune complexes in the serum in SLE and in carriers of hepatitis B antigen. Quantitation by binding to radiolabelled C1q. *Journal of Clinical Investigation*, **54**, 297.

Osterland C.K., Espinoza L., Parker L.P. & Schur P.H. (1975) Inherited C2 deficiency and SLE: studies on a family. *Annals of Internal Medicine*, **82**, 323.

Peltier A.P. (1975) Complement and pathogenesis of rheumatoid and non-rheumatoid synovitis. In *Immunological Aspects of Rheumatoid Arthritis*. *Rheumatology*. Vol. 6, 24. Karger, Basel.

Plotz P.H. (1982) Studies of immune complexes. *Arthritis and Rheumatism*, **25**, 1151–1155.

Ruddy S. & Austen K.F. (1970) The complement system in rheumatoid synovitis. I. An analysis of complement component activities in rheumatoid synovial fluids. *Arthritis and Rheumatism*, **13**, 713.

Rynes R. (1982) Inherited complement deficiency states and SLE. In: *Clinics in Rheumatic Diseases*, Vol. 8, pp. 29–49. Ed: G.R.V. Hughes. Saunders, Philadelphia.

Schrager M.R. & Rothfield N.F. (1976) Clinical significance of serum properdin levels of properdin deposition in the dermal–epidermal junction in systemic lupus erythematosus. *Journal of Clinical Investigation*, **57**, 212.

Schur P.H. (1975) Complement in lupus. In: *Clinics in Rheumatic Diseases*, Ed: N.F. Rothfield. Saunders, Philadelphia.

Talal N. (1975) Animal modes for SLE. In: *Clinics in Rheumatic Diseases*, Vol. 1, p. 485. Ed: N. Rothfield. Saunders, Philadelphia.

Tan E.M., Schur P.H., Carr R.I. & Kunkell H.G. (1966) Deoxyribonucleic acid (DNA) and antibodies to DNA in the serum of patients with SLE. *Journal of Clinical Investigation*, **45**, 1732.

Weisman M. & Zvaifler N. (1975) Cryoglobulins in rheumatoid arthritis. In: *Immunological Aspects of Rheumatoid Arthritis*, Vol. 6, p. 60. Eds: J. Clot & J. Sany. Karger, Basel.

Whaley K., Webb J. & Hughes G.R.V. (1976) Systemic lupus erythematosus in man and animals. *Recent Advances in Rheumatology*, p. 67. Eds: W.W. Buchanan & W.C. Dick. Churchill Livingstone, Edinburgh.

Williams R.C. (1981) Immune complexes: a clinical perspective. *American Journal of Medicine*, **71**, 743−755.

Wilson C.B. & Dixon F.J. (1971) Quantitation of acute and chronic serum sickness in the rabbit. *Journal of Experimental Medicine*, **134**, 7S.

Wilson W.A., Hughes G.R.V. & Lachmann P.J. (1976) Deficiency of factor B of the complement system in sickle cell anaemia. *British Medical Journal*, **i**, 367.

Winchester R.J., Agnello V. & Kunkel H.G. (1970) Gamma globulin complexes in synovial fluids of patients with rheumatoid arthritis. Partial characterisation and relationship to lowered complement levels. *Clinical and Experimental Immunology*, **6**, 689.

Winfield J.B., Koffler D. & Kunkel H.G. (1975) Specific concentration of polynucleotide immune complexes in the cryoprecipitates of patients with systemic lupus erythematosus. *Journal of Clinical Investigation*, **56**, 563.

Zvaifler N.J. (1973) Immunopathology of joint inflammation in arthritis. In: *Advances in Immunology*, Vol. 16, p. 265. Eds: F.J. Dixon & H.G. Kunkel. Academic Press, New York.

Appendix
Immunological Tests
in the Rheumatic Diseases

Clinical and serological similarities between the connective tissue diseases are numerous, and the finding of positive antinuclear (ANF), LE cell or rheumatoid factor tests has limited value in clinical diagnosis. The more commonly used tests are briefly described in this appendix. Table 1 lists the approximate percentage of positive results found in the various conditions.

RHEUMATOID FACTOR

In 1940 Waaler observed that sheep red blood cells coated with antibody were agglutinated by the rheumatoid sera. The factor in serum responsible, so-called rheumatoid factor (RF) has since been defined as an immuno-globulin with antibody activity against human or animal IgG. Although found in up to 80% of rheumatoid arthritis (RA) patients it is also found in a wide variety of other conditions (Table 2). It has a number of properties which have relevance to the pathogenesis of inflammation in RA, in particular its property of interacting with immune complexes.

RFs are defined as antibodies with specificity for antigenic determinants on the Fc fragment of human or animal IgG. While RFs may also be found in other immunoglobulin classes (IgG, IgA, secretory IgA and low molecular weight IgM) the agglutination tests commonly used primarily detect IgM RF (reviewed by Stage & Mannick 1972). Most of the genetic markers on IgG are located on the Fc fragment of IgG (Natvig & Kunkel 1968), and human RFs have been used in the delineation of these markers (Gaarder & Natvig 1970).

Although RF activity is usually directed towards denatured immuno-globulin, reactions with native, apparently unaltered IgG have been demonstrated (Normansell & Stanworth 1968).

The aetiology of rheumatoid factor is unknown, though it appears during the course of chronic human infections, particularly bacterial endo-carditis, and, interestingly, disappears with successful treatment of the endocarditis (Williams & Kunkel 1962). In animals it may be produced experimentally by prolonged immunization with bacteria or with auto-logous gammaglobulins.

Table 1 Laboratory aids in the connective tissue disorders (percentage of cases positive)

Disorder	Rheumatoid factors	ANF	LE cells	DNA antibodies (>30%)	Serum complement
SLE	20–40	98–100	70–80	80–100	N or ↓
Sjøgren's syndrome	75–100	40–70	10–20	10	N
Rheumatoid arthritis	70–80	10–20	5–10	0–5	N[†]
Scleroderma	5–10	40–60*	0–5	0–5	N
Polyarteritis nodosa	0–5	0–5	0–5	0–5	N
Dermatomyositis	0–5	10–20	0–5	0–5	N

* Speckled or nucleolar patterns frequent.
† Serum complement may be raised during acute inflammation as an 'acute phase' reactant.

Table 2 Diseases leading to positive RF tests

Connective tissue disease
Sicca syndrome (Sjøgren's syndrome)
Rheumatoid arthritis
SLE
Scleroderma

Other diseases with immunological features
Chronic liver disease
Sarcoidosis
Paraproteinaemias and mixed cryoglobulinaemia
Recipients of homografts

Chronic infections
Syphilis, leprosy, visceral larva migrans,
bacterial endocarditis, chronic pulmonary tuberculosis

Others
Relatives of RA patients
Increasing age

Tests for RF

IgM RF is detected by various agglutination methods, generally using carrier particles coated with human or animal IgG. The commonly used carriers are latex or bentonite particles or sheep RBCs. The latex test is the most widely used. It is more sensitive, and therefore slightly less specific than the sheep cell agglutination test (SCAT). The reagents required for SCAT are more labile, and absorption of sera prior to testing is necessary to remove heterophile antibodies which might give 'false-positive' reactions in, for example, infectious mononucleosis. The various methods for the detection of RF have been reviewed by Waller (1969).

Clinical significance of RF

IgM RF is found in 70–80% of RA patients, up to 40% of SLE sera, and less frequently in other diseases. In the sicca syndrome up to 100% of patients have RF. Some of the diseases in which RF may be seen are listed in Table 2.

Thus RF is not diagnostic for RA, and indeed some clinicians no longer use RF testing. As a group, however, those with positive IgM RFs tend to have a poorer prognosis, particularly in terms of systemic complications of RA (see Chapter 4).

IgG rheumatoid factor (not detected by the latex and SCAT methods) is found in seronegative as well as in seropositive forms of RA (Torrigiani & Roitt 1967) as well as in psoriatic arthritis (Tapanes, Rawson & Hollander 1972) and may also play a pathogenetic role in RA synovitis (Winchester, Agnello & Kunkel 1969).

IgA rheumatoid factors were seen in 7 of 10 patients with systemic sicca syndrome and only 5 of 59 patients with other connective tissue diseases (Elkon *et al.* 1981).

Biological properties of RF

Some of these are listed in Table 3 and are discussed briefly. It is not known whether the beneficial effects of RA outweigh the pathogenetic. It is known for example that certain viruses coated with antibody retain their infectivity. However, infectivity could be neutralised markedly by the addition of human IgM RFs (Fig. 1) (Notkins 1971). This might have theoretical benefit in RA.

Table 3 Biological properties of RF

Antiglobulin
Virus neutralization
Complement fixation
Chemotaxis
Phagocytosis
Enzyme release

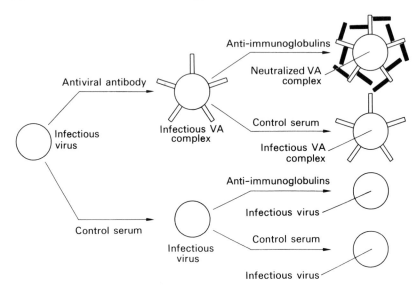

Fig. 1 Neutralization of infectious virus antibody complexes by anti-immunoglobulins. (From Notkins 1971.)

Another effect of RF is on immune complexes and their clearance. By attaching to soluble immune complexes RF increases their size and converts them into complement-fixing ones, necessary for ingestion by neutrophils. For example, normal polymorphs ingest IgM, IgG and C3 from RF-positive synovial fluids and not from RF-negative fluids (Hurd, LoSpalluto & Ziff 1970).

While this may have protective functions, it may also increase chemotaxis and lysosomal enzyme release with a consequent increase in local inflammation (Mannik and Nardelle 1985).

ANTINUCLEAR ANTIBODIES

While the presence of hyperglobulinaemia and false-positive serological tests for syphilis were the earliest recognized immunological abnormalities in SLE, it was the discovery of the LE cell in the 1940s which led to the recognition of the extent of the immunological disturbance in this disease. It is now known that a wide variety of antinuclear antibodies — possibly dozens — exist in SLE (Table 4). The usual immunofluorescent test for antinuclear antibody (ANA) detects the majority of these.

Table 4 Antinuclear and anticytoplasmic antibodies in SLE

Nuclear antigens
DNA — native (double-stranded) — highly specific for SLE
DNA — single-stranded — not specific for SLE
DNA histone (LE cell test)
Nuclear RNA protein ⎫
'Sm' antigen ⎬ 'Extractable nuclear antigen' (ENA)
          ⎭
Histone
Nucleolar RNA (common in scleroderma)

Cytoplasmic antigens
Ribosomes
Cytoplasmic RNA protein
Single-stranded RNA

Other
Double-stranded RNA ⎫
DNA-RNA hybrids   ⎬ ? Viral or human origin

LE cells

The first LE cells were described in a marrow specimen inspected on April 20th 1943 (reviewed by Hargreaves 1969). The report read 'peculiar, rather structureless globular bodies taking purple stain (? artefact)'. This is not diagnostic. The LE cell (Fig. 2) phenomenon results from the presence in the blood of an IgG antibody to DNA-histone complex (also called anti-nucleoprotein) (Holman & Diecher 1959) which reacts with nuclei from many tissues and species. Small amounts of complement are required for LE formation. LE cells are found in 70–80% of SLE patients, though these figures come from centres with a special interest in the LE cell, and the incidence of positive LE cell tests in SLE depends to a great extent on the technical care put into the preparation and reading (Dubois 1974).

The finding of many LE cells in a number of preparations provides strong support for a diagnosis of SLE, though LE cells are not diagnostic and do not distinguish drug and discoid LE from SLE (Table 5).

LE cells may occasionally be detected in a variety of other diseases. In RA they tend to be associated with those cases who also have Sjøgren's syndrome (Whaley *et al.* 1973).

In clinical practice the LE cell test has become redundant as characterization of antinuclear antibodies has become more precise.

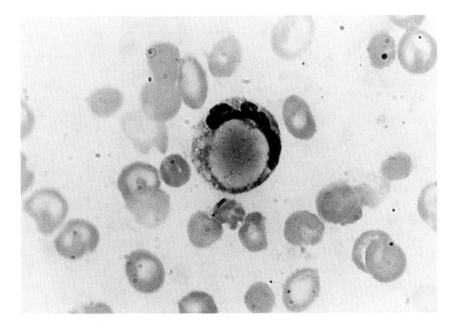

Fig. 2 LE cell.

Table 5 Causes of positive LE cells

Disease	Positive (%)
SLE	70–80%
Drug LE	70–80%
Discoid LE	20%
Chronic active hepatitis	10–15%
RA and Sjøgren's	5–15%
Scleroderma and other CT diseases	Rare
Drug reactions	Occasionally

Antinuclear antibodies

Most, if not all, antinuclear antibodies can be detected by suitable fluorescent antibody techniques (Holborow, Weir & Johnson 1957).

Positive antinuclear antibody (ANA) tests are obtained in 98–99% of all SLE patients, and are the standard screening tests for SLE. Using the indirect immunofluorescence technique, a number of patterns of nuclear fluorescence may be seen. The tissue most commonly used is either human thyroid or rat liver. Although most ANAs are non-species specific, occasional sera react only with human tissue. Polyvalent or class specific antihuman immunoglobulin serum is generally used. Antinuclear antibodies are most commonly IgG but IgM and IgA antibodies are frequently found. Recently there have been reports of increased sensitivity using rapidly dividing cells such as culture cells. These allow detection, for example, of anticentromere antibodies (seen in CREST). However, by definition they detect *qualitatively* different patterns of antinuclear–antigen reactions, and are therefore not of widespread value.

Clinical significance. Positive ANA tests are common in rheumatoid arthritis, progressive systemic sclerosis (Rothfield & Rodnan 1968), Sjøgren's syndrome and fibrosing alveolitis (Turner-Warwick & Haslam 1971). Other diseases with frequently positive ANA tests include the other connective tissue disease, chronic liver disease, Addison's disease, thyroiditis, myasthenia gravis and leukaemia. Positive ANA tests occur with a variety of drugs (Hughes 1982), are more common in relatives of SLE patients (Dubois 1974) and with increasing age (Whaley *et al.* 1973). Positive tests in low titres are extremely common and are diagnostically meaningless.

Patterns of immunofluorescence. The pattern of immunofluorescence obtained by ANA has had limited diagnostic value. Different patterns of nuclear staining which have been observed include homogeneous, shaggy or peripheral, speckled and nucleolar (Figs 3 and 4).

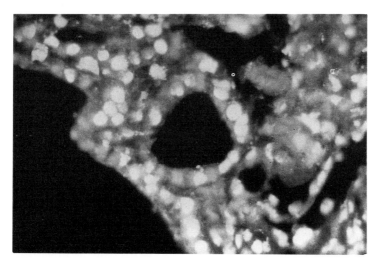

Fig. 3 Diffuse or homogeneous antinuclear fluorescence on human thyroid. (Dr Deborah Doniach, Middlesex Hospital.)

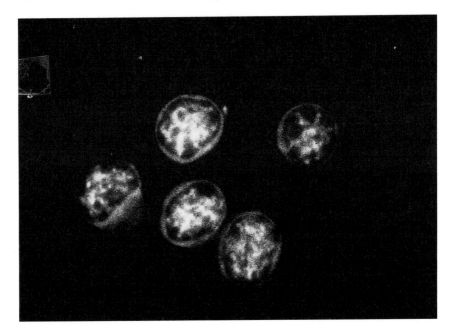

Fig. 4 'Speckled' (or 'reticular' pattern, according to the organ used and the titre of the antibody) antinuclear factor. In this case, lymphoma cells were used. (Dr Deborah Doniach, Middlesex Hospital.)

The visual demonstration of 'patterns' has been overtaken by newer methods for the demonstration of nuclear and cytoplasmic antigens (see below).

Of considerable clinical interest is the observation of an association between a positive ANA-test in Still's disease and the presence of irid-ocyclitis. While it is difficult to link the association on pathogenetic grounds, the finding clearly has important clinical implications.

ANTIDNA ANTIBODIES

These antibodies, first reported in SLE patients in 1957, are of major importance both diagnostically and pathogenetically. As discussed in Chapter 14 there is considerable evidence that the DNA—antiDNA system is quantitatively the most important of the immune complex systems in lupus nephritis (Cochrane & Koffler 1973).

A variety of antiDNA antibodies exists, but they can be broadly divided into three types (Fig. 5): those reacting exclusively with native DNA (highly specific for SLE but uncommon); those reacting exclusively with

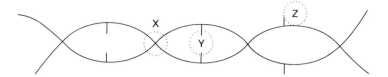

Fig. 5 Hypothetical antigenic groups present on the DNA molecule, X: unique to native DNA. Y: unique to denatured DNA, Z: common to both forms (from Cohen *et al.* 1971).

heat-denatured DNA; and those cross-reacting with both native and heat-denatured DNA. Antibodies reacting with single-stranded DNA are directed against determinants on the deoxyribose backbone of the DNA molecule. They are not seen exclusively in SLE; thus studies using the Farr binding assay (see below) require the exclusion as far as possible, of small 'denatured' strands in the DNA preparation. The use of monoclonal antibodies has helped to demonstrate some of the cross-reactive properties of those antibodies (Shoenfeld *et al.* 1983). The problems of measurement of antiDNA antibodies have been reviewed by Eilat (1986).

The DNA binding (Farr) test

This test has proved most useful in the diagnosis and management of SLE patients (Pincus *et al.* 1969; Hughes 1971, 1975). The technique is based on an immunoassay devised by Farr (1958) and Wold *et al.* (1968) (Fig. 6). The addition of radiolabelled DNA to a serum containing DNA antibodies results in the formation of DNA−antiDNA complexes. These are precipitated

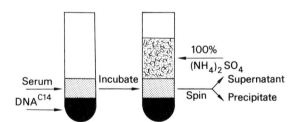

Fig. 6 Farr technique. ^{14}C-labelled DNA is added to test serum. DNA−antiDNA complexes if formed, are precipitated on addition of 100% saturated ammonium sulphate. The amount of radioactivity in the precipitate portion thus measures the antiDNA antibody activity of the serum. (From Hughes *et al.* 1971.)

$$\% \text{ binding activity} \frac{\text{cpm(ppt} - \text{sup)}}{\text{cpm(ppt} + \text{ppt)}} \times 100$$

by the addition of a final dilution of 50% saturated ammonium sulphate. A comparison of radioactivity in the supernate and precipitate gives the so-called 'DNA binding' value. Details of the method are given elsewhere (Pincus *et al.* 1969; Cohen *et al.* 1971; Pincus 1971). A comprehensive symposium has been published on the subject (*Acta Rheumatologica Scandinavica* 1975).

Diagnostic significance of DNA antibodies

The high specificity of antinative DNA antibodies for SLE has been widely confirmed over two decades of clinical practice — indeed antiDNA antibodies are probably the most specific disease marker in this whole subject. Even in conditions in which positive ANF and LE cell tests are found, DNA binding values are generally normal (Fig. 7). Interestingly, normal values are also obtained in the majority of cases of drug-induced lupus.

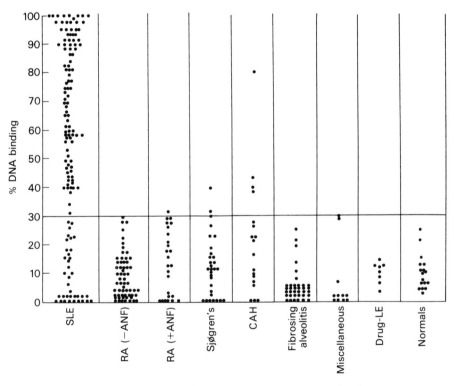

Fig. 7 DNA binding in positive ANF sera. Apart from one value of 80% in a patient with chronic active hepatitis (a second very high value has since been obtained by us in this condition) normal or slightly raised values were obtained (CAH = Chronic active hepatitis). (From Hughes, G.R.V. in *Ninth Symposium of Advanced Medicine*. Pitman 1973.)

Occasional cases of discoid LE do have raised DNA binding values (Davis & Hughes 1974), as do rare cases of chronic active hepatitis and Felty's syndrome.

Monitoring of disease activity

As discussed in Chapter 2 DNA binding and complement estimations are the most important tests in the management of SLE. With the notable exception of some patients with CNS lupus, it is rare for a patient with clinically active SLE to have a normal DNA binding value.

The titre of antibodies usually rises well before a clinical exacerbation of disease, and herein lies one of the problems of the test — there are SLE patients in whom high binding may persist for periods of a year or more without clinical evidence of disease activity. While some of these patients may have 'subclinical' lupus (Edmonds & Hughes 1975), our own approach at present is to treat the finding of an abnormal DNA binding test conservatively unless it is accompanied by clinical activity or a falling complement level. In an attempt to assess the prognostic significance of a rising DNA binding value in the absence of clinical disease activity. Lightfoot & Hughes (1977) studied 32 patients in whom this situation existed. Fourteen patients went on to disease exacerbation. In the group with persistent serological abnormalities, the subsequent period in hospital during disease flares was markedly increased.

Thus despite an overall prognostic tendency, the DNA binding test has limitations in interpretation as an absolute guide to disease activity.

Aetiology of DNA antibodies

It is remarkable that although DNA antibodies are so prominent in SLE, DNA itself is an extremely poor antigen, and experimental attempts to raise antibodies against native DNA have not been successful (Whaley, Hughes & Webb 1976).

In contrast to native DNA, UV-light irradiated DNA is a potent immunogen, and Tan and his colleagues have demonstrated immune complex formation in skin and kidneys of experimental animals using a UV DNA system (Natali & Tan 1972, 1973; Tan 1976).

A third potential aetiological factor may be that of depressed thymic suppressor function in SLE, which could lead to exaggerated humoral responses (reviewed by Hahn 1975).

It is perhaps simpler to regard antiDNA antibodies as a secondary effect of the impaired suppressor T-cell function and exaggerated humoral response seen in SLE.

RNA antibodies

These antibodies, again found predominantly in SLE (Fig. 8), have aroused considerable interest because of evidence that they are directed against double-stranded RNA. Human RNA is predominantly single-stranded, and this has led to suggestion that the antibodies are directed against viral RNA (Talal 1970). Their measurement, while relatively simple (Davis, Cunnington & Hughes 1975), does appear not to have clear clinical usefulness at the present time.

EXTRACTABLE NUCLEAR ANTIGENS

The number of nuclear antigens now characterised is increasing rapidly. A broad pragmatic classification is into those characterized chemically, such as double-stranded DNA, histones and so on, and a second group of nuclear and cytoplasmic antigens which are largely saline extractable (ENAs — Table 6).

In the past decade, largely through the work of Reichlin, Tan and others, the clinical and biological importance of ENAs have become widely appreciated.

Their detection is cheap and easy, and depends on comparison with available known sera (Fig. 9). The method devised by Bunn, Gharavi &

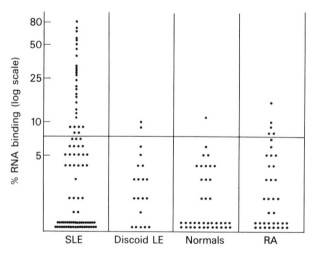

Fig. 8 RNA antibodies using phage double-stranded RNA (log scale). Approximately one-third of SLE sera tested demonstrated raised RNA binding. Of interest was the lack of fluctuation in titres with alteration in disease activity, unlike the case of DNA binding.

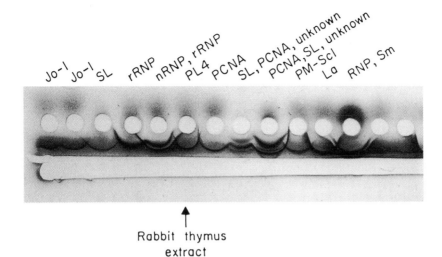

Fig. 9 Method of detecting ENAs (from Hughes 1984). Testing for extractable nuclear antigens by comparing precipitation lines with those of known serum controls (see Tables 7 and 8 for explanation of symbols).

Hughes (1982a) based on the method of Kurata & Tan takes one hour, uses a drop of serum, and brings the measurement of ENA within the scope of all service laboratories.

Over 20 such ENA systems are now recognized, and the more important, with their main clinical associations, are listed in Table 7. More comprehensive reviews are provided elsewhere (Hughes 1984; Bunn, Gharavi & Hughes 1982b).

Insights into the molecular structure of a number of extractable nuclear antigens have come from techniques such as immunoprecipitation using

Table 6 Antinuclear and anticytoplasmic antibodies (from Hughes 1984)

Antigen	Disease association
Group 1: DNA and histones	
Antidouble-stranded DNA	Systemic lupus erythematosus
Antisingle-stranded DNA	Non-specific
Antihistone	Procainamide lupus erythematosus (90%)
Group 2: Non-histone antigens	
Predominantly saline soluble nuclear and cytoplasmic ribonucleoproteins (ENAs)	SLE, myositis, Raynaud's, and 'overlap' syndromes

Table 7 Principal extractable nuclear antigens (from Hughes 1984)

Antigen	Disease association
Sm	SLE (7% in white individuals; 30% in blacks and Chinese)
Ro ('SSA')	SLE Antinuclear antibody negative lupus Sjøgren's syndrome Congenital heart block ?ITP
La ('SSB')	SLE Sjøgren's syndrome
RNP	MCTD (100%) SLE
Scl-70	PSS
Jo-1	Myositis with pulmonary fibrosis
XR/XH	CAH-PBC

SLE = systemic lupus erythematosus; ITP = idiopathic thrombocytopenic purpura;
MCTD = mixed connective tissue disease; PSS = progressive systemic sclerosis; CAH =
chronic active hepatitis; PBC = primary biliary cirrhosis; RA = rheumatoid arthritis.

cells cultured with radiolabelled phosphorus or amino acids to obtain labelled RNA or proteins which can then be precipitated by antibody or 'Western' blotting using nitrocellulose membranes. Some antigens are naked protein but most are soluble ribonucleoproteins, either predominantly nuclear (Sm and RNP) or cytoplasmic (Ro, Jo-1). Some of the antigens exist together in macromolecular complexes. Thus Sm antisera can precipitate both Sm and RNP. Jo-1 has been shown to be directed against histidyl-tRNA synthetase. Possibly antibodies to extractable nuclear antigens may not only prove to be useful probes for cell biologists but may directly influence messenger processes within the cell.

CLINICAL IMPORTANCE OF ENAs

The extractable nuclear antigens have been of value in the clinical assessment of 'overlap' syndromes, in which myositis, Raynaud's phenomenon, rashes, and Sjøgren's syndrome figure prominently. Table 8 lists the frequency of some of the more important associations seen in our patients, including some collaborative data obtained with other centres. Although grey areas abound, some associations between antibody and disease are

Table 8 Disease associations in 1018 sera from different connective tissue diseases (from Hughes 1984)

Antibody system	SLE	MCTD	Primary Sjøgren's syndrome	Myositis	PSS	RA	PBC	CAH	Other
Sm	7	7	—	—	—	—	—	—	—
RNP	23	100	4	14	2·5	—	—	—	—
Ro	24	17	75	8	4	3	6	4	—
La	8	3	42	—	—	—	—	—	—
Jo-1	—	3	—	25	—	—	—	—	—
SL	6	3	—	—	—	—	—	—	—
Pm-Sci	—	—	—	11	—	—	—	—	—
XR	—	—	—	—	—	—	10	11	—
SCL-70	—	—	nd	—	16	—	nd	nd	—
Centromere	2	—	—	—	29	—	8	—	—
Mitochondria	—	—	4	—	—	—	88	2	—

For abbreviations, see Table 7.

notably specific — those between antiRNP and mixed connective tissue disease, antiRo and primary Sjøgren's syndrome (as well as chronic cutaneous lupus erythematosus, see below), antiJo-1 and myositis-pulmonary fibrosis, and antiXR in chronic active hepatitis. Some of these associations will be discussed in more detail.

AntiRNP antibodies

AntiRNP antibodies are found in high titres in a group of patients with Raynaud's phenomenon and synovitis of their finger joints and tendons. Though these patients appear to represent a fairly recognizable subset, the clinical and serological features of the syndrome may change with time, many patients ultimately progressing towards scleroderma and becoming 'seronegative'. AntiRNP antibodies are also seen in systemic lupus erythematosus (23%) and in myositis (14%). Apart from these groups the diagnostic specificity seems high, antiRNP antibodies being found, for example, in only between 2% and 5% of patients with primary systemic sclerosis and 4% of patients with primary Sjøgren's syndrome.

Myositis-associated antibodies

Several antibodies directed against proteins associated with transfer RNA have been detected in myositis. One of these — antiJo-1 — appears highly specific (Table 9). It is rarely found in systemic lupus erythematosus but has been detected in a quarter of patients with polymyositis. This subgroup of patients with polymyositis appears to have a high incidence of pulmonary fibrosis and a relapsing course. To date (though only time will tell) we have not detected antiJo-1 in cases of polymyositis associated with malignancy. The finding that antiJo-1 antibody is directed against the enzyme responsible for catalysing the charging of histidine to its transfer RNA leads one to reflect that some picornaviruses interact with transfer RNA synthetase enzymes. These include Coxsackie viruses, previously implicated by our group in the pathogenesis of some cases of polymyositis.

Table 9 Clinical associations of antiJo-1 antibody

25% of dermatomyositis
Raynaud's and other 'overlap'
Pulmonary fibrosis (no malignancy)

ENA in Sjøgren's syndrome

Recognition that antibodies directed against nuclear and cytoplasmic extracts were found in patients with Sjøgren's syndrome dates back over 30 years. A number of groups of workers recognized that antibodies against two particular antigens — first called Ro and La — were particularly prominent in primary Sjøgren's syndrome. Later, Tan and his colleagues independently reported these antibodies and gave them the titles SS-A and SS-B. SS-A and SS-B are now known to be identical with Ro and La respectively.

Sjøgren's syndrome occupies a central position among the connective diseases. It is found in a significant proportion of patients with other connective tissue diseases and is a common isolated finding in older patients whose sera are found on routine testing to be positive for antinuclear antibody. AntiRo antibodies are found by most groups to be the commonest antinuclear antibody in patients with primary Sjøgren's syndrome, being found in three-quarters of our patients.

ANA-negative lupus

Dermatologists have long recognized that tests for antinuclear antibodies may prove negative in several patients with otherwise typical systemic lupus erythematosus (pleurisy, pericarditis, arthritis, rashes and alopecia). Almost by definition it is impossible to know the incidence of such cases.

Some of these patients with 'antinuclear antibody negative' lupus have recurring photosensitive rashes (sometimes with a characteristic annular appearance — 'chronic cutaneous lupus erythematosus'), Sjøgren's syndrome, an excellent response to antimalarial treatment, and a low incidence of renal disease. Characteristically, only antiRo antibody is detectable — hence the frequently negative conventional test for antinuclear antibody.

In addition to this syndrome antiRo is found in other connective tissue diseases, notably in up to three-quarters of patients with primary Sjøgren's syndrome, and possibly — though yet to be confirmed — in a subset of patients with idiopathic thrombocytopenic purpura (Table 10).

Table 10 Main clinical associations of antiRo antibodies

ANA-negative SLE
Sjøgren's syndrome
Subacute cutaneous LE
Congenital heart block
?Thrombocytopenia

Congenital heart block

Not only in these 'overlap' groups of patients have tests for antiRo antibodies provided a useful additional diagnostic marker. They have already helped to highlight a link between systemic lupus erythematosus and an apparently unrelated condition, congenital heart block. Pregnancy is not usually contraindicated in systemic lupus erythematosus and children of patients with systemic lupus erythematosus are generally healthy; but a rare cardiac abnormality — congenital heart block — is seen in some of their offspring. This condition, with its generally benign prognosis, may be handed down through more than one generation. Studies of mothers of children with congenital heart block have shown that up to one-third had systemic lupus erythematosus or a systemic lupus erythematosus variant and that up to two-thirds had circulating antiRo antibodies.

Scleroderma

'Speckled' and antinuclear patterns of antinuclear antibody have been recognized as common features of patients with scleroderma for many years. The predominant antinuclear antibodies in scleroderma are anti-centromere and antiScl-70 antibodies. Anticentromere antibody (demonstrable particularly well on HEp2 cell preparations with rapidly dividing cells and prominent chromosomes and centromeres but not detected by routine counterimmunoelectrophoresis) is found in up to 80% of patients with CREST syndrome (calcinosis, Raynaud's, oesophagitis, sclerodactyly, and telangiectasia) and 8% of patients with primary biliary cirrhosis.

AntiScl-70 is now recognized as an important prognostic marker pointing to systemic spread in scleroderma.

Antimitochondrial antibodies are the most well-recognized marker in primary biliary cirrhosis. Other antinuclear antibodies are seen, however, and, in future, may come to have some diagnostic importance. One such antibody, designated XR, was found in almost a quarter of patients with chronic active hepatitis.

Much as the titre of antiDNA antibody may change, so also may the titres of other antinuclear antibodies such as antiRNP and antiRo. Furthermore, in our own retrospective studies occasional patients have over the years changèd not only the character of their disease but their antinuclear antibody profile. Only prospective studies will tell how closely these changes parallel each other and how useful changes in antinuclear antibodies will prove in assessing prognosis and management.

REFERENCES

Bunn C.C., Gharavi A.E. & Hughes G.R.V. (1982a) Antibodies to ENA in 173 patients with SLE. *Journal of Clinical and Laboratory Immunology*, **8**, 13−17.

Bunn C.C., Gharavi A.E. & Hughes G.R.V. (1982b) Identification of antibodies to acidic antigens by counter-immunoelectrophoresis − a useful analysis. *Annals of the Rheumatic Diseases*, **41**, 554−555.

Cochrane C.G. & Koffler D. (1973) Immune complex disease in experimental animals and man. In: *Advances in Immunology*, **16**, 186. Eds: F.J. Dixon & H.G. Kunkel. Academic Press, New York.

Cohen S.A., Hughes G.R.V., Noel G.L. & Christian C.L. (1971) Character of antiDNA antibodies in systemic lupus erythematosus. *Clinical and Experimental Immunology*, **8**, 551.

Davis P., Cunnington P. & Hughes G.R.V. (1975) Double stranded RNA antibodies in systemic lupus erythematosus. *Annals of the Rheumatic Diseases*, **34**, 239−243.

Davis P. & Hughes G.R.V. (1974) DNA antibodies in discoid LE. *British Journal of Dermatology*, **91**, 175.

Dubois E.L. (1974) *Lupus Erythematosus*. University of Southern California Press.

Edmonds J.P. & Hughes G.R.V. (1975) Subclinical involvement and serological abnormalities in minimal lupus. Proceedings of the VIII European Rheumatology Congress, Helsinki. *Scandinavian Journal of Rheumatology*, **8**, 42.

Eilat D. (1986) AntiDNA antibodies: problems in their study and interpretation. *Clinical and Experimental Immunology*, **65**, 215−222.

Elkon K.B., Caeiro F., Gharavi A.E. & Hughes G.R.V. (1981) Radioimmunoassay profile of antiglobulins in connective tissue diseases: elevated level of IgA antiglobulin in systemic sicca syndrome. *Clinical and Experimental Immunology*, **46**, 547−556.

Farr R.S. (1958) A quantitative immunochemical measure of the primary interaction between I BSA and antibody. *Journal of Infectious Diseases*, **103**, 239.

Gaarder P.I. & Natvig J.B. (1970) Hidden rheumatoid factors reacting with 'non-a' and other antigens of native autologous IgG. *Journal of Immunology*, **105**, 928.

Hahn B.H. (1975) Cell mediated immunity in systemic lupus erythematosus. In: *Clinics in Rheumatic Diseases*. Ed: N. Rothfield. Saunders, Philadelphia.

Hargreaves M.M. (1969) Discovery of the LE cell and its morphology. *Mayo Clinic Proceedings*, **44**, 579.

Holborow E.J., Weir D.M. & Johnson G.D. (1957) A serum factor in lupus erythematosus with affinity for tissue nuclei. *British Medical Journal*, **ii**, 732.

Holman R. & Diecher H.R. (1959) The reaction of the LE cell factor with deoxyribonucleo-protein of the cell nucleus. *Journal of Clinical Investigation*, **38**, 2059.

Hughes G.R.V. (1971) Significance of antiDNA antibodies in SLE. *Lancet*, **ii**, 861.

Hughes G.R.V. (1975) Antinucleic acid antibodies in SLE — clinical and pathological significance. In: *Clinics in Rheumatic Diseases*. Ed: N. Rothfield. Saunders, Philadelphia.

Hughes G.R.V. (1982) Hypotensive agents, beta-blockers and drug induced lupus. *British Medical Journal*, **284**, 1358–1359.

Hughes G.R.V. (1984) Autoantibodies in lupus and its variants: experience in 1000 patients. *British Medical Journal*, **289**, 339–342.

Hughes G.R.V., Cohen S.A., Lightfoot R.W., Meltzer J.I. & Christian C.L. (1971) The release of DNA into serum and synovial fluid. *Arthritis and Rheumatism*, **14**, 259.

Hurd E.R., LoSpalluto J. & Ziff M. (1970) Formation of leucocyte inclusions in normal polymorphonuclear cells incubated with synovial fluid. *Arthritis and Rheumatism*, **13**, 724.

Lightfoot R.W. & Hughes G.R.V. (1977) Significance of persisting serologic abnormalities in SLE. *Arthritis and Rheumatism*, **19**, 837.

Mannik M. & Nardella F.A. (1985) IgG rheumatoid factors and self association of these antibodies. In: *Clinics in Rheumatic Diseases*, Vol. 11, pp. 551–572. Ed: R.C. Williams. Saunders, Philadelphia.

Natali P.G. & Tan E.M. (1972) Experimental renal disease induced by DNA antiDNA immune complexes. *Journal of Clinical Investigation*, **51**, 345.

Natali P.G. & Tan E.M. (1973) Experimental skin lesions in mice resembling systemic lupus erythematosus. *Arthritis and Rheumatism*, **16**, 579.

Natvig J.B. & Kunkel H.G. (1968) Genetic markers of human immunoglobulins. The Gm and Iny systems. *Series Haematologica*, **1**, 66.

Normansell D.E. & Stanworth D.R. (1968) Interactions between rheumatoid factor and native γG globulins studies in the ultracentrifuge. *Immunology*, **5**, 549.

Notkins A.L. (1971) Infectious virus–antibody complexes: interaction with antiimmuno-globulins, complement and rheumatoid factor. *Journal of Experimental Medicine*, **134**, 41S.

Pincus T. (1971) Immunochemical conditions affecting the measurement of DNA anti-bodies using ammonium sulphate precipitation. *Arthritis and Rheumatism*, **14**, 623.

Pincus T., Schur P.H., Rose J.A., Decker J.L. & Talal N. (1969) Measurement of serum DNA binding activity in SLE. *New England Journal of Medicine*, **281**, 701.

Rothfield N.F. & Rodnan G.P. (1968) Serum antinuclear antibodies in progressive systemic sclerosis (scleroderma). *Arthritis and Rheumatism*, **11**, 607.

Shoenfeld Y., Ranch J. & Massicote H. *et al.* (1983) Polyspecificity of monoclonal lupus antibodies produced by human-human hybridomas. *New England Journal of Medicine*, **308**, 414–420.

Stage D.E. & Mannik M. (1972) Rheumatoid factors in rheumatoid arthritis. *Bulletin on the Rheumatic Diseases*, **23**, 720.

Talal N. (1970) Immunologic and viral factors in the pathogenesis of systemic lupus erythematosus. *Arthritis and Rheumatism*, **13**, 887.

Tan E.M. (1976) The role of UV light in the pathogenesis of SLE. In: *Topics in Rheumatology*. Ed: G.R.V. Hughes. Heinemann, London.

Tapanes F.J., Rawson A.J. & Hollander J.L. (1972) Serum anti immunoglobulins in psoriatic arthritis as compared with rheumatoid arthritis. *Arthritis and Rheumatism*, **15**, 153.

Torrigiani G. & Roitt I.M. (1967) Antiglobulin factors in sera from patients with rheumatoid arthritis and normal subjects. *Annals of the Rheumatic Diseases*, **26**, 334.

Turner-Warwick M. & Haslam P. (1971) Antibodies in some chronic fibrosing lung diseases. I. Non-organ specific autoantibodies. *Clinical Allergy*, **1**, 83.

Waaler E. (1940) On the occurrence of a factor in human serum activating the specific agglutination of sheep blood corpuscles. *Acta Pathologica Microbiologica Scandinavica*, **17**, 172.

Waller M. (1969) Methods of measurement of rheumatoid factor. *Annals of New York Academy of Sciences*, **168**, 5.

Whaley K., Hughes G.R.V. & Webb J. (1976) Systemic lupus erythematosus in man and animals. In: *Recent Advances in Rheumatology*. Eds: W.W. Buchanan & W.C. Dick. Churchill Livingstone, Edinburgh.

Whaley K., Webb J., MacAvoy B.A., Hughes G.R.V., Lee P., MacSween R.N.M. & Buchanan W.W. (1973) Sjøgren's syndrome: 2. Clinical associations and immunological phenomena. *Quarterly Journal of Medicine*, **52**, 513.

Williams R.C. & Kunkel J.G. (1962) Rheumatoid factor, complement and conglutinin aberrations in patients with subacute bacterial endocarditis. *Journal of Clinical Investigation*, **41**, 666.

Winchester R.J., Agnello V. & Kunkel H.G. (1969) The joint fluid gamma globulin complexes and their relationship to intra-articular complement diminution. *Annals of the New York Academy of Science*, **168**, 195.

Wold R.T., Young F.E., Tan E.M. & Farr R.S. (1968) Deoxyribonucleic acid antibody; a method to detect its primary interaction with deoxyribonucleic acid. *Science*, **161**, 806.

Wolfe J.F., Adelstein E. & Sharp G.C. (1978) Disease pattern of patients with PM-1 antibody. *Arthritis and Rheumatism*, **21**, 604 (Abstr.).

Zvaifler N.J. (1973) Immunopathology of joint inflammation in arthritis. *Advances in Immunology*, Vol. 16, p. 265. Eds: F.J. Dixon & H.G. Kunkel. Academic Press, New York.

Index

Page numbers in italic refer to figures, those in bold refer to tables.